Cancer
and the
Adolescent

Cancer and the Adolescent

Second edition

EDITED BY

T. O. B. Eden
Academic Unit of Paediatric Oncology, University of Manchester, Manchester, UK

R. D. Barr
Department of Paediatrics, McMaster University, Hamilton, Ontario, Canada

A. Bleyer
Department of Paediatrics, The University of Texas MD Anderson Cancer Center, Houston, Texas, USA

M. Whiteson
Teenage Cancer Trust, London, UK

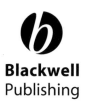

Blackwell
Publishing

© 2005 by Blackwell Publishing Ltd
BMJ Books is an imprint of the BMJ Publishing Group Limited, used under licence

Blackwell Publishing, Inc., 350 Main Street, Malden, Massachusetts 02148–5020, USA
Blackwell Publishing Ltd, 9600 Garsington Road, Oxford OX4 2DQ, UK
Blackwell Publishing Asia Pty Ltd, 550 Swanston Street, Carlton, Victoria 3053, Australia

First published 1996
Second edition 2005

Library of Congress Cataloging-in-Publication Data

Cancer and the adolescent.— 2nd ed. / edited by T. O. B. Eden . . . [et al.].
      p. ; cm.
   Includes bibliographical references and index.
   ISBN-13: 978-0-7279-1810-9 (pbk.)
   ISBN-10: 0-7279-1810-9 (pbk.)
   1. Cancer in adolescence.   2. Tumors in adolescence.
   [DNLM: 1. Neoplasms—therapy—Adolescent—Congresses.   2. Neoplasms—psychology—
Adolescent—Congresses.   QZ 275 C208 2005]   I. Eden, T. O. B.

   RC281.C4C345   2005
   616.99′4′00835—dc22

                                                                                    2005008026

ISBN-13: 978-0-7279-1810-9
ISBN-10: 0-7279-1810-9

A catalogue record for this title is available from the British Library

Set in 9.5/12 pt Meridien by Graphicraft Limited, Hong Kong
Printed and bound in Harayana, India by Replika Press Pvt Ltd

Commissioning Editor: Mary Banks
Editorial Assistant: Mirjana Misina
Development Editor: Veronica Pock
Production Controller: Debbie Wyer

For further information on Blackwell Publishing, visit our website:
http://www.blackwellpublishing.com

Contents

List of contributors

Editors

T. O. B. Eden, Academic Unit of Paediatric Oncology, University of Manchester, Manchester, UK

R. D. Barr, Department of Paediatrics, McMaster University, Hamilton, Ontario, Canada

A. Bleyer, Department of Pediatrics, The University of Texas MD Anderson Cancer Center, Houston, Texas, USA

M. Whiteson, Teenage Cancer Trust, London, UK

Contributors

J. Arbuckle, Western General Hospital, Edinburgh, UK

R. D. Barr, McMaster University, Hamilton, Ontario, Canada

J. M. Birch, Cancer Research UK Paediatric and Familial Cancer Research Group, Royal Manchester Children's Hospital, Manchester, UK

A. Bleyer, The University of Texas MD Anderson Cancer Center and University of Texas Medical School, Houston, Texas, USA

M. F. H. Brougham, Royal Hospital for Sick Children, Edinburgh, UK

L. Brugières, Département de Pédiatrie, Institut Gustave Rousaay, Villejuif, France

T. Budd, Children's Oncology Group, Arcadia, California, USA

R. Cotton, Christie Hospital NHS Trust, Manchester, UK

A. Craft, Department of Child Health, Royal Victoria Infirmary, Newcastle upon Tyne, UK

M. P. Gerrard, Sheffield Children's Hospital, Sheffield, UK

I. Gibson, MP and Chairman of All Party Cancer Group, UK

R. J. Grimer, The Royal Orthopaedic Hospital NHS Trust, Birmingham, UK

R. Hain, Department of Child Health, University of Wales College of Medicine, Penarth, UK

R. Jones, South West Wales Cancer Institute, Singleton Hospital, Swansea NHS Trust, Swansea, UK

R. Kanarek, Teenage Cancer Trust Unit, The Middlesex Hospital, London, UK

M. Leahy, Teenage Cancer Trust Senior Lecturer, Cancer Research UK Clinical Centre, St James's University Hospital, Leeds, UK

R. Leonard, Cancer Institute, Swansea, UK

I. Lewis, St James University Hospital, Leeds, UK

M. Montello, The University of Texas MD Anderson Cancer Center and University of Texas Medical School, Houston, Texas, USA

S. Morgan, Teenage Cancer Trust Unit, St James's University Hospital, Leeds, UK

J. B. Nachman, Department of Pediatrics Hematology/Oncology, Chicago, Illinois, USA

K. L. Neville, Department of Nursing, Kean University, New Jersey, USA

V. Riley, Teenage Cancer Trust Unit, The Middlesex Hospital, London, UK

P. Selby, Cancer Research UK Clinical Centre, St James's University Hospital, Leeds, UK

M. C. Self, North West Cardiff Community Mental Health Team, Cardiff, UK

A. Shah, Non-Communicable Disease Epidemiology Unit, London School of Hygiene and Tropical Medicine, London, UK

L. Shearer, Poole, UK

J. Spinetta, San Diego State University, San Diego, California, USA

D. A. Walker, Faculty of Medicine and Health Sciences, University of Nottingham, Nottingham, UK

W. H. B. Wallace, Royal Hospital for Sick Children, Edinburgh, UK

M. Whiteson, Teenage Cancer Trust, London, UK

K. P. Windebank, University of Newcastle upon Tyne and Royal Victoria Infirmary, Newcastle upon Tyne, UK

J. Whelan, The Meyerstein Institute of Oncology, The Middlesex Hospital, London, UK

M. Woods, Manchester, UK

R. Yates, Statistical Information Team, Cancer Research UK, London, UK

Introduction

Thanks to the Teenage Cancer Trust, attention is at last being focused on the disadvantaged position of teenagers and young adults with cancer. Advances are now being made in their management.

The recognition of their needs, both medical and psychosocial, by the UK National Institute for Clinical Excellence is a key milestone. Work will result in their production of national guideline recommendations for this group of patients.

The third International Conference on Cancer and the Adolescent, organized and sponsored by the Teenage Cancer Trust, has thrown a spotlight on the issues for this cohort of young people. There are common problems for young people with cancer right around the world and we in the UK appear to be in the vanguard of championing their case.

Attention has been drawn to the low level of recruitment into clinical trials and the increasing incidence of cancer in the 16- to 24-years age group, a dearth of specialist facilities and multidisciplinary teams to look after such patients, and the relatively poor outcome for this group. In addition, it is clear that social and financial discrimination is experienced by many of the survivors. It is clearly now time for government as well as charities like the Teenage Cancer Trust to do something much more active. I would personally recommend that governments should offer financial support matching that given by, for example, the Teenage Cancer Trust to ensure that this group of teenage and young adult cancer patients receive the level of care to which they are entitled and which they deserve.

Dr Ian Gibson
MP and Chairman of the All Party Cancer Group

CHAPTER 1

A right, not a privilege!

M. Whiteson

In 1948, when the National Health Service was established in the UK, we were promised health-care 'from the cradle to the grave'. No-one mentioned much about the in-between years. Here, and in many other countries, health-care is provided separately for children and adults. The age at which one becomes an 'adult' in this context varies from 12 to 18 years, and sometimes appears to be an arbitrary line drawn in the sand. In England and Wales this line divides the men from the boys (and the girls from the women) at 16 years. I am not sure why. We make other divisions about other issues; for instance, we may hold a child over 10 to be criminally responsible. In the field of education we separate infants from juniors, and all of them from the secondary stage at 11 years of age, and may even subdivide the 11 to 17/18 age group. In doing this, it is acknowledged that adolescents or teenagers have specific needs and must be dealt with differently.

We all know that the commercial world recognizes these 'in-betweens' and makes a great deal of money by meeting their needs. However, in the medical context, teenagers and young adults are a neglected group and suffer as a result. It is their right to have their special needs recognized and satisfied. This should not be seen as a privilege.

The Teenage Cancer Trust (TCT) was established formally in the early 1990s by a small group of charitably minded individuals who, having set up the first specialist unit for young cancer patients at the Middlesex Hospital, London, realized the yawning gap in the provision of treatment and care for this group of patients.

The vision of TCT is to supply a teen-friendly environment in which an expert and highly specialized team of health-care professionals provide their patients with the very best chance of recovery. TCT units are this and more. They espouse a philosophy of putting the patient first. This is not really a new idea, for, as Professor J. B. Murphy (1857–1916, Professor of Surgery, Northwestern University, Chicago, USA) pointed out some 100 years ago, 'The patient is the centre of the medical universe around which all our work revolves, and toward which all our efforts trend.' Within TCT units, the needs of young people are recognized and respected, and not just their needs as cancer patients. The emphasis is on the quality of life as well as its duration.

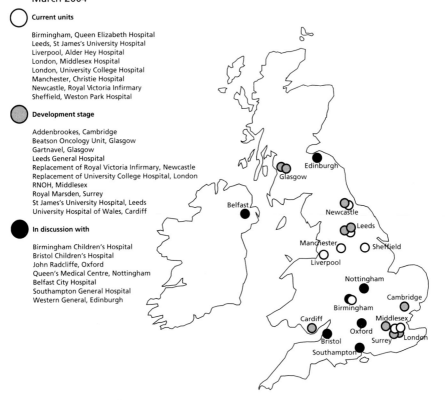

Teenage Cancer Trust Units
March 2004

◯ **Current units**

Birmingham, Queen Elizabeth Hospital
Leeds, St James's University Hospital
Liverpool, Alder Hey Hospital
London, Middlesex Hospital
London, University College Hospital
Manchester, Christie Hospital
Newcastle, Royal Victoria Infirmary
Sheffield, Weston Park Hospital

◉ **Development stage**

Addenbrookes, Cambridge
Beatson Oncology Unit, Glasgow
Gartnavel, Glasgow
Leeds General Hospital
Replacement of Royal Victoria Infirmary, Newcastle
Replacement of University College Hospital, London
RNOH, Middlesex
Royal Marsden, Surrey
St James's University Hospital, Leeds
University Hospital of Wales, Cardiff

● **In discussion with**

Birmingham Children's Hospital
Bristol Children's Hospital
John Radcliffe, Oxford
Queen's Medical Centre, Nottingham
Belfast City Hospital
Southampton General Hospital
Western General, Edinburgh

Fig. 1.1 Distribution of Teenage Cancer Trust units.

We have gone on to establish eight TCT units around the UK and are in the process of developing a further 17 (Fig. 1.1). Setting up these units is a slow process, and it is not the TCT that is causing the delay. Lack of government support, lack of recognition within the medical profession, failure of physicians to cooperate across the age divide, and conservative and unimaginative hospital managements are the main impediments.

In developing these units, we have learned that physically appropriate environments – where architecture and interior design not only provide pleasant surroundings but also add constructively to the well-being of the patient – really make a difference to the quality of patients' lives. In 2003 the TCT unit at Weston Park Hospital, Sheffield, received a commendation from the Commission for Health Improvement for its innovative design and for meeting patients' needs. Additionally, in 2003 the TCT unit at St James's University Hospital, Leeds, was the winner of one of the Department of Health's Health and Social Care Awards – the Cancer New Hope Award.

The growth of a network of units is beginning to allow specialization (and so expertise) within adolescent cancer medicine. There is a definite growth of interest in the field which can only benefit our patients.

We have also extended our sphere of work to support the basic concept of specialized units for youthful cancer patients. We sponsor the Teenage Cancer Trust Multidisciplinary Forum, organize conferences such as the International Conference on Cancer and the Adolescent, and also Find Your Sense of Tumour – a conference for young cancer patients. We are setting up a Family Support service, run an Education and Awareness team for schools and universities – and hope to be appointing the first Chair in Adolescent Cancer Medicine in the world, very shortly.

We consider we have played a considerable part in focusing attention on the needs of this hitherto neglected group of patients, world-wide. Attendance at our international conference has increased from the involvement of five countries to 18 countries, indicating the massive growth in interest. This is one field where the UK (and TCT) is showing the way!

World-wide, cancer service provision for those at such a sensitive and crucial stage of life appears generally inadequate and fails to meet all the needs of the patient. Cancer service provision, we would argue, is about more than treatment: it is also about the quality of care and life both during and after treatment. As in other social structures, this transitional stage of development of young people has to be recognized and our state health services have to make provision built upon good information and must be available to all who require them. Within the UK we appeal to our government and our National Health Service to work with TCT to meet that need.

Some people question whether there is a need for specialized care for adolescent and young adult cancer patients and ask whether teenagers get cancer. The common perception – not only among the general public but sometimes also among professional and political decision-makers – is that children get cancer and adults get cancer, but teenage cancer numbers are insignificant. Yet cancer is the commonest cause of non-accidental death in teens and young adults in both the USA[1] and the UK.[2] In the UK we are just below the European average for 5-year survival rates for children and teenagers with cancer, which leaves much room for improvement.[3]

What are the issues?

Cancer services are delivered by an out-of-date infrastructure that, by and large, fails teenagers and young adults.

- There are difficulties in obtaining reliable statistics.
- Teens and young adults are often subject to late diagnosis.
- Levels of skill and expertise vary between and within treatment centres and we need to know the effect of these variations on outcome.
- Young people have low enrolment in clinical trials.

- They are placed at the crossover between adult and childhood cancers and experience a different distribution of cancers from other age groups.
- This complexity is exacerbated by the usual division of child and adult services. In the UK (and elsewhere, too) the approach to children is generic, across the board, whereas for adults it is specific to the cancer site.
- Different protocols are used by adult and paediatric practitioners for the same diseases – the relative success of these needs to be evaluated.

Cancer patients in their teens and early adulthood tend to be disadvantaged at every stage.

Do we have the information?

Although statistics for this age group are still difficult to obtain, we are beginning to appreciate, contrary to common perception, that there are more young people with cancer in the 15–24 age group than in children aged 0–14 years. It is estimated that around 2000 new diagnoses are made per annum in the teenage and young adult (TYA) group in the UK. Some of those treated successfully for cancer during childhood go on to relapse during adolescence. About 75% of children with cancer are cured, but many continue to require physical and emotional follow-up in the long term. Because of the way we gather information in the UK and other countries, we do not actually know how many young people nationwide will be calling upon our cancer services.

In England and Wales the National Institute for Clinical Excellence is currently studying cancer services for children and young people. The National Public Health Service for Wales[4] has data which suggest that the falling birth rate will result in a change in the population's demographic profile, with increasing numbers in the older age groups projected to 2011. Since the incidence rate of cancer is higher in the 15–24 age group (214 per million) than the 0–14 age group (134 per million), increased survival and a changing demography are likely to result in an increase in absolute numbers of incident and prevalent cancer patients aged 15–24. This suggests an increased need for services both in the short and longer term for the TYA group.

Why has this not been sufficiently considered by the medical profession? Failure to do so has hindered the reorganization of service delivery. Why has the National Health Service not made the necessary infrastructure changes to care appropriately for young cancer patients? Surely this is negligence! In the UK, it has taken a charity – TCT – to show the way and inspire change.

The numbers game

The problems of gathering statistics are, in part, due to the division of TYAs between child and adult services. This is a serious problem and an obstacle to the provision of sound information. It undermines the establishment of appropriate standards and systems of service delivery to the complex group of patients that make up the TYA sector. The work of Birch and colleagues[5] highlights the value of detailed data in assessing the needs of and the provision of services to the hitherto neglected youth with cancer.

In order to fulfil our duty to young cancer patients, both as a profession and as a society, we need more focused information-gathering. The sector of the population with whom we are concerned presents many problems that would be addressed by more reliable information, and this information would also enable us to build structured approaches to treatment and help resolve the unique issues.

It may be too cynical to suggest that failure to identify this group of patients – so that true figures and information are not available – has resulted in the absence of demand for special facilities, treatment, research and funding. Defining this group out of existence might save governments, the National Health Service and the health trusts a great deal of money. You don't have to spend on what doesn't exist.

Late diagnosis

There is much anecdotal evidence and some factual indication regarding the issue of general practitioner delay. Many factors contribute to this impediment to speedy diagnosis and treatment.

- Teenagers themselves! Often they are hesitant or even reluctant to visit the doctor. In the USA it is observed that young adults have the lowest rate of primary care use.[1]
- Young people are under-educated regarding their own health.
- Parents are less involved in their children's personal care at this stage of life.
- Few general practitioners have experience of adolescent and young adult cancers.
- Few general practitioners have cancer in their lexicon of possible diagnoses for young patients (the low profile of teenage cancer may contribute to this).
- There is not a clear pathway of referral, as there is for children. As a result, the locus of referral is something of a lottery. In turn, this influences the levels of experience and expertise that patients will find. We need to know how this affects the outcome.

Clinical trials

Relatively few teenagers and young adults with cancer are enlisted in clinical trials. Overall, the outcome for patients involved in trials tends to be more favourable. Results of clinical trials provide the information base for future treatment. They are the foundation upon which treatment can be improved and standardized. Therefore, once again young cancer patients are disadvantaged.

It is accepted that few TYAs are included in trials. The following factors contribute to their exclusion.

- The pharmaceutical industry dominates in this field. Pharmaceutical companies work on numbers, and we are talking about a relatively small group of patients. It is accepted that within each country the numbers are proportionally small, but world-wide there is a considerable total, enough to justify research. The pharmaceutical industry appears to show little interest in this age group.
- Governments, who are sizeable customers of the pharmaceutical companies, should place requirements on these organizations to test drugs to benefit young people. In the USA the Food and Drug Administration requires drug companies to evaluate their products for children in order to obtain a paediatric licence. This is an encouraging move.
- While eminent clinicians advocate clinical trials for young cancer patients, we in Europe are concerned about a European Union directive, due to come into force in May 2004, which will make clinical trials for children, adolescents and even young adults even less likely than they are now. If implemented, this directive will make trials more costly and the outcome will be that only the pharmaceutical companies will be able to afford to set up trials, and academic trials will be severely curtailed as a result. This can only further limit the involvement of young cancer patients in such research.
- Some of the cancers which TYAs experience are rare and so do not inspire trials.
- Clinicians often see young people as non-compliant, and there may be some validity in this argument – but insufficient to justify not involving them. A concentration of young people in specialist centres such as TCT units would assist in the setting up and management of clinical trials and help mitigate patient resistance.

It is vital that young people with cancer are actively involved in clinical trials, in order to ensure a consistent and enhanced standard of care.

Range of cancer services

The variety of cancers affecting the age group in question includes childhood and adult cancers. Imposing this diversity upon the rigid structure of childhood or adult centres and protocols raises further problems.

It is common practice in the UK for the approach to childhood cancer treatment to be generic while that for adult cancer is site-specific. These systems do not mesh well. As a result, those on the cusp may not get the appropriate approach to treatment. This is often exacerbated by a lack of cooperation between adult and paediatric practitioners. Unfortunately, this is sometimes my experience when working with hospitals in the UK, and having conducted a straw poll via nurses from a number of other countries I conclude that this glass wall exists in those countries too.

But TYA cancer patients should not be limited to either paediatric or adult services – there is another alternative. There is the transitional facility – such as TCT units – where the skills and expertise are focused on their specific needs.

Too many young people with cancer do not have the benefit of access to a specialized teenage unit – this is true abroad, and also here in the UK. We look forward to the day when TCT units and services are the norm, as paediatric services are now. Until then we need to call upon consultants to exhibit a generous degree of cooperation and flexibility and to bridge the discipline and age boundaries.

Generally, service provision for TYAs is supplied in two self-contained structures, with children in the paediatric box and all the rest in the adult box. For some, where there is a TCT unit, an alternative to the rigid two-box system is offered and this works best where practitioners show an elasticity of approach.

In declaring that we offer care from the cradle to the grave, we must ensure that needs are met at all ages. No-one questions paediatric medicine today – nor do they question geriatric medicine – so why do we fail to meet the needs of those at the most sensitive, transitional stage of life?

For teenagers and young people with cancer the appropriate situation is to have specialized staff with specific training in the management of the cancers affecting this age group, and nurses and other staff who have a particular interest in young people who are trained to deal with the medical and psychosocial issues affecting this group of patients.

Ideally (Fig. 1.2), genuinely concerned practitioners will endeavour to accommodate the needs of these patients by blurring the delivery edges. Keeping the patients central, the consultants will bring their particular expertise to the

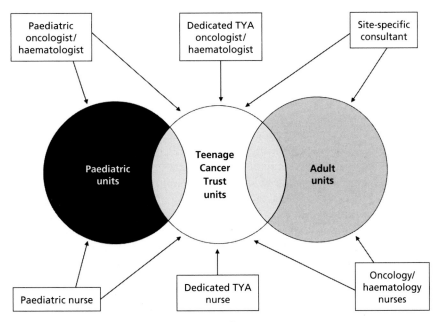

Fig. 1.2 Diagram of professional practitioner flow.

patients, and I envisage that, in all probability, there will always be a need for consultants in certain cancer types to be involved. Nurses specializing in adolescents with cancer will be supplemented by paediatric oncology nurses with an interest in the age group. This will be demanding, particularly where facilities for the very young and for the elderly are miles apart, but some movement in that direction must take place until a critical mass of practitioners specializing in adolescent cancer medicine is built up and we can provide every young person with cancer access to a specialized, age-appropriate facility and team.

Why is this group so special?

I have indicated already some of the particular issues complicating the diagnosis and treatment of young people with cancer. These people are going through a great many changes aside from the impact of their cancer: physical, psychological, emotional, educational and lifestyle alterations.

- *Staff* need different skills when dealing with these patients and also with their parents. Negotiations are far more complex when dealing with TYAs than with small children or fully independent adults. Who makes the decisions – patient or parent? What if they disagree?
- *Physical changes*. While any cancer patient will struggle with physical changes, these are so much more painful for the TYA patient. In our surveys, patients identify their appearance as of more concern than the possibility of death.
- *Fertility* is a vitally important concern for young people. It is a significant possibility that fertility will be impaired or lost as a result of treatment. This can cause major psychological and social damage. When young people are treated in a paediatric setting they are deemed to be children and are not offered advice on fertility. But even in adult centres patients are failed by a lack of fertility counselling.
- *Social relationships*. Peer groups are of primary importance during this period of life. Cancer diagnosis singles out and isolates the young patient. Youth can be a difficult stage to handle without the added complication of cancer. Lack of confidence (despite an often brash image) is not uncommon during the 'in between' years. Both self-perception and expectations can deteriorate. Life-threatening disease, change of image, loss of contact with contemporaries and possible loss of fertility can all undermine the fragile self-assurance of the young patient.

    Many of our patients who have been treated in either children's or adult wards have complained that their friends would not visit them – highlighting their sense of being different – and of isolation. In TCT units, friends are considered important and welcomed into the user-friendly surroundings.
- *Education*. It is the norm within the UK for education to be provided for children in hospital – that is, up to 16 years of age – but it is from that age that education and examinations become more serious and achievements at the 16 to early 20s stage can dictate future life work and lifestyle. There is

rarely any educational provision for 17-year-olds and over who are being treated in adult facilities.

- *Independence*. For this age group generally and for our patients in particular, family issues are complex to handle. Many of our patients will just be gaining independence and their illness will throw them back into dependency. Instead of becoming financially self-supporting, or even a contributor to the family coffers, they become a burden. The equilibrium of normal separation, both emotional and financial, will be unbalanced to the detriment of both parents and youngster.
- *Palliative care* too requires very special expertise when dealing with adolescents and young adults. The issues differ considerably from those relevant to other age groups with cancer, and appropriately trained staff for both patients and their families are necessary.
- *Long-term effects* for young people may be more far-reaching than for older cancer patients. Impaired image, fertility loss, neurological and psychological damage, loss of education and life chances, loss of independence and the sword of Damocles effect can all severely affect their future. Will having had cancer always affect their personal relationships, as it may their financial ones? Will potential partners be deterred from long-term relationships? Many insurers are unwilling to provide insurance (sometimes even holiday insurance) or mortgages for people they see as a risk. Or if they do, the premiums are unsupportable. In the USA it has been noted that the young adult age group is the least likely sector to have medical insurance anyway – they are not able to afford it and are too old to be included under their parents' policies. Having cancer when young can determine a survivor's pattern of life.

And now?

We cannot in all honesty say that cancer services, anywhere, are offering the very best to young people with cancer. There is much that is within our power to do and much that we have yet to learn. We know that having cancer at any age is tough, and to combine it with adolescence and young adulthood makes things even harder. We *can* do something about this – and to fail to do so is to fail our young citizens.

Within the UK we have a great advantage. We have the TCT, which for over 10 years has been highlighting the needs, showing the way, lobbying and bringing about change to reduce the disadvantage experienced by many young cancer patients – while successive governments have done nothing!

Although our government has given lip service to the needs of TYA cancer patients, what have they done? In discussion with colleagues from other countries the same or a worse situation seems to exist for them.

We are not even asking the British government for money. This has to be a first! We will continue, as we have over the years, raising money in pennies and pounds to fund our activities – but we *are* asking them for something!

It is hard to believe, but health trusts can take years to see the needs of their TYA cancer patients as any sort of priority. There are hospitals which, after 10 years of discussions, are still deliberating and denying their young patients the service they need and deserve. These institutions need the push that only the state can give. We are willing to go on providing specialized units, to develop expertise, to work on prevention, to encourage research, to provide staff and to continue many of the support services required, but without the backing of the government – without their requirement that health trusts make appropriate provision for young people with cancer – our work will continue to be uphill and slow.

Is the UK government going to sit on its hands and watch while young people with cancer continue to fall behind in the cancer lottery? There may have been some recent improvement overall in cancer death rates, but not necessarily in the young people with whom we are concerned. Funds have been given to support cancer services, but how much has this benefited TYA patients?

Our patients are dying for government recognition and support. It must be remembered that these young people are citizens of the UK; they are the future and current voters, taxpayers, workers, politicians and parents (as are their families) and cannot continue to be ignored.

The government has a responsibility here – one that it has an obligation to meet. It is time that our work was endorsed by the government. This would help accelerate the development of TCT units and services and hopefully improve patients' quality and chance of life.

Remember, it is our young patients' *right* – not just their *privilege* – to receive the best treatment, care and chance of recovery.

References

1 Albritten K, Bleyer WA. The management of cancer in the older adolescent. *Eur J Cancer* 2003; **39**: 2584–2599.
2 Office for National Statistics. *20th Century Mortality. 2000 Update*. London: ONS, 2000.
3 Gatta G, Corazziari I, Magnani C, *et al*.; EUROCARE Working Group. Childhood cancer survival in Europe. *Ann Oncol* 2003; **14** (Suppl. 5): v119–v127.
4 National Public Health Service for Wales (2003/4). http://www.wales.nhs.uk/sites/documents/368/EXTNPHS0304.pdf
5 Birch JM, Alston RD, Quinn M, Kelsey AM. Incidence of malignant disease by morphological type, in young persons aged 12–24 years in England, 1979–1997. *Eur J Cancer* 2003; **39**: 2622–2631.
6 Gatta G, Capocaccia R, De Angelis R, Stiller C, Coeburgh JW, EUROCARE Working Group. Cancer survival in European adolescents and young adults. *Eur J Cancer* 2003; **39**: 2600–2610.
7 Jeha S. Who should be treating adolescents and young adults with acute lymphoblastic leukaemia? *Eur J Cancer* 2003; **39**: 2579–2583.

Part one
Patterns and perspectives

CHAPTER 2

Patterns of incidence of cancer in teenagers and young adults: implications for aetiology

J. M. Birch

Introduction

Cancer is predominantly a disease of the late middle-aged and elderly, and 65% of all registered cancers (excluding non-melanoma skin cancer) in England are of patients aged 65 years and above. In the year 2000, 0.6% of all cancer registrations were for teenagers and young adults aged 15–24 years.[1] However, cancer is the most common natural cause of death in this age group and is exceeded only by accidents.[2] Since national cancer statistics are published in 5-year age groups, it is not possible to derive figures for younger teenagers. Little is known about the aetiology of cancers in such young people. It is likely that environmental agents account for the great majority of cancers in older age groups, following chronic exposures over many years,[3] but in the young there is no opportunity for such long-term exposure. The mechanisms operating between exposure to a risk factor and the clinical onset of a cancer in the young may therefore be fundamentally different compared with late-onset cancers. In addition, the contributions of the various factors may be proportionally very different and it is likely that genetic susceptibility plays a greater role.

Although a coordinated national approach to the treatment of cancers in younger children was established many years ago,[4] teenage and young adult cancer patients have not benefited from a similar policy.[5] The teenage years and early twenties are a crucially important period in terms of educational, social and career development. Interruption of education, vocational and professional training following the diagnosis of cancer can have a lasting impact on later life. Furthermore, the potential late effects of cytotoxic treatment can have a greater and more lasting impact in the young than in the middle-aged and elderly. Loss of fertility, the development of treatment-induced second malignancies and organ failure are critical considerations in this age group. Furthermore, the types and distribution of malignancies presenting in teenagers and young adults are markedly different compared with those seen in young children as well as in older patients.[6] For all these reasons, the development of specialist services targeted towards teenage and young adult cancer patients is desirable and necessary to improve all aspects of outcome. In order to develop services tailored to the needs of this age group, it is necessary to define the extent and nature of the patient population through precise analyses of relevant population-based data.

Diagnostic classification

Cancer incidence data are usually presented in terms of the primary site according to the International Classification of Diseases (ICD).[7–9] In general, this is satisfactory for the majority of cancers occurring in later life, which are mainly carcinomas, but in young people carcinomas are rare. Therefore, for epidemiological and service planning purposes data on cancers in young people should be presented mainly in terms of morphology.

A classification scheme which is specifically tailored to the teenage and young adult cancer groups has recently been published by our research team.[6] The scheme is largely based on morphology, and diagnostic groups are specified in terms of the International Classification of Diseases for Oncology (ICD-O) morphology and topography codes.[10] We proposed that the classification scheme should be used in future studies of cancers in teenagers and young adults to achieve a standard format for data presentation, to facilitate international comparisons and encourage an interest in research into these cancers. The scheme was applied to national cancer registration data for England for the years 1979–1997 for patients aged 15–24 years. In this age range the main cancers that occurred were lymphomas, leukaemias, bone tumours, central nervous system tumours, germ cell tumours, soft tissue sarcomas and carcinomas. In contrast to older age groups, where carcinomas of the lung, breast, large bowel and prostate account for more than 50% of all cases[1] at these sites, carcinomas represent only 2% of malignancies in 15- to 24-year-olds. However, certain 'adult' cancers are relatively more frequent in this age range. Melanoma and carcinoma of the thyroid represent 8% and 3% of all cancers respectively in 15- to 24-year-olds, but across all ages these cancers make up only 2% and 0.4% of the total.[6]

The classification scheme was subsequently applied to an extended age range, which included younger adolescents, and also presented incidence rates by more detailed morphological type.[11] These incidence rates have now been updated to include national cancer registrations for England up to 2000 and are presented below.

Data and statistical analyses

Anonymized national data on individual registered cancers for the years 1979–1992 were obtained from the Office for National Statistics on CD-ROM.[12] More recent data up to 2000 were supplied directly by the Office for National

Statistics. From 1979 to 1994 data are coded by the ICD-O first edition[13] and the ICD ninth revision[7] and from 1995 onwards by the ICD-O second edition (10) and the ICD tenth revision.[8] National population estimates by single year of age, sex and calendar year were supplied by the Population Estimates Unit of the Office for National Statistics.

Eligible cases included all malignant tumours and non-melanoma skin cancers occurring in England from 1979 to 2000 in young persons aged 13–24 years. *In situ* cancers and neoplasms of uncertain behaviour were excluded, as were non-malignant CNS tumours. Individual cancer registrations were classified by type of cancer, age group (13–14, 15–19, 20–24 years), sex and time period (1979–1985, 1986–1992, 1993–2000). Cancer groups were defined by specific morphology and topography code combinations according to the scheme described by Birch *et al.*[6] Algorithms for selecting tumour groups are given at http://www.biomed2.man.ac.uk/crcpfcrg/CRUKPFCRG/PFCRG.htm. Person years at risk for each subgroup were calculated from the population data. Age group, sex- and diagnostic group-specific annual incidence rates per 100 000 population were calculated. An age-standardized rate was calculated at each time period, using direct standardization to the world population.[9] A combined rate for the entire time span was obtained using a weighted average of the separate standardized rates.[14] The significance of variability by sex, age group and time period was assessed using Poisson regression. Changes in the incidence rate over time were assessed after taking into account variability in cancer rates by age and sex. It was assumed that the changes in incidence rates over time were consistent. All calculations were performed using the statistical package GLIM 4.[15]

Incidence rates by age and group

The study included 31,921 cases of malignant neoplasms, 3009 in the 13- to 14-year age range, 10,856 in 15- to 19-year-olds and 18,056 in 20- to 24-year-olds. The study population comprised a total of 178,082,000 person years at risk, including 28,085,000 in the 13- to 14-year age range, 73,197,000 in the 15- to 19-year age range and 76,800,000 in the 20- to 24-year age range (Table 2.1).

Table 2.2 shows the incidence and percentage distribution of malignant disease among the study population by age group and main diagnostic group. Among 13- to 14-year-olds, highest rates were seen for the leukaemias, with lymphomas second highest, then central nervous system (CNS) tumours and bone tumours. In this age group, soft tissue sarcomas, germ cell tumours, melanoma and carcinomas were relatively uncommon. In comparison with younger teenagers, the most striking difference in the 15- to 19-year-olds was a doubling of the incidence rates for lymphomas, which were the most common malignancies in this age group. Rates for leukaemias, CNS tumours and bone tumours were a little lower than those observed in the 13- to 14-year age group, but increases in rates relative to the younger age group were observed

Table 2.1 Registered cases of cancer by age group, time period and main diagnostic group in England, 1979–2000*

Age group (years)	1979–1985			1986–1992			1993–2000		
	13–14	15–19	20–24	13–14	15–19	20–24	13–14	15–19	20–24
100 Leukaemia	249	575	429	191	546	496	241	523	469
200 Lymphoma	185	1,023	1,258	185	1,007	1,576	256	937	1,506
300 Malignant brain tumours	189	380	401	152	410	507	203	380	491
400 Bone tumours	149	360	172	127	310	222	137	386	222
500 Soft tissue sarcomas	55	237	269	65	228	300	66	214	279
600 Germ cell neoplasms	38	297	825	28	332	1,007	63	410	1,215
710 Malignant melanoma	20	164	405	27	202	664	31	279	752
800 Carcinoma	75	440	1,141	78	341	1,233	84	448	1,436
900 Miscellaneous tumours	21	51	54	17	47	67	26	39	48
1000 Unspecified malignant neoplasms NEC	8	48	83	22	155	341	21	87	188
All	989	3,575	5,037	892	3,578	6,413	1,128	3,703	6,606
Population (1000s)	10,309	26,881	25,377	8,106	23,268	26,758	9,670	23,048	24,665

*Excludes non-malignant CNS tumours and non-melanoma skin cancer.
NEC, not elsewhere classified.

Table 2.2 Cancer incidence rates per 10^5 and percentage distribution for main groups of cancers in young persons aged 13–24 years in England, 1979–2000

	Age group (years)					
	13–14		**15–19**		**20–24**	
	Rate	% all cancers in group	Rate	% all cancers in group	Rate	% all cancers in group
Leukaemia	2.42	22.6	2.25	15.1	1.82	7.7
Lymphoma	2.23	20.8	4.05	27.3	5.65	24.0
Malignant brain tumours	1.94	18.1	1.60	10.8	1.82	7.7
Bone tumours	1.47	13.7	1.44	9.7	0.80	3.4
Soft tissue sarcoma	0.66	6.2	0.93	6.3	1.10	4.7
Germ cell neoplasms	0.46	4.3	1.42	9.6	3.97	16.9
Malignant melanoma	0.28	2.6	0.88	5.9	2.37	10.1
Carcinoma	0.84	7.9	1.68	11.3	4.96	21.1
Miscellaneous tumours	0.23	2.1	0.19	1.3	0.22	1.0
Unspecified malignant neoplasms	0.18	1.7	0.40	2.7	0.80	3.4
Total	10.71		14.83		23.51	

in soft tissue sarcomas, germ cell tumours, melanoma and carcinomas. However, rates for these malignancies were still markedly lower than rates for leukaemia and lymphoma. There were distinct differences in the incidence pattern of cancers seen in the 20- to 25-year age range compared with younger age groups. There was a marked increase in rates of lymphomas, which were the most common malignancies, with a substantial decrease in rates for leukaemias. The ratio of lymphomas to leukaemias was approximately 1:1 in 13- to 14-year-olds, but in 20- to 25-year-olds this had increased to more than 3:1. However, the most striking differences were in the rates for carcinomas, germ cell tumours and melanomas, which were the second, third and fourth most common cancer groups observed in these young adults. In contrast, bone tumours were much less frequent compared with the younger age groups, but there was an increase in the incidence of soft tissue sarcomas. The incidence of CNS tumours was fairly similar across all three age groups. The pattern of malignancies that occur in 20- to 24-year-olds overall is therefore very different compared with the younger teenagers. The 15- to 19-year-olds show a transitional pattern. The incidence of all malignancies combined in the 20- to 24-year age group was more than double that observed in 13- to 14-year-olds.

Table 2.3 shows incidence rates for leukaemia subtypes and for non-Hodgkin's lymphoma (NHL) and Hodgkin's disease (HD). In 13- to 14-year-olds most leukaemias were acute lymphoid leukaemia (ALL), which represented more than two-thirds of all cases. Acute myeloid leukaemia (AML) accounted for nearly all of the remaining cases. Among 15- to 19-year-olds, the pattern was similar, ALL being the most common; AML accounted for most of the

Table 2.3 Incidence of leukaemias and lymphomas per 10^5 in young persons in England, 1979–2000

	Age group (years)		
	13–14	15–19	20–24
Acute lymphoid leukaemia	1.70	1.24	0.65
Acute myeloid leukaemia	0.57	0.73	0.80
Chronic myeloid leukaemia	0.07	0.13	0.23
Other unspecified leukaemias	0.08	0.16	0.14
Non-Hodgkin's lymphoma	0.91	1.22	1.52
Hodgkin's disease	1.32	2.84	4.13

remainder, but there was an increase in rates for AML and a decrease in ALL relative to the younger age group. However, among 20- to 25-year-olds, AML was the most frequent subtype, accounting for nearly 50% of the cases. Chronic myeloid leukaemia (CML) was relatively rare at all ages but showed increasing rates with increasing age. The incidence of CML in 20- to 25-year-olds was more than three times that seen in 13- to 14-year-olds.

In contrast to ALL, rates for NHL increased with increasing age. Only about half of all registered cases were coded to a specific subtype of NHL. The subtypes specified in the data set are inconsistent with the current international classification of lymphomas, as the classification of NHL has changed substantially during the period covered.[16,17] However, in summary, nearly 80% of all cases with a specified subtype across the age range 13–24 years were classified as diffuse, about 10% as follicular/nodular and the remainder as other miscellaneous subtypes. The incidence of HD increased markedly with age, and the incidence among 20- to 25-year-olds was more than three times that seen in 13- to 14-year-olds. HD subclassification was consistent across the time period and was based on the Rye scheme.[18] More than two-thirds of the HD cases were coded to a specified subtype. Of these, more than 70% were nodular sclerosing HD and this proportion did not differ markedly within age groups. Mixed cellularity HD comprised nearly 20% of all specified cases and was somewhat more frequent among 15- to 24-year-olds than in 13- to 14-year-olds. Lymphocyte-predominant HD formed less than 10% of all specified cases but was rather more frequent at younger than older ages. Lymphocyte-depleted HD was infrequent across all age groups.

Table 2.4 presents incidence rates of malignant CNS tumours. The most frequent CNS tumour was astrocytoma; in those with a specified subtype, low-grade astrocytomas were more common than glioblastoma and anaplastic astrocytoma in the 13- to 14-year-olds and 15- to 19-year-olds. However, the difference in rates between low-grade and high-grade astrocytoma was less marked in 15- to 19-year-olds than in the younger age group. In 20- to 25-year-olds, high-grade astrocytomas were more frequent than low-grade variants. Rates for ependymoma did not differ markedly among the age groups,

Table 2.4 Incidence of malignant brain tumours per 10^5 in young persons in England, 1979–2000

	Age group (years)		
	13–14	**15–19**	**20–24**
Astrocytoma	1.04	0.85	0.92
Other glioma	0.27	0.30	0.43
Ependymoma	0.15	0.10	0.11
Medulloblastoma and other PNET	0.30	0.15	0.16
Other and unspecified malignant intracranial and intraspinal neoplasms	0.18	0.20	0.20

PNET, primitive neuroectodermal tumours.

but ependymoma was somewhat more frequent in the youngest group. Medulloblastoma and other primitive neuroectodermal tumours (PNETs) were twice as common in the younger age group as in patients aged 15–24 years. The rates for CNS tumours overall did not differ greatly across age groups, but although rates were only slightly higher in 13- to 14-year-olds than in 20- to 25-year-olds, they constituted 18% of all cases in the younger age group but less than 8% in the older group (Table 2.1).

Table 2.5 presents the incidence of bone tumours and soft tissue sarcomas. Rates for bone tumours were higher among patients aged 13–19 years than among 20- to 25-year-olds. In all three age groups, osteosarcoma was the most frequent tumour, but the proportion of osteosarcoma was lower in 20- to 25-year-olds, with a relatively higher proportion of chondrosarcoma compared with the younger age groups. Ewing's tumour is the second most common type of bone tumour in all three age groups but rates are higher in 13- to 14-year-olds than at older ages and the rate in the 20- to 25-year-olds is only half that seen in the youngest group.

Table 2.5 Incidence of bone and soft tissue sarcoma per 10^5 in young persons in England, 1979–2000

	Age group (years)		
	13–14	**15–19**	**20–24**
Osteosarcoma	0.84	0.77	0.33
Chondrosarcoma	0.04	0.08	0.10
Ewing's tumour	0.52	0.47	0.26
Other bone tumours	0.07	0.11	0.11
Fibromatous neoplasms	0.10	1.17	0.30
Rhabdomyosarcoma	0.28	0.30	0.15
Other and unspecified STS	0.28	0.45	0.66

STS, soft tissue sarcoma.

Table 2.6 Incidence of carcinomas per 10^5 in young persons in England, 1979–2000

	Age group (years)		
	13–14	15–19	20–24
Thyroid carcinoma	0.19	0.42	0.86
Other carcinoma of head and neck	0.20	0.28	0.36
Carcinoma of trachea, bronchus and lung	0.02	0.04	0.13
Carcinoma of breast	0.00	0.06	0.53
Carcinoma of genitourinary tract	0.15	0.36	2.07
Carcinoma of gastrointestinal tract	0.18	0.36	0.71
Carcinoma of other and ill-defined sites NEC	0.10	0.17	0.30

NEC, not elsewhere classified.

Soft tissue sarcomas, although less common than bone tumours, constitute an important group of malignancies in teenagers and young adults. Soft tissue sarcomas represent about 6% of all malignancies in 13- to 14-year-olds. Rates for rhabdomyosarcoma are lower in the 20- to 25-year-olds, but rates for other soft tissue sarcomas increase with age.

Table 2.6 shows incidence rates for carcinomas. In 13- to 14-year-olds and 15- to 19-year-olds, the head and neck forms the most common primary site group for carcinomas, making up 46 and 41% respectively of all carcinomas among these two age groups, but in 20- to 25-year-olds carcinomas of the head and neck region make up only 25% of all carcinomas. The thyroid is by far the most common primary site for carcinomas in the head and neck, and rates for carcinoma of the thyroid steadily increase across the three age groups. Nasopharyngeal carcinoma, which is extremely rare in the population in Britain in general,[1] makes up more than 10% of all carcinomas in 13- to 14-year-olds but represents only 2% among 20- to 25-year-olds, although the rate is similar to that seen in the younger age group.

Carcinomas of the lung, breast, colon, rectum and bladder constitute nearly 50% of all cancers at all ages[1] but are all very rare in teenagers and young adults. However, examples of all of these carcinomas are seen and the rates increase from the 13- to 14-year age group to the 20- to 25-year-olds. The rates for carcinomas of the genitourinary tract show a marked increase across the three age groups. Genitourinary tract carcinomas comprise 18% of all carcinomas in 13- to 14-year-olds but 21 and 42% in the 15- to 19-year-olds and 20- to 25-year-olds respectively. All sites within the genitourinary tract show increases with age but the greatest increases are for invasive carcinoma of the cervix and uterus. The most common sites among carcinomas of the gastrointestinal tract are the colon and rectum in all three age groups. Adrenocortical carcinoma is exceedingly rare but is seen across the 13- to 24-year age range.

Table 2.7 includes incidence rates for germ cell tumours, melanoma and certain tumours that are typically seen in younger children. The most dramatic

Table 2.7 Incidence of germ cell tumours, melanoma and other miscellaneous tumours per 10^5 in young persons in England, 1979–2000

	Age group (years)		
	13–14	**15–19**	**20–24**
Germ cell and trophoblastic neoplasms of gonads	0.33	1.25	3.76
Non-gonadal germ cell neoplasms	0.13	0.17	0.21
Melanoma	0.28	0.88	2.37
Other embryonic tumours NEC	0.16	0.09	0.08
Other specified neoplasms NEC	0.07	0.10	0.14
Unspecified malignant neoplasms NEC	0.18	0.40	0.80

NEC, not elsewhere classified.

increase in rates with age among the adolescent and young adult group occurs in the gonadal germ cell tumours, for which the rate increases from 0.33 per 100,000 in 13- to 14-year-olds to 1.25 in 15- to 19-year-olds and to 3.76 in 20- to 25-year-olds, representing more than an 11-fold increase in rates over the age range. This is entirely due to testicular germ cell tumours. Non-gonadal germ cell tumours are much less frequent than gonadal, and although rates increase across the age groups the trends with age are less dramatic. There is a small decrease in rates with increasing age for intracranial germ cell tumours. Wilms' tumour, neuroblastoma, hepatoblastoma and retinoblastoma have peak incidences in children aged less than 5 years but a small number of cases have been registered in the teenage and young adult age range. Cases of pancreaticoblastoma and pulmonary blastoma are also present. Collective rates for all these tumours are shown in the table as 'Other embryonic tumours NEC'. In addition, it is interesting to note that there are a number of cases of myeloma, which normally occurs in much older patients.

Incidence rates by sex

Examination of the rates of malignancies in males compared with females showed a number of statistically significant differences. In ALL overall, the male to female rate ratio was significantly above 1 ($P < 0.0001$) and the ratio also increased with increasing age. For AML there was a small excess rate among males ($P = 0.04$) but this did not differ by age. In NHL there was a marked excess rate among males in all age groups ($P < 0.0001$), but the male to female ratio fell slightly with increasing age. The pattern of incidence amongst males and females with HD across the three age groups was similar to that seen for NHL, although the male to female ratio was only slightly above 1 ($P = 0.013$).

There was a significantly higher incidence of CNS tumours in males than in females ($P < 0.0001$), which did not differ significantly by age group. Among diagnostic subgroups only, astrocytoma and medulloblastoma/PNET showed significantly higher rates in males ($P < 0.01$ and <0.0001 respectively). An interesting pattern was observed among the bone tumours, where overall there was a significant excess incidence among males ($P < 0.0001$), but the ratio of rates in males and females differed significantly between age groups ($P < 0.001$). In osteosarcoma and in Ewing's tumour there was a reversal of the ratio of incidence in males to females from an excess rate in females aged 13–14 years to an excess in males aged 20–24 years. The most marked change in incidence rates between males and females with increasing age occurred among the gonadal germ cell tumours. In the 13- to 14-year-olds the ratio of incidence in males to females was less than 0.5, but in 20- to 25-year-olds the male to female ratio had increased to over 17 ($P < 0.0001$). Rates for melanoma and carcinoma of the thyroid were markedly higher in females at all ages (in both groups $P < 0.0001$). There was an overall significant excess of females with adrenocortical carcinoma ($P = 0.002$). A significant excess incidence rate of nasopharyngeal carcinoma and carcinoma of the bladder was seen among males (in both groups $P < 0.0001$). Apart from the gender-specific carcinomas (breast, cervix and uterus), there were no other statistically significant differences in incidence rates among males and females in other main diagnostic groups.

Temporal trends in incidence

Table 2.8 and Fig. 2.1 present time trends in incidence rates for the whole age group (13–24 years) for those groups showing a statistically significant trend with time period. Across all diagnostic groups there was a highly significant increase in incidence rates over time (P for trend <0.0001), although there was little difference between the second and third time periods. Rates for

Table 2.8 Temporal trends in rates of cancer in young persons aged 13–24 in England, 1979–2000

	Rates per 10^5 by time period of diagnosis			
	1979–1985	**1986–1992**	**1993–2000**	**P for trend**
Acute myeloid leukaemia	0.67	0.75	0.78	0.03
Non-Hodgkin's lymphoma	1.00	1.42	1.47	<0.0001
Hodgkin's disease	2.95	3.22	3.21	0.01
Astrocytoma	0.75	0.91	1.09	<0.0001
Ewing's tumour	0.31	0.36	0.51	<0.0001
Germ cell tumour	1.88	2.22	2.90	<0.0001
Melanoma	0.95	1.45	1.83	<0.0001
Thyroid carcinoma	0.45	0.51	0.74	<0.0001
Colorectal carcinoma	0.26	0.23	0.37	0.0007
All cancers	15.41	18.23	19.80	<0.0001

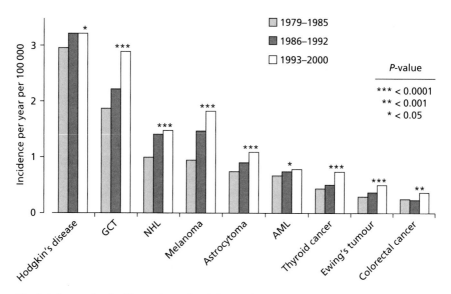

Fig. 2.1 Increasing incidence in England during the past quarter-century of the common malignancies that occur in 13- to 24-year-olds. GCT, germ cell tumours; NHL, non-Hodgkin lymphoma; AML, acute myeloid leukaemia.

leukaemias overall remained stable over the study period, but AML showed a small increase. NHL showed a highly significant increase with time period but the increase over time for HD was less marked (*P* for trend <0.0001 and <0.05 respectively). Rates for all CNS tumours increased over time, but among subgroups of brain tumours only astrocytoma showed a statistically significant increase (*P* < 0.0001). Rates for Ewing's tumour showed a significant increase, which was particularly marked between the second and third time periods (*P* < 0.0001). To what extent this increase in rates for Ewing's tumour may be due to changes in diagnostic practice is uncertain, but there were no comparable decreases in rates of other bone tumours. This observation warrants further investigation. Rates for soft tissue sarcomas overall, and for rhabdomyosarcoma also, did not change, but rates for fibrosarcoma decreased while the incidence of other soft tissue sarcomas increased. The data are not shown but this result is probably due to changes in diagnostic criteria and classification following developments in immunohistochemistry and molecular pathology,[19] as discussed elsewhere.[6]

Marked increases in incidence were also seen for gonadal germ cell tumours (accounted for primarily by testicular tumours), melanoma and carcinoma of the thyroid (in all cases *P* < 0.0001). There was no corresponding significant increase in ovarian germ cell tumours. Colorectal carcinomas showed a significant trend, which was accounted for by an increase between the second and third time periods (*P* < 0.001). Temporal trends in incidence in 15- to 24-year-olds are reported in more detail elsewhere.[6]

Interpretation of incidence patterns

We have established that ICD is not a satisfactory vehicle for presenting data on cancer in teenagers and young adults. Carcinomas are uncommon in this age group and ICD cannot distinguish non-epithelial cancers from carcinomas, or different types of these from each other. Data on cancers in young people are more appropriately presented in terms of morphology. Morphology-based classification systems for the analysis and presentation of data on childhood cancers have been in existence for many years[20,21] and the childhood cancer scheme has been applied to cancer incidence data in adolescents aged 15–19 years.[22] However, a number of the major groups of cancers in children (for example, most embryonic tumours) are so rare as to be irrelevant in teenagers and young adults. Conversely, carcinomas are inappropriately subdivided in the childhood classifications.[23] In an attempt to overcome these problems, one study has used a combination of the childhood classification groups and ICD site groups,[24] but this leads to a lack of clarity and coherence in the data. Birch *et al.* have developed a classification system which has been specifically tailored to the teenage and young adult age range,[6] based primarily on morphology. This classification scheme has now been applied to national data for England on almost 32,000 cancers in young persons aged 13–24 years. Detailed data, as presented above, are of importance in assessing service requirements and in the delivery of services designed to meet the needs of this vulnerable age group. Observation of detailed patterns of incidence can also provide pointers to aetiology and identify areas for future research. Classification of cases for analysis which takes account of biological similarities and differences is of critical importance if advances in knowledge and understanding are to be made.

Aetiological factors

There is accumulating epidemiological evidence that childhood precursor B-cell ALL, which demonstrates a characteristic peak in incidence between the ages of 2 and 6 years, is aetiologically linked to delayed exposure to infections in early childhood, resulting in delayed immune stimulation. There is also strong evidence that an initial mutational event occurs *in utero* and predisposes the child to the subsequent development of leukaemia in early life.[25–29] Space–time clustering patterns in childhood leukaemia also support a role for infections.[30] The decrease in incidence rates in ALL with increasing age following the childhood peak to young adulthood suggests that aetiological factors and/or mechanisms may also change with age. Nevertheless, infections may play an important role in the aetiology of leukaemia in teenagers and young adults, but whereas in young children mainly indirect mechanisms have been proposed, in these older age groups a directly transforming virus may be more likely.[31]

With respect to AML, the increased risk following exposure to certain thera-peutic agents used to treat an initial malignancy,[32] i.e. chemical induction of AML, suggests the possibility of a role for environmental chemical exposures in a proportion of cases in young people in general. Higher rates for AML were seen with increasing age among teenagers and young adults and there was some evidence of an increase in incidence rates over time. The possibility that these patterns of incidence might be due, at least in part, to postnatal exposures to environmental chemical agents should be given some consideration.

Viruses may also be involved in the aetiology of both NHL and HD. An increased risk of NHL has been observed in association with HIV1, HTLV1 and Epstein–Barr virus (EBV). *Helicobacter pylori* infection of the stomach is associated with gastric lymphoma. While these are all relatively rare occurrences and probably account for only a small proportion of total NHL, a role for other viruses and indirect mechanisms involving common infections remain a possibility.[33] EBV infection is aetiologically linked to a proportion of HD, particularly the mixed cellularity subtype. Epidemiological studies have demonstrated that the magnitude of the risk and proportion of cases attributable to EBV infections varies with age, sex, ethnicity and the level of material deprivation. EBV infection is extremely common and other unknown modifying factors are likely to be of importance in the aetiology of HD in teenagers and young adults.[34,35]

The decline in incidence of PNETs, the increase in high-grade astrocytomas and the decrease in low-grade astrocytomas with increasing age may reflect a change in aetiological mechanisms in these tumours. A possible role of polyoma viruses, including simian virus 40 (SV40), JC and BK viruses in CNS tumours, has been the subject of much speculation. Viral DNA sequences have been detected in human brain tumours, including PNETs, ependymomas, high- and low-grade astrocytomas and meningiomas.[36–38] In addition, space–time clustering has been detected in astrocytomas and ependymomas in older children.[39] The presence of space–time clustering is consistent with an infectious aetiology. Furthermore, there are similar temporal trends in the incidence of brain tumours in children, teenagers and young adults.[6,40] It follows that there may be shared aetiological factors for certain brain tumours across these age groups. Hypotheses relating to viral exposures should be investigated.

The increasing ratio of male to female cases across the three age groups 13–14, 15–19 and 20–24 years suggests that the onset of osteosarcoma and Ewing's tumour may be associated with the adolescent growth spurt, which occurs earlier in females than in males. Dietary and hormonal factors may be relevant. The possibility of a viral aetiology for osteosarcoma has also been considered and SV40-like sequences have been detected in osteosarcoma tissue in several studies.[41–44] In the most recent of these studies, the frequency of SV40-like sequences in peripheral blood cells from osteosarcoma patients was compared with that in normal, healthy controls and was found to be substantially increased in the osteosarcoma patients.[44] Space–time clustering has been reported in childhood soft tissue sarcomas.[45] It would be of considerable interest to determine whether soft tissue sarcomas in teenagers and young adults exhibit space–time clustering.

The very marked temporal increase in the incidence of testicular germ cell tumours in young men has been reported previously. The aetiology of testicular germ cell tumours is uncertain but genetic and hormonal factors, including *in utero* exposure to oestrogen, appear to be implicated.[46] A recent cohort study of young men in Sweden found a positive association between height at 18 years and the incidence of testicular cancer which was not accounted for by gestational age and birth weight. The authors concluded that factors influencing postnatal growth, such as diet and growth-related genes, might underlie the association.[47] The incidence trends for melanoma of the skin have also been discussed previously. Melanoma of the skin shows associations with socio-economic factors, skin and hair colouring, certain heritable syndromes and, in particular, patterns of sun exposure.[46]

The pattern of carcinomas in teenagers and young adults differs greatly from that seen at older ages. Carcinomas of the head and neck, including the thyroid and nasopharynx, make up nearly 30% of carcinomas in the 13- to 24-year age range. The temporal increase in carcinoma of the thyroid in young people has been discussed elsewhere.[6] The highest incidence rates for nasopharyngeal carcinoma are found in parts of the Far East, where it occurs in association with EBV infection. The rare cases of nasopharyngeal carcinoma in young people in Western developed countries may also be associated with EBV, and this should be explored, but it is likely that other cofactors are involved.[48] Carcinoma of the cervix and uterus, although typical of older age groups, is relatively frequent in young adult females and appears to be closely linked with sexually transmitted infections, including herpes simplex virus type 2 and human papilloma virus.[46] Other carcinomas seen in teenagers and young adults which typically occur in later life may be strongly associated with genetic predisposition at young ages, as discussed below.

Genetic predisposition and genetic susceptibility

Cancer occurs mainly in the late middle-aged and the elderly and at the molecular level involves multiple, serially accumulated genetic changes following decades of exposure to carcinogens, such as tobacco smoke. The occurrence of cancer at young ages, where the opportunity for such chronic environmental exposures does not exist, strongly suggests that individuals are genetically predisposed to developing certain cancers or are genetically susceptible to the carcinogenic effects of environmental agents. In such individuals, the number of genetic changes required to achieve malignant transformation at the cellular level is reduced and/or metabolic processes are modified. In many instances gene–environment interactions will be involved.

Genetic factors appear to be of aetiological importance in CNS tumours in young people, and brain tumours occur in association with a number of cancer predisposition syndromes characterized by germ-line mutations in cancer-associated genes.[49] Of particular relevance to teenage and young adult cases of high-grade astrocytoma is the possibility that these may arise in patients with germ-line TP53 mutations.[50,51] Anaplastic astrocytoma shows a peak incidence in the fourth decade of life and glioblastoma is rare before the age of 30 years.[52] However, in individuals with germ-line TP53 mutations these tumours tend to arise at much earlier ages.[51,53] Brain tumours, notably medulloblastoma among patients with germ-line mutations of the APC gene, are often diagnosed in older children, teenagers and young adults.[54] The unusually early age of onset of brain tumours in familial cancer syndromes may represent a combination of genetic susceptibility and environmental exposure. The detection of SV40 viral sequences in tumours from patients with germ-line TP53 mutations is of interest in this context.[55] It appears that genetic factors may be important in the aetiology of both osteosarcoma and Ewing's tumour. Osteosarcoma is frequently seen in families with germ-line TP53 mutations and cases are usually diagnosed during the teens and twenties.[53,56] Evidence for genetic susceptibility to Ewing's tumour comes from the striking variation in incidence with ethnic origin. Ewing's tumour is extremely rare among black Africans and among African-Americans.[57] In common with osteosarcoma, soft tissue sarcomas are a principal component of the cancer predisposition syndrome associated with germ-line TP53 mutations, and in such patients soft tissue sarcomas are frequently diagnosed at young ages.

Carcinoma of the breast is extremely rare in the teenage and young adult age range, but is of particular interest since a recent study detected pathogenic alterations in breast cancer susceptibility genes (including BRCA1, BRCA2 and TP53) in 20% of a large series of women with breast cancer diagnosed under the age of 30.[58] It is possible that a similarly high rate of mutations in susceptibility genes associated with colorectal carcinoma might also be found among very young patients. Genes of interest in these patients include APC and the mismatch repair genes.[59] The frequency of mutations in relevant genes among these very early-onset cases of common carcinomas should be determined.

Conclusions

Descriptive data provide a basis for service planning and also offer a stimulus for studies of aetiology. Furthermore, detailed analyses of incidence patterns by geographical region and demographic factors together with the determination of variations in incidence in time and space will provide additional insights into aetiology and suggest possible lines of investigation. The chronic occupational and social exposures, including cigarette smoking, which are responsible for the majority of late-onset cancers, are unlikely to be prime causes of cancers in young people. In some circumstances exposure to such environmental agents may be involved in aetiology, but other cofactors, such as genetic susceptibility and hormonal factors, may predominate. The possibility that environmental agents may target different organs and tissues in the growing child, leading to different cancers in teenagers and young adults compared with older adults, should be considered. In a number of cancers occurring in young people, the most promising areas for investigation include the roles of specific viruses, other infections, dietary factors, and their influence on growth and development and inherited predisposition. Little is known about the aetiology of cancer in this fascinating age group and carefully targeted research in this field should produce rewarding results.

Acknowledgements

Jillian M. Birch is a Cancer Research UK Professorial Research Fellow. Data presented in this chapter were contributed by the nine regional cancer registries in England and were supplied by the National Cancer Intelligence Centre, London (Director, Dr M. J. Quinn). Statistical analyses were carried out by Dr R. D. Alston.

References

1 Office for National Statistics. *Cancer statistics registrations: registrations of cancer diagnosed in 2000, England. Series MB1 No. 31.* London: Office for National Statistics, 2003.
2 Office for National Statistics. *Twentieth century mortality. Mortality in England and Wales by age, sex, year and underlying cause: year 2000 update.* London: Office for National Statistics, 2002.
3 World Health Organization. The causes of cancer. In: Stewart BW, Kleihues P, eds. *World Cancer Report.* Lyon: IARC Press, 2003: 22–28.
4 Ablett S, ed. *Quest for Cure – the UK Children's Cancer Study Group: The First 25 Years.* London: UKCCSG/Trident Communications, 2002.
5 Bleyer WA. Cancer in older adolescents and young adults: epidemiology, diagnosis, treatment, survival and importance of clinical trials. *Med Pediatr Oncol* 2002; **38**: 1–10.
6 Birch JM, Alston RD, Kelsey AM, Quinn MJ, Babb P, McNally RJQ. Classification and incidence of cancers in adolescents and young adults in England 1979–1997. *Br J Cancer* 2002; **87**: 1267–1274.
7 World Health Organization. *International Classification of Diseases, Injuries and Causes of Death,* 9th edn. Geneva: World Health Organization, 1975.
8 World Health Organization. *International Statistical Classification of Diseases and Related Health Problems – Tenth Revision.* Geneva: World Health Organization; 1992.
9 Parkin DM, Whelan SL, Ferlay J, Teppo L, Thomas DB, eds. *Cancer Incidence in Five Continents, Vol. VIII.* IARC Scientific Publications, No. 155. Lyon: IARC, 2002.
10 Percy C, Van Holten V, Muir C, eds. *International Classification of Diseases for Oncology (ICD-O),* 2nd edition. Geneva: World Health Organization, 1990.
11 Birch JM, Alston RD, Quinn M, Kelsey AM. Incidence of malignant disease by morphological type, in young persons aged 12–14 years in England, 1979–1997. *Eur J Cancer* 2003; **39**: 2622–2631.
12 Quinn MJ, Babb PJ, Jones J, Baker A, Ault C. Cancer 1971–1997. *Registrations of cancer cases and deaths in England and Wales by sex, age, year, health region and type of cancer* (CD-ROM). London: Office for National Statistics, 1999.
13 World Health Organization. *International Classification of Diseases for Oncology,* 1st edition. Geneva: World Health Organization, 1976.
14 Blair V, Birch JM. Patterns and temporal trends in the incidence of malignant disease in children: I. Leukaemia and lymphoma. *Eur J Cancer* 1994; **30**: 1490–1498.

15 Francis B, Green M, Payne C. *The GLIM system, Release 4 Manual*. Oxford: Clarendon Press, 1993.

16 Harris NL, Jaffe ES, Diebold J *et al*. The World Health Organization Classification of Neoplastic Diseases of the Hematopoietic and Lymphoid Tissues. Report of the Clinical Advisory Committee Meeting, Airlie House, Virginia, Nov. 1997. *Ann Oncol* 1999; **10**: 1419–1432.

17 Jaffe ES, Harris NL, Stein H, Vardiman JW, eds. *The World Health Organization Classification of Tumours. Pathology and Genetics of Tumours of Haematopoietic and Lymphoid Tissues*. Lyon: IARC Press, 2001.

18 Lukes RJ, Craver L, Hall T, Rappaport H, Ruben P. Report of the nomenclature committee. *Cancer Res* 1996; **26**: 1311.

19 Weiss SW, Goldblum JR. *Enzinger and Weiss's Soft Tissue Tumors*. 4th edn. St Louis: Mosby, 2001.

20 Birch JM, Marsden HB. A classification scheme for childhood cancer. *Int J Cancer* 1987; **40**: 624–629.

21 Kramárová E, Stiller CA. The International Classification of Childhood Cancer. *Int J Cancer* 1996; **68**: 759–765.

22 Smith MA, Gurney JG, Ries LA. Cancer in adolescents 15–19 years old. In: Ries LA, Smith MA, Gurney JG *et al*., eds. *SEER Pediatric Monograph, United States STEER Program 1975–1997*. NIH Publication No. 99–4649. Bethesda (MD): National Cancer Institute, 1999.

23 Fritschi L, Coates M, McCredie M. Incidence of cancer among New South Wales adolescents: which classification scheme describes adolescent cancers better? *Int J Cancer* 1995; **60**: 355–360.

24 Gatta G, Capocaccia R, De Angelis R, Stiller C, Coebergh JW and the EUROCARE Working Group. Cancer survival in European adolescents and young adults. *Eur J Cancer* 2003; **39**: 2600–2610.

25 Greaves MF. Speculations on the cause of childhood acute lymphoblastic leukaemia. *Leukaemia* 1998; **2**: 120–125.

26 Kinlen LJ. Epidemiological evidence for an infective basis in childhood leukaemia. *Br J Cancer* 1995; **71**: 1–5.

27 Smith MA, Simon R, Strickler HD *et al*. Evidence that childhood acute lymphoblastic leukaemia is associated with an infectious agent linked to hygiene conditions. *Cancer Causes Control* 1998; **9**: 285–298.

28 Gale KB, Ford AM, Repp R *et al*. Backtracking leukaemia to birth: identification of clonotypic gene fusion sequences in neonatal blood spots. *Proc Natl Acad Sci USA* 1997; **94**: 13950–13954.

29 Wiemels JL, Cazzaniga G, Daniotti M *et al*. Prenatal origin of acute lymphoblastic leukaemia in children. *Lancet* 1999; **354**: 1499–1503.

30 Birch JM, Alexander FE, Blair V *et al*. Space-time clustering patterns in childhood leukaemia support a role for infection. *Br J Cancer* 2000; **82**: 1571–1576.

31 International Agency for Research on Cancer. *Human Immunodeficiency Viruses and Human T-Cell Lymphotropic Viruses. IARC Monographs on the Evaluation of Carcinogenic Risks to Humans, Vol. 87*. Lyon: IARC Press, 1996.

32 Bhatia S, Yasui Y, Robison LL *et al*. High risk of subsequent neoplasms continues with extended follow-up of childhood Hodgkin's disease: report from the Late Effects Study Group. *J Clin Oncol* 2003; **21**: 4386–4394.

33 Baris D, Zahm SH. Epidemiology of lymphomas. *Curr Opin Oncol* 2001; **12**: 383–394.

34 Glaser SL, Lin RJ, Stewart SL *et al*. Epstein–Barr virus-associated Hodgkin's disease: epidemiologic characteristics in international data. *Int J Cancer* 1997; **70**: 375–382.

35 Flavell KJ, Biddulph JP, Powell JE *et al*. South Asian ethnicity and material deprivation increase the risk of Epstein–Barr virus infection in childhood Hodgkin's disease. *Br J Cancer* 2001; **85**: 350–356.

36 Weggen S, Bayer TA, von Deimling A *et al*. Low frequency of SV40, JC and BK polyomavirus sequences in human medulloblastomas, meningiomas and ependymomas. *Brain Pathol* 2000; **10**: 85–92.

37 Del Valle L, Gordon J, Assimakopoulou M *et al*. Detection of JC virus DNA sequences and expression of the viral regulatory protein T-antigen in tumors of the central nervous system. *Cancer Res* 2001; **61**: 4287–4293.

38 Del Valle L, Gordon J, Enam S *et al*. Expression of human neurotropic polyomavirus JCV late gene product agnoprotein in human medulloblastoma. *J Natl Cancer Inst* 2002; **94**: 267–273.

39 McNally RJQ, Cairns DP, Eden OB *et al*. An infectious aetiology for childhood brain tumours? Evidence from space-time clustering and seasonality analyses. *Br J Cancer* 2002; **86**: 1070–1077.

40 McNally RJQ, Kelsey AM, Cairns DP *et al*. Temporal increases in the incidence of childhood solid tumours seen in North West England (1954–1998) are likely to be real. *Cancer* 2001; **92**: 1967–1976.

41 Lednicky JA, Stewart AR, Jenkins III JJ, Finegold MJ, Butel JS. SV40 DNA in human osteosarcomas shows sequence variation among T-antigen genes. *Int J Cancer* 1997; **72**: 791–800.

42 Mendoza SM, Konishi T, Miller CW. Integration of SV40 in human osteosarcoma DNA. *Oncogene* 1998; **17**: 2457–2462.

43 Carbone M, Rizzo P, Procopio A *et al*. SV40-like sequences in human bone tumors. *Oncogene* 1996; **13**: 527–535.

44 Yamamoto H, Nakayama T, Murakami H *et al*. High incidence of SV40-like sequences detection in tumour and peripheral blood cells of Japanese osteosarcoma patients. *Br J Cancer* 2000; **82**: 1677–1681.

45 McNally RJQ, Kelsey AM, Eden OB *et al*. Space-time clustering patterns in childhood solid tumours other than central nervous system tumours. *Int J Cancer* 2003; **103**: 253–258.

46 Quinn M, Babb P, Brock A, Kirby L, Jones J. *Cancer Trends in England and Wales 1950–1999*. Studies on Medical and Population Subjects No. 66. London: Office for National Statistics, 2001.

47 Rasmussen F, Gunnell D, Ekbom A, Hallqvist J, Tynelius P. Birth weight, adult height and testicular cancer: cohort study of 337,249 Swedish young men. *Cancer Causes Control* 2003; **14**: 595–598.

48 Griffin BE. Epstein–Barr virus (EBV) and human disease: facts, opinions and problems. *Mutat Res* 2000; **462**: 395–405.

49 Kleihues P, Cavenee WK. Familial tumour syndromes involving the nervous system. In: *World Health Organization Classification of Tumours. Pathology and Genetics of Tumors of the Nervous System*. Lyon: IARC Press, 2000: 215–242.

50 Li Y-J, Sanson M, Hoang-Xuan K *et al*. Incidence of germ-line p53 mutations in patients with gliomas. *Int J Cancer* 1995; **64**: 383–387.

51 Chen P, Iavarone A, Fick J *et al*. Constitutional p53 mutations associated with brain tumors in young adults. *Cancer Genet Cytogenet* 1995; **82**: 106–115.

52 Kleihues P, Cavenee WK. Astrocytic tumours. In: *World Health Organization Classification of Tumours. Pathology and Genetics of Tumors of the Nervous System.* Lyon: IARC Press, 2000: 9–54.

53 Birch JM, Blair V, Kelsey AM *et al.* Cancer phenotype correlates with constitutional TP53 genotype in families with the Li-Fraumeni syndrome. *Oncogene* 1998; **17**: 1061–1068.

54 Hamilton SR, Liu B, Parsons RE *et al.* The molecular basis of Turcot's syndrome. *N Engl J Med* 1995; **332**: 839–847.

55 Malkin D, Chilton-MacNeill S, Meister LA, Sexsmith E, Diller L, Garcea RL. Tissue-specific expression of SV40 in tumors associated with the Li-Fraumeni syndrome. *Oncogene* 2000; **20**: 4441–4449.

56 Birch JM. The Li-Fraumeni syndrome and the role of the TP53 mutations in predisposition to cancer. In: Eeles RA, Easton DF, Eng C, Ponder BA. *Genetic Predisposition to Cancer*, 2nd edn. London: Edward Arnold, 2004: 141–154.

57 Parkin DM, Kramárová E, Draper GJ *et al.*, eds. *International Incidence of Childhood Cancer, Vol. II.* World Health Organization, IARC Scientific Publications, No. 144. Lyon: IARC Press, 1998.

58 Lalloo F, Varley J, Ellis D *et al.* Prediction of pathogenic mutations in patients with early-onset breast cancer by family history. *Lancet* 2003; **361**: 1101–1102.

59 Fearnhead NS, Wilding JL, Bodmer WF. Genetics of colorectal cancer: hereditary aspects and overview of colorectal tumorigenesis. *Br Med Bull* 2002; **64**: 27–43.

CHAPTER 3

Lack of participation of older adolescents and young adults with cancer in clinical trials: impact in the USA

A. Bleyer, T. Budd and M. Montello

Introduction

A patient newly diagnosed with cancer between 15 and 30 years of age is more likely to be thrust into a state of limbo – both medically and socially – than either a child or older adult with cancer. Thus, it is no surprise that patients with cancer in this age group are less likely to find their way into a clinical trial that seeks to improve their chances of survival than either younger or older patients. And indeed this has been shown to be so in the USA, where only about 1% of these patients are entered into treatment trials compared with approximately 60% of patients less than 15 years of age and 3–5% of older adults.[1–3] This report summarizes the status of participation of older adolescents and young adults in clinical trials in the USA and addresses the impact this deficit has had on this age group and how the effect is likely to occur in other countries.

The deficit in adolescent and young adult participation in cancer clinical trials

Figure 3.1 shows the number of patient entries in national cancer treatment trials sponsored by the National Cancer Institute during 1997–2003 as a function of patient age. The cancer treatment trial participation rate among 15- to 19-year-olds was approximately half of the corresponding rate in those younger than 15 years old. In 20- to 29-year-olds, it was approximately 15% of the rate in children. Among older patients, the trial participation rate was higher (between 3% and 5% overall), but still much lower than in children.

Management at dedicated cancer centres

More than 90% of children aged less than 15 years with cancer are managed at institutions that participate in National Cancer institute (NCI)-sponsored

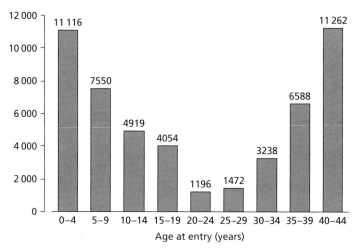

Fig. 3.1 Entries of 51 395 patients below 45 years of age into US national cooperative group treatment trials sponsored by the Cancer Therapy Evaluation Program (CTEP) of the National Cancer Institute Division of Cancer Treatment and Diagnosis during 1997–2003 inclusive.

clinical trials, and 55–65% of these young patients are entered into clinical trials. In contrast, only 20–35% of 15- to 19-year-olds with cancer are seen at such institutions, and only about 10% are entered into a clinical trial.[4,5] Among 20- to 29-year-olds, the participation rate is even lower, fewer that 10% being seen at member institutions of the cooperative groups, either paediatric or adult, and only about 1% entering clinical trials either of the paediatric or adult cooperative groups.

Race/ethnicity
Figure 3.2 shows the race/ethnicity-specific accruals for each 5-year age interval from 15 to 40 years of age, relative to the average for those aged 0 and 15 years of age.[2] The accrual pattern is similar among all racial/ethnic groups. With the lower rates of inclusion in non-Hispanic whites, Hispanics, African-Americans, Asians, American Indians, Alaskan natives, and Hawaiian and other Pacific Islanders, in terms of overall participation by ethnicity, Hispanic patients have less than one-fifth the rate seen in white patients, African-Americans have one-tenth, and Asians, native Indians and Alaskan natives each have about 1% (Fig. 3.2).[2]

Gender
The nadir in clinical trial participation rate at 20–30 years of age is apparent in both females and males, although it is considerably more striking in females (Fig. 3.2). The lower participation rate is apparent in all of the ethnicities/races specified above.

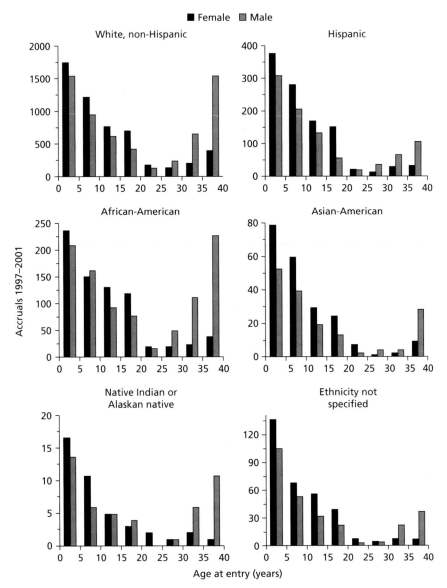

Fig. 3.2 Accrual of patients under 45 years of age to cooperative group treatment trials by race/ethnicity as a function of age at entry during 1997–2001 inclusive.

Residence

Geographically, this gap has been observed throughout the USA and is in striking contrast to the uniform accrual of a majority of patients less than 15 years of age in virtually all metropolitan and rural areas across the country.[5] Although minority group adolescent patients have a lower participation rate than younger patients, regardless of ethnicity or race, their deficit is qualitatively and quantitatively similar to that apparent in the majority group.[3] This equity exists despite minority group under-representation in visits to physician offices.[6]

Individual types of cancer

With one exception, all of the individual types of cancer that have been evaluated for age-dependent clinical trial participation have shown a similar pattern. These include non-Kaposi's sarcomas (osteosarcoma, Ewing's sarcomas, synovial cell sarcoma, rhabdomyosarcoma, other soft tissue non-rhabdomyosarcomas),[7] brain tumours, leukaemia,[8] lymphoma and breast cancer (Fig. 3.3).

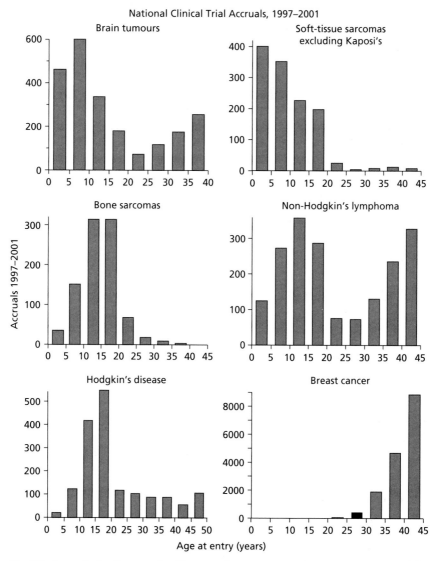

Fig. 3.3 Accrual of patients under 45 years of age to cooperative group treatment trials by cancer type as a function of age at entry during 1997–2001 inclusive.

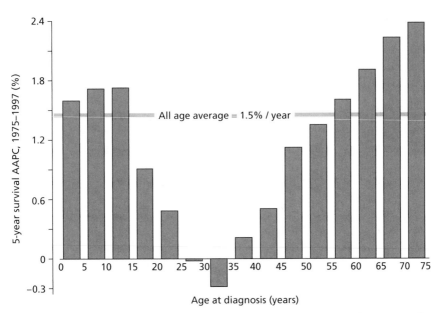

Fig. 3.4 Average annual percentage change in the 5-year survival rate of patients with invasive cancer who were in the US SEER registry from 1997 to 2001.

Impact of the deficit in clinical trial participation in the USA

Mortality and survival trends in the USA in 15- to 45-year-olds pale in comparison with the gains made in younger and older persons.[1-3] This is particularly true for 20- to 30-year-olds but it is also apparent for 15- to 19-year-olds.[4]

Survival improvement

The average annual improvement in the 5-year survival rate during the past quarter-century exceeded 1.5% per year both in children younger than 15 years and in adults older than age 50 (Fig. 3.5).[1] In 15- to 25-year-olds, the improvement averaged less than 0.5%, with no perceptible improvement at all in patients aged 20–30 years (Fig. 3.4). Whereas this trend has partially been corrected during the past decade in 25- to 45-year-olds, the survival deficit has actually worsened among 15- to 25-year-olds.

Mortality rate reduction

The cancer mortality rate among 15- to 45-year-olds has correspondingly lagged behind the reduction seen in children and older adults (Fig. 3.5).[1] To compound matters, the absolute incidence of cancer in 25- to 35-year-olds has increased at a faster rate than in children and adults.

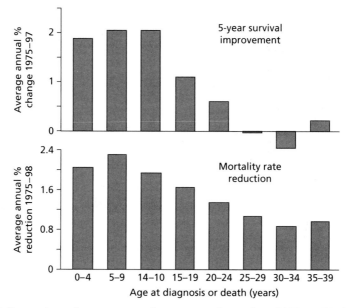

Fig. 3.5 Comparison of average annual percentage change from 1975 to 1997 in the 5-year survival rate (US SEER) of patients with invasive cancer (upper panel) and the average annual reduction from 1975 to 1998 in the national cancer mortality rate (lower panel).

Gender and ethnicity/race

These ominous trends in mortality and survival among 15- to 45-year-olds are apparent in both males and females, with males sustaining a greater deficit than females (Fig. 3.6), and in all ethnicities examined to date, including non-Hispanic whites, Hispanics, African-Americans and Asians.

Cancer deaths versus other causes of mortality

In the USA, cancer is the leading cause of non-accidental death among adolescents and young adults. Among 20- to 39-year-olds, cancer causes more deaths than suicide, heart disease, human immunodeficiency virus infection, cerebrovascular disease and cirrhosis.[9] In females, deaths due to cancer occur at more than twice the frequency of the second leading cause of death due to disease. In 15- to 19-year-olds, cancer is the fourth leading cause of all deaths, following accidental injuries, suicide and homicide.

Individual types of cancer

The trends have been found in sarcomas,[5] lymphomas, brain tumours (astrocytomas, ependymoma and other gliomas), breast cancer and leukaemia.[8] Young adults with leukaemia did not have a nadir in outcome improvement but they have had a worse mortality rate relative to incidence than any other

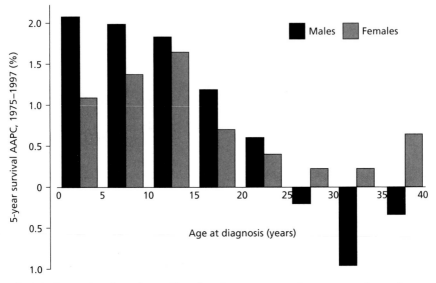

Fig. 3.6 Comparison in males and females of average annual percentage change from 1975 to 1997 in the 5-year survival rate with invasive cancer (US SEER).

age group.[8] The opposite pattern, in which a peak in outcome improvement instead of a nadir occurs during young adulthood, was apparent in patients with Kaposi's sarcoma (Fig. 3.4).

In 1975 the overall 5-year survival rate was estimated to be 64% among patients who were 15–19 years of age when diagnosed. By 1990, the 5-year survival rate had increased to 76%. The corresponding survival rates for patients younger than 15 years of age were 55% in 1975 and 75% in 1990. Thus, the relative improvement in the 5-year survival rate was considerably greater in younger patients (absolute increase 20%, relative increase 36%) than in older adolescents (absolute increase 12%, relative increase 19%), as shown in Fig. 3.4. If this trend is projected from 1990 to 2000, the 5-year survival rate should have reached 80% in 15- to 19-year-olds and 85% in younger patients. This would result in an inversion of superiority from a 10% advantage of the older age group in 1975 to a 5% disadvantage compared with the younger patients in 2000. A similar reversal can be projected to have occurred for 20- to 29-year-olds, although the difference in improvement would not be as dramatic.

The worst outcomes among the common cancers in 15- to 19-year-olds are in acute myeloid leukaemia (AML), acute lymphoid leukaemia (ALL) and the sarcomas, particularly rhabdomyosarcoma, Ewing's sarcoma and osteosarcoma. With the exceptions of thyroid carcinoma, melanoma and germ cell tumours, the remaining common cancers in older adolescents are associated with a worse prognosis than is found with the same cancers in younger age groups.

The mortality burden is a function of the survival and incidence rates. In particular, more than 80% of the US national cancer mortality burden among 15- to 19-year-olds is due to four malignancy groups: sarcomas, leukaemia/lymphomas, CNS tumours and germ cell tumours. Leukaemia is the primary contributor to the cancer mortality burden in 15- to 19-year-olds. Although thyroid carcinoma and melanoma are among the more common cancers in this age group, because of their high cure rates they contribute little to the overall cancer mortality burden.

Analysis of reasons for the clinical trial participation deficit

The reasons for the gap in trial participation are to a large extent unknown and undoubtedly multifactorial. The reasons that were identified at an NCI-sponsored workshop on the topic and further developed in subsequent evaluations[10] are summarized in Table 3.1.

Table 3.1 Potential barriers to participation of older adolescents and young adults in clinical trials

Continuity of care and philosophy
- In the USA, young adults and older adolescents have the lowest rate of primary care use of any age group.
- Adolescents and young adults are also more likely than younger children to lack a usual source of care. Without a primary physician who knows the patient, there may be reluctance to trust the medical establishment and the clinical trial enterprise.
- Physicians and other health-care professionals are poorly trained, or unwilling, to care for adolescents.
- Adolescents and young adults are not 'supposed to' have cancer. Clinical suspicion is low and symptoms are often attributed to physical exertion, fatigue, trauma and stress.
- Adolescents and young adults have a strong sense of invincibility. Out of denial, they may delay seeing a physician for symptoms. Even when seen, they may give poor historical information, especially to a physician untrained to read between the lines of a teenager's history.

Economic, insurance-based factors
- In the USA, young adults are the most uninsured and the most under-insured age group. Nearly half of all 15- to 19-year-olds lose the health-care insurance provided by their parents and do not acquire adequate coverage at their next destination in life, whether at an institution of higher learning or via an employer.
- Treating physicians may be reluctant to use clinical trials because of the time, cost and effort involved, not only on their part (and that of their team) but also on the part of the patient and family.
- Health insurance organizations may deter referral of adolescents and young adults to a centre or cooperative group, or enrolment onto a clinical trial. Attendees had little direct evidence for this factor.

Continued

Provider bias

- Coping with an older adolescent or young adult is difficult. Adding the additional burden of clinical trial participation is more difficult to achieve for the adolescent than for younger or older patients.
- Treating physicians may be reluctant to use clinical trials because they perceive the patient as likely to be non-compliant (or non-adherent) to the protocol requirements. The patient is perceived to have enough difficulty in complying with the treatment plan and keeping up their lives without the additional burden of protocol obligations.
- Oncologists (surgeons, radiotherapists, medical oncologists and gynaecologists) in private practice may retain these patients rather than refer them to a tertiary-care facility or cooperative group member institution.
- Providers may be biased against clinical trials in adolescents. Reasons may include the historically better results compared with older and younger patients, and the need to explain and obtain consent for study entry from both patient and family.
- Family practitioners, gynaecologists and internists may not regard multimodal therapy as important in young adults or older adolescents as they do in younger or older patients. Reasons may include the perceived better results obtained in this age group in comparison with older patients and the higher rate of single-modality therapy normally applied to patients in this age range.
- Providers may be unaware of opportunities for clinical trial participation for adolescents and young adults with cancer.

Patient/family preferences

- Patients and/or parents are more inclined to refuse referral to a cooperative group member institution or to be entered into a clinical trial.
- Patients and/or parents may be unaware of opportunities for clinical trial participation for adolescents and young adults with cancer.

Provider age policies

- The age policies of hospitals may prevent patient access to clinical trials that are under way at the institution. Children's hospitals may have upper age limits that deny the older patient or deny the treating physician who does not have clinical privileges. The reverse may be true for younger patients accessing clinical trials primarily intended for adult patients.
- The clinical trial itself may have age limits that prohibit entry of an otherwise eligible patient.

Cooperative group limitations

- Paediatric cooperative group and adult cooperative group clinical trials may not allow entry of adolescent and young adults because of restrictive eligibility criteria.
- A clinical trial may not be available.
- Adult cooperative groups may lack treatment protocols for the youngest patients.
- Paediatric cooperative groups may lack treatment protocols for older patients.
- Clinical trials for the types of cancer that predominate among adolescents and young adults may not be a priority of the cooperative group enterprise.

A factor that does *not* explain the discrepancy is the participation of minority adolescent patients in clinical trials. In the USA, minority children and adolescents with cancer have equal or higher rates of entry into national clinical trials.[5]

One of the most important factors is the place of treatment, since fewer patients in the 15- to 30-year age group are referred to dedicated, comprehensive cancer centres than in any other age group, with the possible exception of the most elderly age group (over age 85). In the USA and Canada, more than 90% of children younger than 15 years with cancer are treated at institutions that participate in NCI-sponsored clinical trials. In contrast, only about 20% of 15- to 19-year-olds are treated at such institutions, and only about 10% are entered into a clinical trial. Among 20- to 29-year-olds the inclusion rate is even lower, with fewer than 10% treated at member institutions of the cooperative groups, either paediatric or adult, and only about 1% of 20- to 25-year-olds are entered into clinical trials of the paediatric or adult cooperative groups.

For acute lymphoblastic leukaemia, one of the most common cancers in the adolescent and young adult age group, a striking difference has been reported from both France and the USA. In both countries, the use of a paediatric treatment regimen resulted in a better outcome – nearly twice the event-free and overall survival rates – compared with the same young adult age group (16–21 years) treated in adult leukaemia trials.[11,12] In Children's Cancer Group trials in the period from 1989 to 1995, 196 patients aged 16–21 years had a 6-year event-free survival of 64%, whereas for 103 patients aged 16–20 years in Cancer and Leukemia Group B trials during the period from 1988 to 1998 the 6-year event-free survival was only 38%.[12] A suggestion that this was apparently so had been reported earlier in the USA for both ALL and AML.[13] On the other hand, a population-based study of 15- to 29-year-olds with acute leukaemia in England and Wales showed no difference between patients treated in national clinical trials and patients not entered, or between patients treated at teaching hospitals and patients treated at non-teaching hospitals, in contrast to the figures for younger patients.[14] This observation appears to be exceptional, however, in that subsequent national AML trials in the UK have shown some of the best results reported to date.[15] At the University of Texas M.D. Anderson Cancer Center, results of treatment of AML in adults improved substantively after treatment tested in paediatric trials was introduced into the institution's trials involving adult patients.[16]

The lower clinical trial participation rate by young adults in the USA and Canada may help explain the lower than expected improvement in their outcome relative to both younger and older patients. Studies of younger children have certainly shown a survival advantage over children enrolled in clinical trials for ALL,[17] non-Hodgkin's lymphoma,[18] Wilms' tumour[19] and medulloblastoma.[20]

In its Tumor Registries, the American College of Surgeons has tracked 15- to 19-year-old patients who were referred to centres participating in Children's Cancer Group (CCG) or Pediatric Oncology Group (POG) trials. Patients aged 15–19 years who were treated at CCG and POG sites with ALL,

AML, osteosarcoma or Ewing's sarcoma had better 5-year survival rates than did those treated elsewhere.[21] There were no differences in the 5-year rates for patients with Hodgkin's disease or testicular carcinoma, both of which are associated with an excellent outcome, or with brain tumours, cancers that are associated with some of the worst prognoses.

The spectrum of cancers among adolescents and young adults is different from that at any other age. There is no discipline in medicine devoted to this group. Neither paediatric oncologists nor oncologists who care for adult patients are trained – certainly not optimally – for this set of diseases. Moreover, even those diseases that appear to be the same often have biological differences in this age group. Adolescents have different forms of leukaemia than either younger or older persons. Acute lymphoblastic leukaemia, for example, changes dramatically after age 10–12. Breast cancer before age 30–40 is different from breast cancer in older women.

Adolescents have not historically been considered a separate entity but have been treated on either paediatric or adult protocols. A problem in dividing adolescents between treatment protocols is that doing so makes it difficult to know which treatments are most effective for the age group. It does not make sense to have one *best* treatment (for adolescents) on the paediatric unit and another *best* treatment on the adult unit for the same disease and age group.

Programmes to increase clinical trial participation of older adolescents and young adults with cancer in North America: the Adolescent and Young Adult Initiative

Attempting to meet these needs is the goal of the Adolescent and Young Adult Initiative of the Children's Oncology Group and the National Cancer Institute of the USA (Table 3.1). 'The Initiative', now 4 years old, aims to bring advances in cancer education, prevention and treatment – including educational, social and emotional development – to a segment of the North American population that has fallen behind the progress that has been achieved in younger and older patients.

M.D. Anderson physicians are also developing institutional policies and protocols that ensure that adolescent cancer patients with the same disease receive the same medical treatment. For example, under consideration is a modification of the treatment protocols for acute lymphoblastic leukaemia. Currently, there are two protocols: one for children and one for adults. In place of this traditional division, doctors are considering instituting three protocols based on trends in the disease and current treatment successes: a protocol for patients younger than 10 years of age, one for patients aged 10–40, and one for those more than 40 years old. With the present protocols, cure rates are very high until patients reach the age of 10, when the rates begin dropping. The intention is to keep patients younger than 10 and older than 40 on the current protocols and design a third protocol for those in between. This may be relatively easier to do at the cancer centre because more than a decade ago the adult leukaemia programme adopted the Pediatric Oncology Group strategy with high-dose cytosine arabinoside and high-dose methotrexate to treat their patients. In AML, a decision has been made to place all patients, regardless of age, on a regimen derived from a prior Children's Cancer Group study.

Summary

Cancer in adolescents and young adults has unique features in addition to the special medical, physical, psychological and social needs of patients in this age group. The spectrum of malignant diseases in this age group is different from that in any other period of life, and it is strikingly different from the pattern in older persons. More people 15–25 years of age are diagnosed with cancer than during the first 15 years of life. During the last 25 years, the incidence of cancer in this age range has increased faster and the reduction in cancer mortality has been lower than in younger or older patients. The improvement in the 5-year cancer survival rate from the mid-1970s to the early 1990s was significantly lower for adolescents and young adults than improvements noted in both younger and older age groups, especially in comparison with results of the national paediatric cooperative cancer groups. Thus, the 5-year outcome in 15- to 19-year-olds with leukaemias and sarcomas is not only worse than in younger patients but also lower in this population at large than in patients of the same age treated at former Children's Cancer Group and Pediatric Oncology Group institutions.

The most highly correlated single factor that accounts for the deficit is lack of participation in clinical treatment trials. And most disquietingly, fewer than 1% of 15- to 25-year-olds with cancer in the USA are being entered into clinical trials, in contrast to 60–65% of younger patients and 2–4% of older patients. Thus, cancer during adolescence and early adult life is a new frontier in oncology that merits specific resources, solutions and a national focus. The availability of and increased participation in clinical trials is paramount if the battle to overcome the deficits of cancer in young adults and older adolescents is to be won. To address the survival deficit will require broad support to increase clinical trial participation among 15- to 29-year-olds.

Cancer in adolescents and young adults is the new frontier in oncology, now that the outcome of cancer in younger and older persons has surpassed that seen in adolescent and young adult patients. Though it was once an advantage to have cancer during the adolescent and young adult years, it is now a detriment, as children and older adults have benefited more in survival prolongation and mortality reduction. Adolescents and young adult patients are now left behind, orphaned in the world of cancer care delivery.

A new discipline seems in order: adolescent and young adult oncology. This age group deserves trained care providers, specialized clinics, inpatient units and – probably most importantly – dedicated research strategies that are not available for either paediatric or adult care programmes.

References

1 Bleyer A, Montello M, Budd T, Kelahan A, Ries L. US cancer incidence, mortality and survival. Young adults are lagging further behind. 2002, http://www.asco.org/ac/1,1003,_12-002511-00_18-0016-00_19-001907,00.asp (select *Slide Presentation* for additional information).

2 Bleyer A, Budd T, Montello M. Cancer in older adolescents and young adults: a new frontier. *POGO News*, Fall 2002, pp. 8–11.

3 Albritton K, Bleyer A. The management of cancer in the older adolescent. *Eur J Cancer* http://authors.elsevier.com/sd/article/S0959804903008098, 2003; **39**: 2548–2599.

4 Bleyer WA. The adolescent gap in cancer treatment. *J Registry Manage* 1996; **23**: 114–115.

5 Bleyer WA, Tejeda H, Murphy SM *et al.* National cancer clinical trials: children have equal access; adolescents do not. *J Adolesc Health* 1997; **21**: 366–373.

6 Ziv A, Bouler JR, Slap GB. Utilization of physician offices by adolescents in the U.S. *Pediatrics* 1999; **104**: 35–42.

7 Bleyer A, Montello M, Budd T, Saxman S. Young adults with sarcoma: lack of clinical trial participation and lack of survival prolongation. *Proc Am Soc Clin Oncol* 2003; **22**: 816.

8 Bleyer A, Montello M, Budd T. Young adults with leukemia in the United States: lack of clinical trial participation and mortality reduction during the last decade. *Proc Am Soc Clin Oncol* 2004; **23**: 586.

9 Jemal A, Thomas A, Murray T *et al.* Cancer statistics, 2002. *CA Cancer J Clin* 2002; **52**: 23–47.

10 Bleyer A. Older adolescents with cancer in North America: deficits in outcome and research. *Pediatr Clin North Am* 2002; **49**: 1027–1042.

11 Boissel N, Auclerc MF, Lheritier V *et al.* Should adolescents (15–20y) with ALL be treated as old children or young adults? Comparison of the French FRALLE-93 and LALA-94 trials. *J Clin Oncol* 2003; **2**: 774–870.

12 Stock W, Sather H, Dodge RK *et al.* Outcome of adolescents and young adults with ALL: a comparison of Children's Cancer Group (CCG) and Cancer and Leukemia Group B (CALGB) regimens [abstract]. *Blood* 2000; **96**: 467a.

13 Nachman J, Sather HN, Buckley JD *et al.* Young adults 16–21 years of age at diagnosis entered onto Children's Cancer Group acute lymphoblastic leukemia and acute myeloblastic leukemia protocols. Results of treatment. *Cancer* 1993; **71** (10 Suppl.): 3377–85.

14 Stiller CA, Benjamin S, Cartwright RA *et al.* Patterns of care and survival for adolescents and young adults with acute leukemia – a population-based study. *Br J Cancer* 1999; **79**: 658–665.

15 Webb DK, Harrison G, Stevens RF *et al.* Relationships between age at diagnosis, clinical features, and outcome of therapy in children treated in the Medical Research Council AML 10 and 12 Trials for Acute Myeloid Leukemia. *Blood* 2000; **98**: 1714–1720.

16 Kantarjian HM, O'Brien S, Smith TL *et al.* Results of treatment with Hyper-CVAD, a dose-intensive regimen, in adult acute lymphocytic leukemia. *J Clin Oncol* 2000; **18**: 547–561.

17 Meadows AT, Kramer S, Hopson R *et al.* Survival in childhood acute lymphocytic leukemia. Effect of protocol and place of treatment. *Cancer Invest* 1983; **1**: 49–55.

18 Wagner HP, Dingeldein-Bettler I, Berchthold W *et al.*, for the Swiss Pediatric Oncology Group (SPOG). Childhood NHL in Switzerland: incidence and survival in 120 study and 42 non-study patients. *Med Pediatr Oncol* 1995; **24**: 281–286.

19 Lennox EL, Stiller CA, Morris-Jones PH, Wilson-Kinnier LM. Nephroblastoma: treatment during 1970–3 and the effect on survival of inclusion in the first MRC trial. *Br Med J* 1979; **2**: 567–569.

20 Duffner K, Cohen ME, Flannery JT. Referral patterns of childhood brain tumors in the state of Connecticut. *Cancer* 1982; **50**: 1636–1640.

21 Rauck AM, Fremgen AM, Menck HR *et al.* Adolescent cancers in the U.S.: a national cancer data base (NCDB) report. *J Pediatr Hematol Oncol* 1999; **21**: 308, 1.

CHAPTER 4

Adolescents and cancer: perspectives from France

L. Brugières

Introduction

The attention of French oncologists was drawn to adolescents and young adults with cancer in 1998 by a group of young adults who met on the occasion of a patients' meeting organized by the French National League against Cancer.[1] They explained the difficulties for teenagers being treated in an adult ward with elderly cancer patients without any social, educational or psychological support. They decided to found an association whose aims are to urge clinicians to take these problems into account and to create specific wards for teenagers with facilities adapted to their needs.

In France, as in many other countries, there are no systematic recommendations for the treatment of adolescents with cancer. Whereas most children under 15 are referred to a paediatric oncology centre and treated according to the French Society of Pediatric Oncology (SFCE) protocols,[2] patients aged between 15 and 20 are treated either in paediatric oncology centres or in adult oncology centres (in cancer centres, general hospitals or private clinics). The treatment of the older group depends on the place of referral since there are very few common protocols for children and adults (except for Burkitt's lymphoma and Ewing's tumour). Recognition by French paediatric oncologists of the needs of adolescents with cancer resulted in the raising to 18 years for the upper limit of age for inclusion in most paediatric studies.

Facilities for adolescents of paediatric cancer centres

A recent survey in 21 of 34 paediatric centres of the SFCE revealed that the upper age of admission for new patients was 15 years in one centre, 17 years in two centres, 18 years in 11 centres, 20 years in five centres and 25 years in one centre. In two centres there are some beds devoted to adolescents. Interestingly, in a similar survey performed 5 years ago, the upper age limit of admission was 15 in eight centres. The increase in the number of paediatric oncology centres treating adolescents reveals the awareness by paediatric oncologists of the problems faced by adolescents with cancer. However, only ten of the 21 centres treated more than ten new patients older than 15 years in 2003 and only four centres treated patients older than 20 years. Probably fewer than 80% of cancer patients aged 15–20 are treated in paediatric oncology centres.

In six large cancer centres there is systematic referral from adult to paediatric wards of patients under 18, especially for bone tumours and soft tissue sarcomas. In eight centres there are regular meetings of a multidisciplinary paediatric team with adult oncologists, participating especially for brain tumours and sarcomas. In two additional centres, the teams fully involve both paediatric and adult oncologists.

Education for patients who attend secondary schools is organized with voluntary teachers in ten of the 21 centres, and with qualified teachers from the French Department of Education and primary school teachers in five centres. Most of the centres offer their patients various artistic or leisure activities. In three centres, an activity coordinator organizes these activities; five centres offer their patients free access to computers and the Internet.

From this rapid survey, we conclude that most French paediatric centres treat adolescents with cancer. However, very few of them have all the facilities needed for this age group.

Epidemiology of cancer in adolescents in France

In order to study the incidence and survival rates of cancer in adolescents in France, we collected data from the network of French Cancer Registries (FRANCIM), covering 10% of the French population.[3] All cases of cancer in patients aged 15–19 over a 10-year period (1988–1997) were taken into account for the analysis, except cases of basal cell carcinoma. A total of 699 cases were registered. The overall incidence rate was 172.9 per million. Of these, 23% were lymphomas, 12% leukaemia, 12% germ cell tumours, 11% central nervous system tumours, 10% bone tumours, 8% soft tissue sarcomas and 19% carcinomas. These incidence and distribution data are quite similar to the data published previously for this age group from the USA and England.[4,5] In both sexes, there is some indication of rising trends over time, with an annual increase in incidence of 3% over the 10-year period, especially for melanomas, thyroid carcinomas, Hodgkin's disease and malignant germ cell tumours.

Gatta and colleagues have described cancer survival in European adolescents and young adults in a recent paper from the EUROCARE working group.[6] In this study, 5-year survival for all cancer was 73.1% for males and 78.8% for females, with notable variation among countries. Survival for French patients (73.1% in males and 82.6% in females) was very close to the European averages. The most striking result of this study was the difference in survival for several tumour types, such as acute lymphoblastic leukaemia (ALL), non-Hodgkin's lymphomas and bone tumours in adolescents compared with data obtained for children aged 0–14 years.[7] These differences might be due either to differences in treatment or to differences in the biological behaviour of cancer in adolescents compared with children.

Impact of therapeutic protocols

Several studies performed in France and in other countries tend to show that therapeutic protocols might be at least partly responsible for these differences. Boissel and colleagues[8] recently published the outcome for patients aged 15–20 treated for ALL in two contemporary French protocols, the paediatric FRALLE-93 and the adult LALA-94, between September 1994 and May 2000. Even though the initial characteristics were similar in the two groups (median white blood cell count, B-/T-cell lineage, CD10 negative ALL, poor-risk cytogenetics) except for age (15.9 years for FRALLE, 17.9 years for LALA), there were differences in complete remission rates (94% for FRALLE and 83% for LALA) and in 5-year disease-free survival rates (72% for FRALLE and 49% for LALA, $P = 0.0004$). These differences are probably explained by differences in therapeutic protocols, which were more intensive for paediatric patients than for adults.

Another study performed in osteosarcoma patients aged 15–20 in two departments of the Institut Gustave Roussy between 1982 and 1998 showed a 20% difference in 5-year event-free survival (EFS) between patients treated in the paediatric department (71%, 35) and those treated in the adult department (48%, 33 patients). As the initial characteristics of the patients were similar, the differences in EFS were attributed to differences in therapeutic protocols.[9]

The awareness of the specific problems of adolescents with cancer led to a national initiative sponsored by the French National League Against Cancer to evaluate the special needs of these patients, to create working groups aiming to establish guidelines of treatment for this age group independent of the site of care, and to develop specialized adolescent and young adult cancer units. Such a unit with ten beds for patients aged 13–20 with cancer has been open since November 2003 at the Institut Gustave Roussy in Villejuif and a unit for young adults aged 18–30 should open at the same institute before the end of 2004. Several other paediatric and adult centres in France are planning to open such units within a few months (or years). This initiative is aiming to concentrate expertise and resources devoted to this age group in order to improve therapeutic results and to create a suitable environment to take care of patients diagnosed with cancer during adolescence, thus improving their quality of life during and after treatment.

References

1 Ligue Nationale Contre le Cancer. *Les Malades Prennent la Parole*. Paris: Ramsay, 1999.
2 Sommelet D. French pediatric oncology: past, present and future. *Arch Pediatr* 2004; **11**: 81–84.

3 Desandes E, Lacour B, Sommelet D *et al.* Cancer incidence among adolescents in France. *Pediatr Blood Cancer* 2004; **43**: 742–748.

4 Stiller C. Epidemiology of cancer in adolescents. *Med Pediatr Oncol* 2002; **39**: 148–155.

5 Bleyer AW. Cancer in older adolescents and young adults: epidemiology, diagnosis, treatment, survival and importance of clinical trials. *Med Pediatr Oncol* 2002; **38**: 1–10.

6 Gatta G, Capocaccia R, De Angelis R *et al.* Cancer survival in European adolescents and young adults. *Eur J Cancer* 2003; **39**: 2600–2610.

7 Gatta G, Corazziari, Magnani C *et al.* Childhood cancer survival in Europe. *Ann Oncol* 2003; **14** (Suppl.): v119–v127.

8 Boissel N, Aucler MF, Lherithier V *et al.* Should adolescents with acute lymphoblastic leukemia be treated as old children or young adults? Comparison of the French FRALLE-93 and LALA-94 trials. *J Clin Oncol* 2003; **21**: 774–780.

9 Le Deley MC, LeCesne A, Brugières L *et al.* Localized osteosarcoma of young and adult patients: the experience of the Institut Gustave Roussy over a 16-year period [abstract]. *Med Ped Oncol* 2001; **3**: 188.

CHAPTER 5

Care of teenagers with cancer: a North American perspective

R. D. Barr

The challenges that face adolescents with cancer have been described comprehensively[1] but the solutions remain largely elusive. Problems begin with access to care, an issue not limited to those with malignant diseases in this age group. Even in the much-vaunted Canadian health-care system,[2] which claims to provide universal access (as well as 'first dollar coverage'), difficulties abound. The position of the Canadian Pediatric Society's Adolescent Health Committee has been summarized succinctly:[3] 'Adolescence begins with the onset of physiologically normal puberty, and ends when an adult identity and behaviour are accepted. This period of development corresponds roughly to the period between the ages of 10 and 19 years, which is consistent with the World Health Organization's definition of adolescence. Those responsible for providing health care to adolescents must allow sufficient flexibility in this age span to encompass special situations such as the emancipated minor or the young person with a chronic condition leading to delayed development or prolonged dependency.'

At its core this problem of access involves the setting of variable and arbitrary upper and lower age limits for admission to paediatric and adult health-care facilities respectively. These thresholds are inconsistent between provinces, among regions and even within a single institution. In an apposite example,[3] one children's hospital did not admit patients with major trauma over the age of 16 years but provided inpatient services for patients with serious mental health problems up to 19 years of age. Since injuries and suicide are the commonest causes of death in teenagers[4] (cancer being the next in line),[5] the inconsistencies are obvious.

In a national survey undertaken by the Treatment and Outcome Surveillance System (TOSS) of the Canadian Childhood Cancer Surveillance and Control Program (CCCSCP), waiting times from the onset of symptoms to diagnosis and treatment of cancer were compared in adolescents (15–19 years) and children (0–14 years) over a recent 5-year period (1995–2000). The survey included almost 3000 subjects. From the onset of the symptoms to first treatment, adolescents waited twice as long as children (a median of 2 months versus 1 month, $P < 0.01$); this particular survey was limited to paediatric institutions. A similar review was carried out comparing the use of paediatric and adult oncology centres. Adolescents treated in adult facilities were significantly older and more likely to have epithelial tumours. The time from onset of symptoms to first treatment in this group exceeded 3 months, significantly longer than in their counterparts treated in paediatric centres ($P = 0.02$). Also of note was the lower enrolment of adolescents in clinical trials at adult oncology centres compared with those at paediatric institutions ($P < 0.01$).

These findings exhibited regional (geographical) variation that may reflect, in part, the point of first contact with the health-care system. Adolescents were more likely to be referred to an adult centre if seen first by a general practitioner. While the national average for the proportion of adolescents with cancer accessing paediatric institutions in this survey was only one-third (very similar to that reported from the United States),[6] the proportion was twice as high in the prairie provinces. An earlier report from Ontario, Canada's most populous province, provides further information on this matter.[7] Again, the minority of adolescents were referred to paediatric oncology centres. The largest diagnostic group was, as predicted, patients with malignant lymphomas. Given the evidence that adolescents with non-Hodgkin's lymphoma who were treated at member institutions of the children's collaborative study groups in North America (now amalgamated as the Children's Oncology Group, to which all Canadian paediatric oncology centres belong) had survival rates superior to those of adolescents treated elsewhere,[7] this finding (by the Pediatric Oncology Group of Ontario) is particularly worrying.

What of the impact made by a diagnosis of cancer, by the disease and by its treatment in adolescence? In addressing this question, the self-assessed health status of adolescents in the general population offers an important comparison. As teenagers confront the transitional period between childhood and adult life, they establish a self-concept – some sense of who they are. Self-concept consists of two important elements: self-esteem (an assessment of one's own worth) and mastery (the extent to which one feels in control of important aspects of one's life).[8]

In the longitudinal component of the National Population Health Survey undertaken by Statistics Canada,[8] the well-recognized rise in self-concept through the adolescent years was found to be limited to boys. However, regardless of sex or age group, adolescents' level of self-perceived health in 1994–95 was the strongest predictor of their self-perceived health status 6 years later in 2000–01. Furthermore, a strong self-concept bore a direct relationship to physical activity and was related inversely to the risk of obesity.[8]

Somewhat surprisingly, in the Canadian Community Health Survey undertaken by Statistics Canada in 2000–01,[9] which included a sample of more than 12,000 adolescents, 30% of those in this age group described their health as no better than good (on a Likert scale of excellent, very good, good, fair, poor). Self-perceived health among adolescents correlated positively with their families' socio-economic status, as has been reported previously.[10] Negative correlations were revealed between self-perceived health and daily smoking or episodic heavy drinking. Physical inactivity, poor dietary composition and obesity were all independently similarly associated with poor self-perceived health.

Small wonder, then, that the impact of cancer on adolescents can be so devastating.[11,12] Beginning with the processes of informed consent and assent, dealing with the newly diagnosed teenager poses particular challenges,[13–15] which places special demands on the physician–patient relationship.[16]

Compliance has been defined by Haynes and Sackett at McMaster University as the extent to which patients' behaviour coincides with medical and health advice.[17,18] Poor compliance with anti-neoplastic therapy is a major issue in the care of the adolescent with malignant disease,[19–24] being more common than in both younger and older patients. The prevalence may be as high as 60% in teenagers with cancer.[19] It is unrelated to socio-economic status but is more common in dysfunctional families[25] and in adolescents with poor self-concept.[26] Compliance decreases with increasing duration of therapy[27,28] and is overestimated by physicians.[29] Self-reports and proxy reports of compliance are surprisingly well supported by measured cytotoxic drug levels.[27]

A recent authoritative review of compliance in adolescents with cancer, performed by colleagues at the Hospital for Sick Children in Toronto, provides useful information on methods of assessment, risk factors and predictors, interventional strategies and check-lists for physicians.[30]

Faced with issues such as these, the health-care team must provide comprehensive support to the adolescent who is wrestling with cancer and its treatment. Strategies such as structured programmes of school reintegration, with emphasis on normalization,[31,32] and the establishment of peer groups, including those in the setting of camping experiences,[33] have much to offer in this regard. As an example of the latter, Camp Trillium (based in Ontario, and now the biggest camp for children and adolescents with cancer in the world) provides opportunities tailored specifically to the teenage group. Coping is further enhanced[34] by adolescent hopefulness, defined as 'the degree to which an adolescent possesses a comforting, life-sustaining belief that a personal and positive future exists'.[35] Providing comprehensive support to the adolescent with cancer is particularly difficult in the context of palliative care;[36] even the best paediatric institutions are woefully inadequate[37] in such provision.

For adolescent survivors of cancer, other hurdles await in the form of transitions in care.[35] These may be categorized as transition from on-treatment to off-treatment, from off-treatment to post-treatment and from paediatric care to adult care. With respect to the first, it is now common practice at the conclusion of active treatment to review the adolescent's experience from the time of diagnosis to the conclusion of therapy, to reassess prognosis, to emphasize the short-term focus on surveillance and monitoring for early relapse, and to pave the way for longer-term follow-up. The second transition should be a planned move to 'aftercare' in which long-term follow-up pays particular attention to the detection and management of late effects of therapy. Customarily this occurs about 2 years after the completion of active treatment. The importance of this continuing care has been emphasized recently in a report from the Institute of Medicine of the National Academy of Sciences in the USA,[38] by whom the provincial network established in Ontario for the purpose of after-care is recognized as an exemplary model.

The final transition, from paediatric to adult care, poses the greatest difficulty, yet, if accomplished successfully, offers opportunities for health education and promotion in the context of long-term follow-up. Barriers to this transition have been considered in detail.[39] The process has been described by the American Society for Adolescent Medicine as 'the purposeful, planned movement of adolescents and young adults with chronic physical and medical conditions from child-centered to adult-oriented healthcare systems'.[40] But who will service these needs and in what facilities? In Canada, the National Training Initiative in Adolescent Health is a comprehensive multidisciplinary programme that may contribute to the solution but substantial obstacles to implementation remain (Table 5.1). Nevertheless, successful models in other diseases are worthy of emulation (Table 5.2).

When the dust has settled and the adolescents have completed the difficult process of active treatment and have moved on to become young adult survivors, often accomplishing the 'final transition', what health behaviours do they exhibit? These fall into two categories: health promotion and health risk behaviours. In a study undertaken by the CCCSCP, a national retrospective cohort was established of 891 subjects who were diagnosed with a primary cancer before the age of 20, in the decade 1981–1990, and who had survived at least 5 years from diagnosis. Most of the cancers had occurred in adolescence. They were compared with more than 1000 population controls in five health behaviours: three in health promotion (strenuous physical activity at least three times weekly, and regular physical and dental examinations)

Table 5.1 Barriers to paediatric–adult transition

Failure to acknowledge the need for transition
Financial constraints on provision of specialized services
Inadequate education of community-based practitioners
Insufficient acceptance by adolescents of responsibility for their health
Unevenness of long-term care practices

Adapted from MacLean et al. (1996).[41]

Table 5.2 Examples of successful transitions from paediatric to adult care*

Cystic fibrosis
Haemophilia and related disorders
Congenital heart disease

*Either in combined clinics or in separate institutions.

and two health risks (smoking and binge-drinking).[42] Only 25% of survivors participated in regular strenuous physical activity, but this was no different from the control group. Being male and having better self-perceived health were factors associated with this form of health promotion. While survivors underwent more frequent clinical examinations, this may have reflected, in part, the impact of long-term follow-up strategies. Being female, not working and having lower self-esteem were variables that correlated with the frequency of clinical examinations.

When compared with controls, survivors were less likely to smoke or engage in binge-drinking. Nevertheless, 20% were smokers and this group had lower educational levels and lower self-perceived health than the non-smokers. This proportion and profile are similar to those reported from the USA in the Childhood Cancer Survivor Study.[43] In this study the proportion of survivors who were binge-drinkers (30%) was lower than among controls. This survivor group had lower educational levels than the non-binge-drinking group. It is perhaps noteworthy that the Canadian Study of Park[8] and studies in the USA[44,45] have identified higher self-concept to be associated with a reduced rate of risky behaviour among adolescents in the general population.

Given these differences in health behaviours, it is reasonable to enquire about health-care utilization by survivors of cancer in early life. Again, a study from the CCCSCP sheds light on this issue.[46] In this national survey of more than 2000 survivors and a similar number of population controls, after adjustment for the number of physical health problems and self-perceived general health, survivors reported more health-care visits than controls. But the difference was limited to 'specialty practitioners' (oncologists, haematologists, endocrinologists and neurologists) – a designation that excluded general internists. This finding may reflect, in large measure, the advice given to long-term survivors regarding the management of risks associated with their disease and its treatment. The only clinical characteristic associated with the increased visits was organ dysfunction on discharge. Physical health problems and self-perceived general health were associated more strongly with the frequency of health-care visits than any other variable examined.

However, as noted by the authors of the study,[46] 'the odds of survivors reporting more health-care visits than controls were increased for two groups of children: those whose parents either reported poorer mental health or more than high school education'. The frequency of visits also diminished with increasing age of the survivors, perhaps reflecting reduced parental influence over time. But the Childhood Cancer Survivor Study revealed that adult survivors of cancer in childhood have knowledge deficits with respect to their diagnosis and treatment, and only a small minority were anxious about potential harmful late effects.[47]

With all these issues to consider in the care of adolescents with cancer, it is evident that a comprehensive assessment of health-related quality of life (HRQL), self-reported by these individuals, would provide a reliable overview of their health status. In a study of all adolescent survivors (age 15–19 years) of cancer in childhood (0–14 years), at McMaster Children's Hospital, a response rate of 67% was achieved.[48] The study sample, consisting of equal numbers of males and females, was assessed with the Health Utilities Index, a generic multi-attribute, preference-based measure of HRQL developed at McMaster University.[49] Overall, only 15–20% reported no morbidity. The attributes of health affected predominantly were emotion, cognition and pain. Females had significantly poorer HRQL than males in the cancer survivor group and also in the adolescent population controls. The HRQL of male survivors overall was no different from that of their counterparts in the general population.

In a cross-Canada study, undertaken by the CCCSCP (E. Maunsell, L. M. Pogany, K. N. Speechley, A. Shaw, M. Barrera, in preparation), involving more than 1000 adult survivors of cancer in childhood and adolescence and more than 1000 controls, the SF-36, a generic health profile measure of HRQL, was used. The burden of morbidity was greater in the survivor group as a whole than in the control population. However, only those who had had bone or central nervous system tumours were assessed as having 'clinically meaningful differences'.

While adolescents with cancer have been described as a 'lost tribe',[50] evidence is being accumulated on the health-care needs of this population that should lead to improvements in their health outcomes in the foreseeable future.

References

1 Michelagnoli MP, Pritchard J, Phillips MB. The care of the adolescent with cancer. *Eur J Cancer* 2003; **39**: 2571–2695.

2 Naylor CD. The Canadian health care system: a model for America to emulate? *Health Econ* 1992; **1**: 19–37.

3 MacDonald NE. Adolescent access to health care. *Paediatr Child Health* 2003; **8**: 551–552.

4 Federal, Provincial and Territorial Advisory Committee on Population Health. Toward a Healthy Future. Second Report on the Health of Canadians. Health Canada, 1999. www.hc-sc.gc.ca/hppb/phdd/report/toward/.

5 Geran L, Tully P. Leading causes of death at different ages, Canada, 1999. Cat. No. 84F0503XPB. Ottawa: Statistics Canada, Health Statistics Division, 2002.

6 Rauck AM, Fremgen AM, Hutchison CL *et al*. Adolescent cancers in the United States: a national cancer database (NCDB) report [abstract]. *J Pediatr Hematol Oncol* 1999; **21**: 310.

7 Greenberg ML, Barr RD, DiMonte B, McLaughlin E, Greenberg C. Childhood cancer registries in Ontario, Canada: lessons learned from a comparison of two registries. *Int J Cancer* 2003; **105**: 88–91.

8 Park J. Adolescent self-concept and health into adulthood. Health Reports, Statistics Canada 2003 (Suppl.): 41–52.

9 Tremblay S, Dahinten S, Kohen D. Factors related to adolescents' self-perceived health. Health Reports, Statistics Canada 2003 (Suppl.): 7–16.

10 Vingihs E, Wade TJ, Adlaf E. What factors predict students' self-rated physical health? *J Adolesc* 1998; **21**: 83–97.

11 Lewis IJ. Cancer in adolescence. *Br Med Bull* 1996; **52**: 887–897.

12 Barr RD. On cancer control and the adolescent. *Med Pediatr Oncol* 1999; **32**: 404–410.

13 Leikin SL. Beyond proforma consent for childhood cancer research. *J Clin Oncol* 1985; **3**: 420–428.

14 Koocher GP, De Maso DR. Children's competence to consent to medical procedures. *Paediatrician* 1990; **17**: 68–73.

15 Dorn LD, Susman EJ, Fletcher JC. Informed consent in children and adolescents: age, maturation and psychological state. *J Adolesc Health* 1995; **16**: 185–190.

16 King NMP, Cross AW. Children as decision makers: guidelines for pediatricians. *J Pediatr* 1989; **115**: 10–16.

17 Haynes RB, Sackett DL, Taylor DW. *Compliance in Health Care*. Baltimore: Johns Hopkins University Press, 1979: 516.

18 Haynes RB, McDonald H, Garg AX Montague P. Interventions for helping patients to follow prescriptions for medications. *Cochrane Database Syst Rev* 2002; Issue 2.

19 Smith SD, Rosen D, Trueworthy RC, Lowman JT. A reliable method for evaluating drug compliance in children with cancer. *Cancer* 1979; **43**: 169–173.

20 Festa RS, Tamaroff MH, Chasalow F, Lanzkowsky P. Therapeutic adherence to oral medication regimens by adolescents with cancer. I. Laboratory assessment. *J Pediatr* 1992; **120**: 807–811.

21 Tamaroff MH, Festa RS, Adesman AR, Walco GA. Therapeutic adherence to oral medication regimens by adolescents with cancer. II. Clinical and psychological correlations. *J Pediatr* 1992; **120**: 812–817.

22 Tebbi CK. Treatment compliance in childhood and adolescence. *Cancer* 1993; **71** (Suppl. 10): 3441–3449.

23 Kyng AHA, Kroll T, Duffy ME. Compliance in adolescents with chronic diseases. *J Adolesc Health* 2000; **26**: 379–388.

24 Sawyer SM, Aroni RA. Sticky issue of adherence. *J Paediatr Child Health* 2003; **39**: 2–5.

25 Rapoff MA, Bernard MU. Compliance with pediatric medical regimens. In: Cramer JA, Spilker B, eds. *Patient Compliance in Medical Practice and Clinical Trials*. New York: Raven Press, 1991: 73.

26 Litt IF. Know myself – adolescents' self-assessment of compliance behavior. *Pediatrics* 1985; **75**: 693–696.

27 Tebbi CK, Cummings KM, Zevon MA *et al.* Compliance of pediatric and adolescent cancer patients. *Cancer* 1986; **58**: 1179–1184.

28 Fletcher RH. Patient compliance with therapeutic advice: a modern view. *Mt Sinai J Med* 1989; **56**: 453–458.

29 Sackett DL. Helping patients follow the treatments you prescribe. In: Sackett DL, Haynes RB, Guyatt GH, eds. *Clinical Epidemiology: A Basic Science for Clinical Medicine*. Boston: Little Brown, 1991: 249.

30 Gesundheit B, Greenberg ML, Malkin D *et al.* Drug compliance by adolescent cancer patients. In: Bleyer WA, Barr RD, eds. *Cancer in Adolescents and Young Adults*. Heidelberg: Springer-Verlag. (In press).

31 Chekryn J, Deegan M, Reid J. Normalising the return to school of the child with cancer. *J Assoc Pediatr Oncol Nurses* 1986; **3**: 20–24.

32 Glasson JE. A descriptive and exploratory pilot-study into school re-entrance for adolescents who have received treatment for cancer. *J Adv Nursing* 1995; **22**: 753–758.

33 Balen R, Fielding D, Lewis I. An activity week for children with cancer: who wants to go and why? *Child Care Health Develop* 1998; **24**: 169–177.

34 Poncer PJ. Inspiring hope in the oncology patient. *J Psychosoc Nurs Ment Health Serv* 1994; **32**: 33–38.

35 Hinds PS. Inducing a definition of 'hope' through the use of grounded theory methodology. *J Adv Nursing* 1984; **9**: 357–362.

36 George R, Hutton S. Palliative care in adolescents. *Eur J Cancer* 2003; **39**: 2662–2668.

37 Wolfe J, Grier HE, Klar N *et al*. Symptoms and suffering at the end of life in children with cancer. *N Engl J Med* 2000; **342**: 326–333.

38 Hewitt M. Weiner SL, Simone JV, eds. *Childhood Cancer Survivorship. Improving Care and Quality of Life*. Washington (DC): National Academies Press, 2003: 120.

39 Viner R. Bridging the gaps: transition for young people with cancer. *Eur J Cancer* 2003; **39**: 2684–2687.

40 Blum R, Garell D, Hodgman C *et al*. Transition from child-centred to adult health-care systems for adolescents with chronic conditions. A position paper of the Society for Adolescent Medicine. *J Adolesc Health* 1993; **14**: 570–576.

41 MacLean WE, Foley GR, Ruccione K, Sklar C. Transitions in the care of adolescent and young adult survivors of childhood cancer. *Cancer* 1996; **78**: 1340–1344.

42 Pogany L, Shaw A, Maunsell E *et al*. Health behaviors of young adult survivors of childhood cancer: Comparison with population controls. *Qual Life Res.* (In press).

43 Emmons K, Li FP, Whitton J *et al*. Predictors of smoking initiation and cessation among childhood cancer survivors: a report from the Childhood Cancer Survivor Study. *J Clin Oncol* 2002; **20**: 1608–1616.

44 McCaleb A, Edgil A. Self-concept and self-care practices of healthy adolescents. *J Pediatr Nursing* 1994; **9**: 233–238.

45 Gordon-Rouse KA, Ingersoll GM, Orr ADP. Longitudinal health endangering behavior risk among resilient and non-resilient early adolescents. *J Adolesc Health* 1998; **23**: 297–302.

46 Shaw A, Pogany A, Mery L *et al*. Use of health care services by survivors of childhood and adolescent cancer in Canada. *Can Med Assoc J.* (In press).

47 Kadan-Lottick NS, Robison LL, Gurney JG *et al*. Childhood cancer survivors' knowledge about their past diagnosis and treatment: Childhood Cancer Survivor Study. *J Am Med Assoc* 2002; **287**: 1832–1839.

48 Barr R, Grant J, Davidson A *et al*. Health related quality of life in adolescent survivors of cancer in childhood [abstract]. *Med Pediatr Oncol* 2003; **41**: 271.

49 Furlong, WJ, Feeny DH, Torrance GW, Barr RD. The Health Utilities Index (HUI®) system for assessing health-related quality of life in clinical studies. *Ann Med* 2001; **33**: 375–384.

50 Michelagnoli MP, Pritchard J, Phillips MB. Adolescent oncology – a homeland for the 'lost tribe'. *Eur J Cancer* 2003; **39**: 2571–2572.

Part two
Advances

CHAPTER 6

Leukaemia

J. Nachman

Introduction

There are significant differences in the presenting features, immunopheno-typic distribution, leukaemic cell cytogenetics, treatment toxicity and outcome for patients with acute lymphoblastic leukaemia (ALL) aged 1–9 years compared with those over 10 years of age.[1] Older patients have an inferior event-free survival (EFS) and overall survival compared with patients under 10 years of age.[2–11] It is not clear from the literature whether there are significant differences between patients aged 10–15 years and those aged 16–21 years.

Young adults (16–21 years of age at diagnosis) with ALL may be treated in either adult or paediatric ALL trials or receive off-protocol treatment from community-based oncologists. In the USA, very few older teenagers are treated in clinical trials sponsored by the National Cancer Institute. In England and Wales, between 1984 and 1994, 80% of ALL patients younger than 14 years were entered in a clinical trial compared with only 36% for patients aged 15–29 years.[12]

In studies from England, there were no outcome differences noted for adolescents treated in teaching or non-teaching hospitals.[13] There was also no outcome difference for adolescents entered or not entered in national clinical trials, though that dates from a time when overall outcome was inferior to what is now seen.

Recently, adult and paediatric cooperative groups have compared outcomes for young adult ALL patients (15 or 16–21 years of age). In comparisons of outcome data from the Children's Cancer Group (COG) and the Cancer And Leukemia Group B (CALGB),[14] and the FRALLE and LALA groups in France,[15] young adults treated in paediatric trials had significantly better EFS than those treated in adult cooperative group trials. These findings have led to intensive speculation concerning the reasons for the better outcome for young adults treated in paediatric trials. Factors under consideration include differences in protocols, actual drug dose intensity achieved, compliance and supportive care.[16] This chapter reviews the epidemiology, biology and treatment outcome for adolescents 16–21 years of age with ALL in an attempt to explain the different outcomes.

Clinical, biological and epidemiological characteristics of ALL patients aged 16–21 years at diagnosis

In the early paediatric ALL trials very few patients aged 16–21 years were enrolled, so that most analyses performed that compared older and younger patients used the age cut-off of 1–9 and 10+ years. In more recent Children's Cancer Group (CCG) trials, the accrual rate for patients 16–21 years of age has increased significantly. Therefore, we can now compare the features and outcomes for 16- to 21-year-old patients with the 1- to 9- and 10- to 15-year age groups with some reliability. The following data are derived from the CCG-1900 series of ALL trials conducted between 1995 and 2002.[17] The incidence of T-cell ALL was significantly greater in the 16+ age group compared with the 1- to 9-year age group (23.2% versus 12.8%, $P = 0.008$), but there was no significant difference in the incidence of T-cell immunophenotype when the 16- to 21-year group was compared with the 10- to 15-year age group (23.2% versus 24.2%). Since T-cell ALL is associated with higher white blood cell counts (WBC), lymphomatous features and higher haemoglobin levels at diagnosis, we performed separate age-group comparisons for B- and T-lineage patients. For patients with B-lineage ALL, patients over 16 years of age at diagnosis had an increased incidence of negativity for CALLA (common acute lymphoblastic leukaemia antigen), a lower incidence of lymphomatous features (enlarged liver, spleen and/or nodes) and an increased incidence of haemoglobin greater than 11 g when compared with children aged 1–9 years at diagnosis. Interestingly, there was no difference in presenting WBC among the two groups. T-cell patients over 16 years of age had a higher incidence of WBC greater than 50×10^9/litre and haemoglobin greater than 11 g and a lower incidence of lymphomatous features compared with patients aged 1–9 years. There were no significant differences in presenting features between patients aged 10–15 and those aged 16–21 years for patients with either B- or T-lineage disease.

The incidence of Ph+ (Philadelphia chromosome-positive) ALL gradually increases with age at diagnosis. In a Medical Research Council (MRC) study, the incidence of Ph+ ALL was 1.3% for patients aged 1–9, 3.9% for those 10–19 and 12.2% for those aged 20–29 years.[18] Older patients with B-precursor ALL have a significantly lower rate of the (12:21) translocation and of high hyperdiploidy compared with younger patients.[18] Leukaemic blasts from patients aged over 10 years have been reported to manifest significantly increased *in vitro* drug resistance to prednisone (PDN) and daunorubicin when compared with younger patients.[19]

Treatment outcome for adolescents with ALL: general

It is clear that patients over 10 years of age with ALL have a worse outcome than patients aged 1–9 years at diagnosis. In a series of publications from the major paediatric groups which looked at outcome based on various accepted prognostic factors, 5-year EFS ranged from 74 to 87% for patients aged 1–9 years compared with 55 to 79% for patients over 10 years of age.[2–11] Very few paediatric groups have sufficient numbers of patients to examine outcome in patients aged 16–21 years at diagnosis.

BFM-type therapy in CCG

In 1979, the American CCG ran a pilot trial of therapy based on the BFM-76/79 protocol for patients with a presenting WBC over 50×10^9/litre and no lymphomatous features.[20] Therapy consisted of four-drug induction utilizing vincristine, prednisone, L-asparaginase (L-ASP) and daunorubicin. Intrathecal (IT) cytosine arabinoside was given on day 1 and IT methotrexate was given on day 14 (subsequently moved to day 7). Induction was followed by a consolidation phase which included two 2-week courses of cyclophosphamide, cytosine arabinoside and 6-mercaptopurine in conjunction with IT methotrexate and cranial radiation therapy. The intensive induction and consolidation was referred to as Protocol I. An 8-week interim maintenance phase consisted of oral 6-mercaptopurine and oral methotrexate. A delayed reinduction–reconsolidation course was then administered (delayed intensification, DI). A 3-week, four-drug reinduction was given with adriamycin replacing daunorubicin and dexamethasone replacing prednisone. In the 2-week reconsolidation course, 6-thioguanine replaced 6-mercaptopurine. Maintenance therapy consisted of monthly pulses of vincristine and prednisone, daily oral 6-mercaptopurine and weekly oral methotrexate. IT methotrexate was given every 3 months. Boys received 3 years of therapy and girls received 2 years of therapy. The CCG-modified BFM regimen is shown more fully in Table 6.1.

Treatment outcome for adolescents with ALL: CCG

In 1984, age had not been clearly recognized as a prognostic factor in childhood and adolescent ALL. CCG conducted a clinical trial for patients with ALL who were 1–21 years of age and had WBC less than 50×10^9/litre, which evaluated the contributions of Protocol I and DI to outcome.[21] In addition, patients were randomized to receive IT methotrexate alone or IT methotrexate and cranial radiation therapy as central nervous system (CNS) therapy. The study design is shown in Table 6.2.

For younger patients, arms containing a DI phase proved superior to those without a DI phase, and IT methotrexate alone provided similar CNS protection to IT methotrexate and cranial radiation therapy. There was no difference in outcome for arms 3A and 4A, implying that intensive induction consolidation was unnecessary for younger patients. In contrast, for patients over 10 years of age, arm 4B (full BFM plus cranial radiation therapy) provided a better EFS than all of the other regimens. Full BFM produced a long-term EFI of 71%; the other regimens produced EFS ranging from 57 to 64%.

Table 6.1 CCG modified BFM therapy (CM-BFM)

Induction	PRED	60 mg/m^2 p.o. days 1–28 (b.i.d. or t.i.d.) then taper
	VCR	1.5 mg/m^2 i.v. days 1, 8, 15, 22
	DNR	25 mg/m^2 i.v. days 1, 8, 15, 22
	L-ASP	6000 U/m^2 i.m. 3 times per week × 3 weeks beginning on day 3
	I/T ARA-C	Day 1 (age-adjusted dosing)
	I/T MTX	Day 8 (age-adjusted dosing)
Consolidation	PRED	Taper
	CPM	1000 mg/m^2 i.v. days 0, 14
	6-MP	60 mg/m^2 p.o. days 0–27
	ARA-C	75 mg/m^2 i.v. days 1–4, 8–11, 15–18, 22–25
	I/T MTX	Days 1, 8, 15, 22
	RT	1800 cGy cranial for no CNS disease at diagnosis
		2400 cGy cranial + 600 cGy spinal for CNS disease at diagnosis
Interim maintenance (8 weeks)	6-MP	60 mg/m^2 q.d. p.o. days 0–41
	MTX	15 mg/m^2 q.w. p.o. days 0, 7, 14, 21, 28, 35
Delayed intensification (7 weeks)	*Reinduction (4 weeks)*	
	DEX	10 mg/m^2 p.o. q.d. days 0–20, then taper for 7 days
	VCR	1.5 mg/m^2 i.v. days 0, 7, 14
	DOX	25 mg/m^2 i.v. days 0, 7, 14
	L-ASP	600 U/m^2 i.m. days 3, 5, 7, 10, 12, 14
	Reconsolidation (3 weeks)	
	CPM	1000 mg/m^2 i.v. day 28
	6-TG	60 mg/m^2 p.o. q.d. days 28–41
	ARA-C	75 mg/m^2 subq.v./i.v. days 29–32, 36–39
	I/T MTX	Days 29, 36
Maintenance (12-week cycles)	VCR	1.5 mg/m^2 i.v. days 0, 28, 56
	PRED	60 mg/m^2 p.o. q.d. days 0–4, 28–32, 56–60
	6-MP	75 mg/m^2 p.o. days 0–83
	MTX	20 mg/m^2 p.o. days 7, 14, 21, 28, 35, 42, 49, 56, 63, 70, 77
	I/T MTX	Day 0

PRED, prednisolone. VCR, vincristine. DNR, daunorubicin. L-ASP, asparaginase. I/T ARA-C, intrathecal cytosine arabinoside. I/T MTX, intrathecal methotrexate. CPM, cyclophosphamide. 6-MP, 6-mercaptopurine. ARA-C, cytosine arabinoside. RT, radiotherapy. DEX, dexamethasone. DOX, doxorubicin. 6-TG, 6-thioguanine. MTX, oral methotrxate. b.i.d., twice daily. t.i.d., three times daily. cGy, centiGray. CNS, central nervous system. q.d., each day. q.w., each week. subq.v./i.v., subcutaneous or intravenous.

Table 6.2 Study design for CCG clinical trial for patients with ALL, 1–21 years of age and with white blood cell count less than 50×10^9/litre, evaluating the contributions of Protocol I and DI to outcome

Arm	Protocol I	DI	CRT
1A	No	No	No
1B	No	No	Yes
2A	Yes	No	No
2B	Yes	No	Yes
3A	No	Yes	No
3B	No	Yes	Yes
4A	Yes	Yes	No
4B	Yes	Yes	Yes

DI, delayed intensification. CRT, cranial radiation therapy.

From 1989 onward, ALL patients older than 10 years of age were considered at high risk of relapse and standard therapy for those patients became CCG-modified BFM plus cranial radiation therapy for patients without lymphomatous features. Patients with lymphomatous features were treated with either CCG-modified BFM or a different multidrug intensive regimen referred to as the NY regimen.

The pilot trial of BFM-type therapy for high-risk patients with ALL conducted by the CCG revealed that the day-7 bone marrow response had prognostic significance.[22] Patients with fewer than 25% blasts in the day-7 marrow had an EFS of approximately 70% compared with approximately 40% for patients with more than 25% blasts in the day-7 marrow.

The CCG-1882 Protocol, conducted between 1989 and 1995, included patients aged 1–9 with WBC greater than 50×10^9/litre and patients over 10 years of age with any WBC. Patients with lymphomatous features of any age were treated in a separate CCG-1901 trial. Approximately 90% of the 16- to 21-year-old patients with ALL were entered on CCG-1882; the remainder were treated on CCG-1901. In CCG-1882, standard therapy for both rapid and slow early responders consisted of CCG-modified BFM therapy with IT methotrexate and cranial radiation therapy for CNS-directed treatment. For rapid responders, we compared intensive IT methotrexate without cranial radiation therapy with standard IT methotrexate plus cranial radiation therapy. A new treatment programme, augmented BFM, was developed as the experimental arm for patients showing a slow response to induction therapy. Augmented BFM was designed to increase the amount of vincristine steroid and L-ASP given during the first year and to include an escalating dose of intravenous methotrexate without leucovorin rescue. The 'Capizzi MTX' combination (vincristine and intravenous methotrexate on day 1 followed by L-ASP on day 2 with courses repeated at 10-day intervals) had proved effective in the treatment of relapsed ALL. Capizzi MTX was also attractive because

Table 6.3 Augmented BFM therapy (A-BFM)

Induction	PRED	60 mg/m^2 p.o. days 1–28 (b.i.d. or t.i.d.) then taper
	VCR	1.5 mg/m^2 i.v. days 1, 8, 15, 22
	DNR	25 mg/m^2 i.v. days 1, 8, 15, 22
	L-ASP	6000 U/m^2 i.m. 3 times per week × 3 weeks beginning on day 3
	I/T ARA-C	Day 1 (age-adjusted dosing)
	I/T MTX	Day 8 (age-adjusted dosing)
Consolidation	CPM	1000 mg/m^2 i.v. days 0, 28
(9 weeks)	ARA-C	75 mg/m^2 subq.v./i.v. days 1–4, 8–11, 29–32, 36–39
	6-MP	60 mg/m^2 p.o. days 0–13, 28–41
	VCR	1.5 mg/m^2 i.v. days 14, 21, 42, 49
	L-ASP	6000 U/m^2 i.m. days 14, 16, 18, 21, 24, 25, 42, 44, 46, 49, 51, 53
	I/T MTX	Days 1, 8, 15, 22
	RT	1800 cGy cranial for no CNS disease at diagnosis 2400 cGy cranial + 600 cGy + spinal for CNS disease
Interim maintenance I	VCR	1.5 mg/m^2 i.v. days 0, 10, 20, 30, 40
(8 weeks)	MTX	100 mg/m^2 i.v. days 0, 10, 20, 30, 40 (escalate by 50 mg/m^2/dose)
	L-ASP	15000 U/m^2 i.m. days 1, 11, 21, 31, 41
Delayed intensification I	*Reinduction (4 weeks)*	
(8 weeks)	DEX	10 mg/m^2 p.o. q.d. days 0–20, then taper for 7 days
	VCR	1.5 mg/m^2 i.v. days 0, 14, 21
	DOX	25 mg/m^2 i.v. days 0, 7, 14
	L-ASP	600 U/m^2 i.m. days 3, 5, 7, 10, 12, 14
	Reconsolidation (4 weeks)	
	CPM	1000 mg/m^2 i.v. day 28
	6-TG	60 mg/m^2 p.o. days 28-41
	ARA-C	75 mg/m^2 subq.v./i.v. days 29–32, 36–39
	I/T MTX	Days 29, 36
	VCR	1.5 mg/m^2 i.v. days 42, 49
	L-ASP	6000 U/m^2 i.m. days 42, 44, 46, 51, 53
Interim maintenance II	See 'Interim maintenance I', except additional I/T MTX on days 0, 20, 40	
Delayed intensification II	See 'Delayed intensification I'	
Maintenance	VCR	1.5 mg/m^2 i.v. days 0, 28, 56
(12-week cycles)	PRED	60 mg/m^2 p.o. q.d. days 0–4, 28–32, 56–60
	6-MP	75 mg/m^2 p.o. days 0–83
	MTX	20 mg/m^2 p.o. days 7, 14, 21, 28, 35, 42, 49, 56, 63, 70, 77
	I/T MTX	Day 0

PRED, prednisolone. VCR, vincristine. DNR, daunorubicin. L-ASP, asparaginase. I/T ARA-C, intrathecal cytosine arabinoside. I/T MTX, intrathecal methotrexate. CPM, cyclophosphamide. 6-MP, 6-mercaptopurine. ARA-C, cytosine arabinoside. RT, radiotherapy. DEX, dexamethasone. DOX, doxorubicin. 6-TG, 6-thioguanine. MTX, oral methotrxate. b.i.d., twice daily. t.i.d., three times daily. subq.v./i.v., subcutaneous or intravenous. cGy, centiGray. CNS, central nervous system. q.d., each day.

Table 6.4 CM-BFM versus A-BFM: doses of chemotherapy in the first year

	CM-BFM	A-BFM
Vincristine	15	30
L-Asparaginase	15	53
Cytoxan	3	4
Cytosine arabinoside	24	32
Intravenous methotrexate	0	10
Dexamethasone courses	1	2

Rev Clin Exp Hematol 2003; 7.3.

of the increased exposure to vincristine and L-ASP. The CCG BFM consolidation consisted of two courses of cyclophosphamide, cytosine arabinoside and 6-mercaptopurine given at 14-day intervals. The majority of patients had the second course of consolidation held for periods of 7–10 days because of significant neutropenia. We therefore incorporated 2 weeks of vincristine (weekly × 2) and L-ASP (three times/week × 2 weeks) into each consolidation course. A second Capizzi MTX phase (interim maintenance) and a second DI phase were added before maintenance. The augmented BFM treatment programme is shown in Table 6.3. A comparison of the doses of drug administered during the first year of therapy for standard and augmented BFM is shown in Table 6.4.

For rapid responders, there was an early significant difference in EFS favouring the IT methotrexate and cranial radiation therapy arm.[23] However, with longer follow-up the EFS curves actually crossed, such that at 10 years there was a slightly better EFS for patients receiving intensified IT methotrexate alone. For adolescents, patients receiving intensified IT methotrexate had markedly fewer bone marrow relapses compared with patients receiving cranial radiation and IT methotrexate. The EFS for adolescents showing a rapid early response who received intensified IT methotrexate alone for CNS prophylaxis was 72.3 ± 3.3% at 10 years. For slow early responders, augmented BFM produced a highly significant improvement in EFS compared with CCG standard BFM (9-year EFS was 70.2% for augmented BFM and 47.1% for standard BFM, $P = 0.0006$).[24] The difference in outcome was less striking for patients over 10 years of age. Eight-year EFS was 68.7 ± 4.8% for augmented BFM versus 54.5 ± 5.2% for standard BFM ($P = 0.06$).

A total of 196 patients 16–21 years of age were entered in either CCG-1882 ($n = 175$) or CCG-1901 ($n = 21$). These patients had an 8-year EFS of 64%. This was not significantly different from the outcome for patients aged 10–15 years. Following completion of the 1882/1901 studies, it was decided that patients with lymphomatous features should receive BFM-type therapy.

Thus, between 1996 and 2002, adolescents with ALL were entered on the CCG-1961 study. For rapid responders, patients were randomized to receive standard BFM; standard BFM with a second interim maintenance and DI;

augmented BFM with one DI; or full augmented BFM (second interim maintenance and DI phase). For slow early responders, patients were randomized to receive augmented BFM with or without idarubicin and cyclophosphamide in reinduction courses. In a preliminary analysis, augmented BFM with one DI phase provided the best results for rapid-responder patients.

Comparison of outcome for patients 16–21 years of age with ALL treated on adult and paediatric protocols

In a comparison of patients treated in CCG and Cancer and Leukemia Group B (CALGB) between 1989 and 1995, patients treated on CCG protocols (n = 196) had a significantly better EFS than those treated on CALGB protocols (n = 103): 64% versus 38%.[14] French investigators studied adolescents aged 15–20 years treated in paediatric (FRALLE) and adult (LALA) trials. A total of 94% of patients treated on the FRALLE protocol achieved remission compared with 83% on the LALA protocols. Five-year EFS was 67% for adolescents treated on the FRALLE protocol versus 41% for adolescents treated on the LALA protocol.[15] When comparing drug therapy between paediatric and adult trials, patients treated on the paediatric protocols received significantly more vincristine, steroid and L-ASP compared with those patients treated on adult protocols.

Toxicity of therapy in adolescents

In the American series of trials adolescents have a higher incidence of steroid/L-ASP-induced diabetes mellitus compared with younger children. Pancreatitis is also more common in adolescents. Prolonged steroid administration is associated with the development of avascular necrosis (AVN). Until 1989, adolescents with ALL were treated on multiple different protocols based primarily on presenting WBC, and no mention of AVN is found in the report of these trials. In 1989, more than 90% of adolescents with ALL (excluding those with lymphomatous features) were entered in the CCG-1882 study (high-risk ALL). In this trial, patients received 28 days of continuous prednisone during induction and one or two 21-day courses of dexamethasone during delayed intensification. Patients also received monthly 5-day pulses of prednisone during maintenance. Numerous cases of AVN were reported, almost exclusively in adolescents. AVN was diagnosed in 111 out of 1409 patients treated in CCG-1882.[25] The incidence was significantly higher for patients over 10 years of age than for younger patients: 14.2% versus 0.9% ($P < 0.0001$). In older patients, the incidence was higher for girls than for boys: 17.4% versus 11.7% ($P = 0.03$). Older patients receiving two 21-day courses of dexamethasone had an incidence of AVN of 23.2 ± 4.8%. AVN was invariably diagnosed within 3 years of diagnosis, involved weight-bearing bones in 94% of patients and was multifocal in 74%.

Based on these findings, patients with high-risk ALL entered in the next CCG-1961 study between 1996 and 2002 who received two courses of dexamethasone received it intermittently on days 0–7 and 14–21. Preliminary analysis suggests that discontinuous dexamethasone has decreased the incidence of AVN.

Why do adolescents with ALL have a worse outcome?

There are a number of factors which may contribute to the inferior outcome for adolescents with ALL. The low incidence of so-called favourable cytogenetics, in particular the 12/21 translocation (TEL-AML-1) and a hyperdiploid karyotype and the higher incidence of the Philadelphia chromosome, may play a role.[19]

The dose of vincristine is 'capped' in paediatric ALL protocols; that is, the maximum dose given is 2 mg regardless of the patient's body surface area. Patients with a body surface area greater than 1.33 m^2 therefore receive a lower dose per square metre than patients with a body surface area of less than 1.33 m^2. The greater the patient's body surface area the greater the disparity in dose. A recent study has shown that the 'area under the curve' (a measure of drug exposure) for vincristine is significantly less for patients with body surface area greater than 1.5 m^2.[26] However, compared with those with a smaller body surface area, it is unclear whether adolescents can tolerate uncapped vincristine doses, particularly in the vincristine-intensive augmented BFM regimen. Adolescents have a relatively high incidence of peripheral neuropathy when treated with intensive vincristine.

Compliance with oral medication may be another issue for adolescents with ALL. Parents usually supervise younger patients in taking their steroids, 6-mercaptopurine and methotrexate. Many adolescents assume responsibility for their own oral medications. Steroids are particularly unpleasant for teenagers (acne, changes in body image, mood disturbances) and may result in more non-compilance.

Conclusions

Outcomes for adolescents with ALL are clearly worse than those for patients less than 10 years of age. There seems to be little difference in presenting features or outcome for ALL patients 16–21 years of age compared with those aged 10–15 years at the time of diagnosis. There may be a disproportionate benefit for early treatment intensification for younger compared with older patients.

Adolescents 16–21 years of age have a better outcome when treated in paediatric versus adult clinical trials, which may relate to the fact that adolescents with ALL treated on paediatric trials receive significantly more vincristine, steroids and L-ASP than those treated in adult cooperative trials. In the USA, there are plans for the COG, CALGB and Southwestern Oncology Group (SWOG) to use a common treatment programme for young adults with ALL. AVN is a unique toxicity in adolescents with ALL. The use of discontinuous dexamethasone in DI phases may reduce the incidence of AVN, but the anti-leukaemic efficacy of discontinuous dexamethasone remains to be determined.

References

1 Nachman J, Sather HN, Buckley JD *et al*. Young adults 16–21 years of age at diagnosis entered on Children's Cancer Group ALL and acute myeloblastic leukemia protocols. *Cancer* 1993; **71**: 3377–3385.

2 Pui CH, Boyett JM, Rivera GK. Long-term results of Total Therapy studies 11, 12 and 13A for childhood acute lymphoblastic leukemia at St. Jude Children's Research Hospital. *Leukemia* 2000; **14**: 2286–2294.

3 Schrappe M, Reiter A, Zimmermann M *et al*. Long-term results of four consecutive trials in childhood ALL performed by the ALL-BFM study group from 1981 to 1995. *Leukemia* 2000; **14**: 2205–2222.

4 Maloney KW, Shuster JJ, Murphy S *et al*. Long-term results of treatment studies for childhood acute lymphoblastic leukemia: Pediatric Oncology Group studies from 1986–1994. *Leukemia* 2000; **14**: 2276–2285.

5 Gaynon PS, Trigg ME, Heerema NA *et al*. Children's Cancer Group trials in childhood acute lymphoblastic leukemia: 1983–1995. *Leukemia* 2000; **14**: 2223–2233.

6 Harms DO, Janka-Schaub GE on behalf of the COALL Study Group. Co-operative study group for childhood acute lymphoblastic leukemia (COALL): long-term follow-up of trials 82, 85, 89 and 92. *Leukemia* 2000; **14**: 2234–2239.

7 Kamps WA, Veerman AJP, van Wering ER *et al*. Long-term follow-up of Dutch Childhood Leukemia Study Group (DCLSG) protocols for children with acute lymphoblastic leukemia, 1984–1991. *Leukemia* 2000; **14**: 2240–2246.

8 Eden OB, Harrison G, Richards S *et al*. Long-term follow-up of the United Kingdom Medical Research Council protocols for childhood acute lymphoblastic leukaemia, 1980–1997. *Leukemia* 2000; **14**: 2307–2320.

9 Silverman LB, Declerck L, Gelber RD *et al*. Results of Dana-Farber Cancer Institute Consortium protocols for children with newly diagnosed acute lymphoblastic leukemia (1981–1995). *Leukemia* 2000; **14**: 2247–2256.

10 Chessels JM, Hall E, Prentice HG *et al*. The impact of age on outcome in lymphoblastic leukemia; MRC UKALL X and XA compared: a report from the MRC Pediatric and Adult Working Parties. *Leukemia* 1988; **12**: 413–473.

11 Irken G, Oren H, Gulten H *et al*. Treatment outcome of adolescents with acute lymphoblastic leukemia. *Ann Hematol* 2002; **81**: 641–645.

12 Benjamin S, Kroll ME, Cartwright A *et al*. Haematologists' approaches to the management of adolescents and young adults with acute leukaemia. *Br J Haematol* 2003; **111**: 1045–1050.

13 Stiller C, Benjamin S, Cartwright RA *et al*. Patterns of care and survival for adolescents and young adults with acute leukaemia: a population-based study. *Br J Cancer* 1999; **79**: 658–665.

14 Stock W, Sather H, Dodge RK *et al*. Outcome of adolescents and young adults with ALL: a comparison of Children's Cancer Group (CCG) and Cancer and Leukemia Group B (CALGB) regimens. *Blood* 2000; **96**: 467a.

15 Boissel N, Auclerc MF, Cheritier V *et al*. Should adolescents with acute lymphoblastic leukemia be treated as older children or young adults? Comparison of the French FRALLE-93 and LALA-94 trials. *J Clin Oncol* 2003; **21**: 774–780.

16 Schiffer CA. Differences in outcome in adolescents with acute lymphoblastic leukemia: a consequence of better regimens? Better doctors? Both? *J Clin Oncol* 2003; **21**: 760–761.

17 Chessels JM, Swansbury GJ, Reeves B *et al.* Cytogenetics and prognosis in childhood acute lymphoblastic leukemia: results of MRC UKALL X. *Br J Hematol* 1997; **99**: 93–100.

18 Pieters R, den Boer ML, Durian M *et al.* Relation between age, immunophenotype and *in vitro* drug resistance in 395 children with acute lymphoblastic leukemia: implications for treatment of infants. *Leukemia* 1998; **12**: 1344–1348.

19 Tubergen DG, Gilchrist GS, O'Brien RTO *et al.* Improved outcome with delayed intensification for children with acute lymphoblastic leukemia and intermediate presenting features: a Children's Cancer Group phase III trial. *J Clin Oncol* 1993; **11**: 527–537.

20 Gaynon PS, Bleyer WA, Steinherz PG *et al.* Day 7 marrow response and outcome for children with acute lymphoblastic leukemia and unfavorable presenting features. *Med Ped Oncol* 1990; **18**: 273–279.

21 Schrappe M, Reiter A, Wolf-Dieter L *et al.* Improved outcome in childhood acute lymphoblastic leukemia despite reduced use of anthracyclines and cranial radiotherapy: results of trial ALL-BFM 90. *Blood* 2000; **95**: 3310–3322.

22 Nachman J, Sather HN, Cherlow JM *et al.* Response of children with high-risk acute lymphoblastic leukemia treated with and without cranial irradiation: a report from the Children's Cancer Group. *J Clin Oncol* 1998; **16**: 920–930.

23 Nachman JB, Sather HN, Sensel MG *et al.* Augmented post-induction therapy for children with high-risk acute lymphoblastic leukemia and a slow response to initial therapy. *New Engl J Med* 1998; **338**: 1663–1671.

24 Mattano LA, Sather HN, Trigg ME, Nachman JB. Osteonecrosis as a complication of treating acute lymphoblastic leukemia in children: a report from the Children's Cancer Group. *J Clin Oncol* 2002; **18**: 3262–3272.

CHAPTER 7

Advances in treatment for non-Hodgkin's lymphoma

M. P. Gerrard

Introduction

Non-Hodgkin's lymphoma (NHL) accounts for around 7% of all childhood cancers. The annual incidence is approximately 10 per million, with around 100 new cases of NHL in children under 15 diagnosed each year in the UK. NHL is more common in older children, particularly during the second decade of life, and it is infrequent in children under 3 years of age. The incidence of NHL increases with age from 5.9 cases per million in children aged 5–9 years to 15.3 cases per million in teenagers aged 15–19 years. This contrasts with the decline in incidence of acute lymphoblastic leukaemia, which is 58.2 per million in children aged 5–9 years and 12.9 per million between 15 and 19 years of age. The incidence of NHL appears to have been increasing over the last 30 years. Data from the National Cancer Institute SEER programme[1] show that the annual incidence, which was 10.7 cases per million for older teenagers between 1975 and 1979, has increased steadily since then. The latest figures from 1990–1995 show an incidence of NHL in this age group of 16.3 cases per million. Histological subtype varies with age also, more cases of diffuse large-cell lymphoma being seen in teenagers and young adults compared with younger children, the majority of whom have Burkitt's or lymphoblastic lymphomas.

Survival for children aged less than 15 years has improved steadily over the last 25 years. Data from the United Kingdom Children's Cancer Study Group (UKCCSG)[2] show that currently more than 80% of children aged less than 15 years with NHL survive compared with 55% in 1977. This improvement in survival has not been seen to the same extent in older teenagers and young adults. The SEER data show that the 5-year survival rate for 15- to 19-year-old patients diagnosed between 1975 and 1984 was around 55% and in patients diagnosed between 1985 and 1994 it had improved to just under 70%.

There has been significant progress in treating NHL in children and young people over the last 20 years. Outcome was improved in the early 1980s by intensifying treatment for patients with non-localized disease in whom standard chemotherapy regimens appeared to be of limited value. Since then, stratification of treatment based on histological and then immunophenotypic characteristics has become standard. A number of recent and ongoing studies investigate the possibility of reducing the incidence of sequelae, both early and late, in addition to continuing to attempt to improve the outcome for the small number of children who fail first-line treatment.

Pathological classification

There have been several different classification systems applied to paediatric NHL. This can make the interpretation of results of reported studies difficult because of subtle differences in the terminology used by different groups. It can lead to misunderstanding between clinicians and pathologists. Many groups now classify cases using the REAL classification[3,4] and this does seem to be assisting with the comparison of results between studies. However, difficulties remain, particularly in differentiating subcategories of B-cell lymphoma, such as Burkitt's lymphoma and Burkitt-like lymphoma.[5] To discriminate between mature B-cell subtypes, it may be that morphology needs to be complemented by molecular genetic and cytogenetic studies. However, whether these differences have any clinical significance is not clear. Details of the main subtypes of lymphoma seen in children and adolescents are shown in Table 7.1.

Staging

There are several staging classification systems, but the most widely used is the St Jude scheme, which is based on the Ann Arbor staging system for Hodgkin's disease. This separates patients with limited disease (i.e. a single mass with or without regional node involvement) from those with extensive thoracic or

Table 7.1 Histological subtypes of non-Hodgkin's lymphoma

Histology	Percentage of total	Immunophenotype	Clinical presentation	Cytogenetics
Burkitt or Burkitt-like	40–50	B cell	Abdomen Head and neck, marrow CNS	t(8;14)(q24;q32) t(2;8)(p11;q24) t(8;22)(q24;q11)
Diffuse large cell	15–20	B cell	Nodes, abdomen, bone, mediastinum	
Lymphoblastic	25–30	T cell 90% Pre-B cell 10%	Mediastinum, marrow, skin, bone, nodes	t(1;14), t(11;14)
Anaplastic large cell	10–15	CD30+ (Ki 1) T cell 70% Null cell 20% B cell 10%	Nodes, skin, lung, mediastinum	t(2;5)(p23;q25)

intra-abdominal tumour (stage III). Patients with bone marrow and/or central nervous system (CNS) disease are classified as stage IV. Bone marrow involvement in excess of 25% is by convention described as leukaemia rather than lymphoma. However, it is not clear whether these arbitrary definitions are biologically distinct.

Lymphoblastic lymphoma

Lymphoblastic lymphomas account for between 25 and 30% of NHL seen in children and young people. These are predominantly tumours of thymocyte (T-cell) origin. The majority of patients with lymphoblastic lymphoma present with an anterior mediastinal mass, which may be associated with the superior vena cava syndrome. This results in symptoms of dyspnoea, wheezing, stridor, dysphagia, or swelling of the head and neck. Pleural effusions may be present and involvement of lymph nodes, usually above the diaphragm, can be a prominent feature. There may also be involvement of bone, skin, bone marrow, CNS, liver, kidneys, spleen, and occasionally other sites, such as Waldeyer's ring and the testis. Localized lymphoblastic lymphoma is considerably less frequent than extensive disease, but may involve lymph nodes, bone or subcutaneous tissue. Most lymphoblastic lymphomas are positive for TdT and have a T-cell immunophenotype. A small proportion (10–15%) has non-T immunological characteristics (for example, the cALLA-positive precursor B-cell phenotype). Chromosomal abnormalities are not well characterized in patients with lymphoblastic lymphoma. T-cell lymphomas with a mature phenotype (peripheral T-cell lymphomas) may occur at any of the sites where T cells are found – that is, in almost all organs of the body, but particularly in lymph nodes and at surfaces prone to invasion by microorganisms or foreign bodies.

Treatment

Localized disease

Several standard chemotherapeutic regimens will produce at least 65–70% event-free survival (EFS) in patients with limited stage disease. In addition, many groups report survival in excess of 80% using leukaemia-type regimens.[6–9] It appears that lymphoblastic lymphomas also require maintenance or 'continuation' chemotherapy, as do children with acute lymphoblastic leukaemia, but it is not clear how much treatment they require. Link and colleagues[8] reported that patients given 6 months of maintenance treatment in addition to the standard 3 months of CHOP-based chemotherapy had fewer relapses. However, there were only a few patients with localized lymphoblastic disease included in this study.

Extensive disease

All effective treatment regimens for advanced-stage lymphoblastic NHL have been based on treatment designed for the treatment of acute lymphoblastic

Table 7.2 Recent T-lymphoblastic NHL studies

First author	Year	n	Regimen	Radiotherapy	EFS
Tubergen[10]	1995	252	LSA2L2 or ADCOMP	Local	67%
Amylon[11]	1999	195	POG ± HD L-Asp	None	78% with Asp
					64% without Asp
Reiter[12]	2000	101	BFM 90	Cranial	90%
Mora[13]	2003	87	LSA2L2	Local	75%

leukaemia. Most recent reports on patients with stage III or IV lymphoblastic NHL have long-term survival rates of 70–90%.[10-13] For details see Table 7.2. A Paediatric Oncology Group study[11] showed an improved EFS in patients randomized to receive sequential high-dose asparaginase (78% versus 64% in the control group). Currently, the best published results for advanced-stage disease have been reported from the Berlin-Frankfurt-Munster (BFM) group.[12] In the study NHL-BFM 90, patients were stratified according to stage. Patients with stage III and IV received, after consolidation, an eight-drug block of treatment over 7 weeks and cranial radiotherapy (12 Gy for prophylaxis). With a median follow-up of 4.5 years, the estimated EFS at 5 years for 137 patients with lymphoblastic lymphoma was $82 \pm 5\%$. For 105 evaluable patients with T-cell disease, EFS at 5 years was 90% (CI 82–100%). Among the patients with T-cell disease there was one early death, eight tumour failures (within the first year from diagnosis) and one secondary acute myeloid leukaemia. All eight patients who failed therapy died. Following on from this study, a number of European groups, including the BFM group, the Société Française d'Oncologie Pédiatrique (SFOP), the UKCCSG, the Associazione Italiana di Ematologia e Oncologia Pediatrica (AEIOP) and the Nordic Organisation of Pediatric Hematology and Oncology (NOPHO) have developed a cooperative European study which is scheduled to open in 2004. This study, based on the BFM 90 backbone, will test whether dexamethasone or prednisolone is superior during induction, and also whether maintenance treatment can be reduced from 24 to 18 months for all patients. In addition, those with localized disease will receive less intensive consolidation therapy. This study will aim also to examine whether lack of very early response to treatment is of prognostic value. The continuing challenge in the treatment of lymphoblastic lymphoma is to identify risk factors for treatment failure. In the BFM 90 study there were 101 patients evaluable for local response at day 33, and there was no difference in outcome for those achieving a complete response by this time compared with those who had achieved a partial response only. EFS was 95% in those achieving complete response and 89% in those who had a partial response. Only two patients had a reduction in primary tumour size less than 70% at this stage in treatment. It appears that identifying the patients who are at risk of relapse must be done at an earlier stage in treatment to have any possibility of modifying treatment in an attempt to reduce the risk of treatment failure.

Large-cell lymphoma

This includes a heterogeneous group of tumours and accounts for 20–25% of childhood NHL. Diffuse large-cell histology is more common in older teenagers and young adults than at younger ages. The two pathological types of large-cell lymphoma described in the REAL and WHO classifications are anaplastic large-cell and diffuse large-cell. Most diffuse large-cell lymphomas are treated using the regimens used in the treatment of Burkitt and Burkitt-like lymphomas, and survival of around 80% is expected.[14] Anaplastic large-cell lymphoma includes entities that were previously classified as malignant histiocytosis, peripheral T-cell lymphoma and even Hodgkin's disease. Currently, treatment for anaplastic large-cell lymphoma is also similar to that used for extensive B-cell NHL[15–17] (Table 7.3). Analysis of cases of anaplastic large-cell lymphoma treated by several European groups[18] showed that patients can be stratified into risk categories based on disease sites and histology (Table 7.4). The presence of mediastinal and/or pulmonary involvement is an adverse factor, as is lymphohistiocytic histology or skin involvement (except in those where this is the only site of disease and complete resection is possible). Patients with no skin, mediastinal or pulmonary involvement and non-lymphocytic histology had a better outcome. The ALCL 99 study is a European intergroup study examining whether, for standard risk patients, CNS disease control can be achieved with systemic methotrexate only. CNS involvement at presentation is rare, as is CNS relapse. In addition, for the high-risk patients, the study is examining whether the addition of vinblastine improves outcome. The rationale for this is that long-lasting remissions have been reported in relapsed patients treated with vinblastine as a single agent.[19]

Table 7.3 Recent studies on anaplastic large-cell lymphoma

First author	Year	n	Regimen	Disease-free survival, 3–5 years
Brugières[15]	1998	82	HM89 and HM 91 Methotrexate, cyclophosphamide, doxorubicin, vincristine and prednisone No intrathecal therapy	66% 94% (stages 1 and 2) 55% (stages 3 and 4)
Seidemann[16]	2001	89	BFM 90 Dexamethasone, ifosfamide, cyclophosphamide, etoposide, cytarabine, doxorubicin, methotrexate Intrathecal therapy	76%
Williams[17]	2002	72	NHL 9002 Prednisolone, cyclophosphamide, methotrexate, etoposide, cytarabine, doxorubicin Intrathecal therapy	63%

Table 7.4 Prognostic grouping in anaplastic large cell lymphoma[18]

Group	Features
A	Completely resected disease
B (good risk)	No skin or mediastinal involvement Non-lymphohistiocytic variant
C (poor risk)	Skin lesions (other than Group A) Mediastinal and/or lung involvement Lymphohistiocytic variant
D	CNS involvement

Peripheral B-cell lymphomas

This group of diseases includes Burkitt and Burkitt-like histology as well as diffuse large-cell lymphoma. Results of treatment for localized disease are excellent with limited treatment.[8,20–22] Because of this, it is a continuing challenge to determine whether treatment can be reduced further for good risk groups. The outlook for children and young people with advanced B-cell lymphoma has improved significantly with the use of short intensive chemotherapy. However, results remain poor for those who fail to respond to current standard treatment or who relapse following treatment. The SFOP group have, in successive studies since 1981, shown that dose intensification could improve outcome.[22–24] In addition, they confirmed that treatment time could be reduced without affecting survival. Other groups, including BFM,[21,22]

Table 7.5 Recent peripheral B-cell lymphoma studies

First author	Year	n	Regimen	Duration (months)	Toxic deaths	EFS 2 years stage 3	EFS 2 years stage 4/ B ALL
Patte[23]	1986	114	LMB 81	12	11	73%	50% 46%
Patte[24]	1991	201	LMB 84	3–6	14	80%	71% 65%
Reiter[20]	1995	108	BFM 86	4	1	73%	71% 78%
Reiter[21]	1998	249	BFM 90	4	6	88%	73% 74%
Patte[22]	2001	442	LMB 89	4	8	91%	87% 87%

EFS, event-free survival. B ALL, B-cell acute lymphoblastic leukaemia.

Table 7.6 FABLMB prognostic grouping[27]

Group	Extent of disease
A (low risk)	Completely resected stage I or completely resected abdominal stage II
B (intermediate risk)	All cases not eligible for Group A or Group C
C (high risk)	Any CNS involvement and/or bone marrow involvement with ≥ 25% blasts CNS involvement includes: Any L3 blasts in cerebrospinal fluid Cranial nerve palsy (not explained by extracranial tumour) Clinical spinal cord compression Isolated intracerebral mass Parameningeal extension: cranial and/or spinal

UKCCSG[25] and CCG,[26] have reported similar results. Results from these studies are summarized in Table 7.5. Based on the results from the SFOP 89 study, the CCG and UKCCSG, together with SFOP, developed the FABLMB 96 study. This stratified treatment, based on the extent of disease, into three groups, as reported by SFOP. For details see Table 7.6. The study ran from May 1996 to June 2001 and preliminary results were reported at the American Society of Clinical Oncology meeting in 2003.[27–29] Over 1100 patients were entered in the study. The results for patients in Group A confirmed the excellent results seen in SFOP LMB89 for this group using very limited chemotherapy following surgery. There was only one treatment failure in the group of 136 patients. For Group B patients the study sought to assess whether treatment intensity could be reduced. There were four treatment arms, with reduced doses of cyclophosphamide and/or doxorubicin in three arms. The standard arm was as used in the LMB 89 study. There were 760 patients included in this group, the majority (66%) having stage III disease. There were 8% with non-resected stage I, 20% with non-abdominal stage II, and 6% with stage 4 (marrow) disease. There was no difference in outcome between the four treatment arms, confirming that some reduction in the intensity of treatment was possible for this group of patients, with an EFS in excess of 90%. For Group C the study also sought to discover whether treatment intensity could be reduced by using lower doses of cytarabine and etoposide, and also whether three of the four maintenance courses could be eliminated. There were 242 patients included in this group. The 3-year EFS and overall survival were 79 ± 2.7 and $83 \pm 2.5\%$ respectively. The EFS 3 years from randomization was $84 \pm 2.7\%$ combined, $79 \pm 4.2\%$ in the reduced intensity arm and $90 \pm 3.1\%$ in the standard arm. Patients with B-cell (L3) leukaemia without CNS involvement had an excellent outcome, with a 3-year EFS and overall survival of 87 ± 3.1 and $90 \pm 2.7\%$ respectively. This was significantly better than results for the group of CNS-positive patients, in whom EFS and OS were 71 ± 4.4 and $76 \pm 4.1\%$ ($P = 0.002$ and $P = 0.002$ respectively). The outcome for CNS-positive patients with FABLMB 96 was similar to that seen in SFOP LMB 89 despite no cranial irradiation being given.

Late effects of treatment

Although the majority of children and young people with NHL are cured with current treatment, there are significant sequelae. These include cardiac toxicity, the risk of infertility and second malignancies, and psychosocial adjustment difficulties. Many studies, including those detailed above, involve specific long-term follow-up to monitor for these late effects. Infertility risks and management are the subject of another chapter in this book and will not be covered here. Zebrack and colleagues[30] reported recently their results from a study of adult survivors of lymphoid malignancy, including acute lymphoblastic leukaemia and Hodgkin and non-Hodgkin lymphoma. The study compared 5736 survivors with 2565 sibling controls, and showed a 1.7-fold increase in the incidence of depression and somatic distress syndromes among survivors compared with the control group. Exposure to intensive chemotherapy was the only factor that clearly predicted the increased risk of depression.

Cardiac toxicity is a potential consequence of anthracycline chemotherapy. It is estimated that there are 250,000 survivors of childhood cancer world-wide, of whom 50% have received an anthracycline. Anthracyclines such as doxorubicin and daunorubicin are used in the majority of successful NHL treatment regimens. There is no safe single or cumulative dose. There is a linear correlation between the total cumulative dose of anthracycline and the incidence and severity of cardiac damage. A recently reported follow-up study of patients receiving anthracycline failed to show a definite protective benefit for the use of enalapril.[31] However, very prolonged follow-up is required to monitor these patients and to determine the benefits or otherwise of any intervention.

The development of a second malignancy is a devastating late consequence of treatment of childhood cancer. Leung and colleagues[32] reported a study which followed 497 patients with NHL treated at St Jude's Hospital between 1970 and 1997. A second malignant disease occurred in 16 of them (3.2%). In seven this was acute myeloid leukaemia. The estimated cumulative incidence rate was 2.1% ± 0.7% at 10 years and 4.8 ± 1.3% 20 years after the diagnosis of first malignancy. The highest risk at 20 years (10.9 ± 3.6%) was seen in patients with lymphoblastic lymphoma. The incidence of second malignancy appears to be protocol-dependent, but also genetic susceptibility may be involved.

In conclusion, there have been major advances in treatment for NHL in children and young people over the last 20 years. It is precisely because the expectation of cure is high that there is a need to attempt to minimize the cost of treatment, both in the short term, with excellent supportive care, and in the long term. The use of innovative methods of treatment, such as monoclonal antibodies and apoptosis-inducing agents, holds out the prospect of cure with less toxicity. Because NHL remains a rare disease and because survival is expected in the majority, future advances will inevitably require continuation of the international collaboration that has been a feature of the last 10 years.

References

1 Percy CL, Smith MA, Linet M *et al.* Lymphomas and reticuloendothelial neoplasms. In: Ries LA, Smith MA, Gurney JG *et al.*, eds. Cancer incidence and survival among children and adolescents: United States SEER Program 1975–1995. Bethesda (MD): National Cancer Institute, SEER Program 1999. NIH Pub. No. 99–4649.

2 United Kingdom Children's Cancer Study Group. Annual Report. Leicester: UKCCSG, 2004.

3 Harris NL, Jaffe ES, Diebold J *et al.* World Health Organization classification of neoplastic diseases of the hematopoietic and lymphoid tissues: report of the Clinical Advisory Committee meeting – Airlie House, Virginia November 1997. *J Clin Oncol* 1999; **17**: 3835–3849.

4 Harris NL, Jaffe ES, Stein H *et al.* A revised European, American classification of lymphoid neoplasms: a proposal from the International Lymphoma Study Group. *Blood* 1994; **84**: 1361–1392.

5 Lones MA, Auperin A., Raphael M *et al.* Mature B-cell lymphoma/leukemia in children and adolescents: intergroup pathologist consensus with the revised European–American Lymphoma Classification. *Ann Oncol* 2000; **11**: 47–51.

6 Patte C, Kalifa C, Flamant F *et al.* Results of the LMT81 protocol, a modified LSA2L2 protocol with high dose methotrexate, on 84 children with non-B-cell (lymphoblastic) lymphoma. *Med Ped Oncol* 1992; **20**: 105–113.

7 Anderson JR, Jenkin RD, Wilson JF *et al.* Long-term follow-up of patients treated with COMP or LSA2L2 therapy for childhood non-Hodgkin's lymphoma: a report of CCG-551 from the Children's Cancer Group. *J Clin Oncol* 1993; **11**: 1024–1032.

8 Link MP, Shuster JJ, Donaldson SS *et al.* Treatment of children and young adults with early-stage non-Hodgkin's lymphoma. *N Engl J Med* 1997; **337**: 1259–1266.

9 Grenzebach J, Schrappe M, Ludwig WD *et al.* Favorable outcome for children and adolescents with T-cell lymphoblastic lymphoma with an intensive ALL-type therapy without local radiotherapy. *Ann Hematol* 2000; **80** (Suppl. 3): B73–B76.

10 Tubergen DG, Krailo MD, Meadows AT *et al.* Comparison of treatment regimens for pediatric lymphoblastic non-Hodgkin's lymphoma: a Children's Cancer Group study. *J Clin Oncol* 1995; **13**: 1368–1376.

11 Amylon MD, Shuster J, Pullen J *et al.* Intensive high-dose asparaginase consolidation improves survival for pediatric patients with T cell acute lymphoblastic leukemia and advanced stage lymphoblastic lymphoma: a Pediatric Oncology Group study. *Leukemia* 1999; **13**: 335–342.

12 Reiter A, Schrappe M, Ludwig WD *et al.* Intensive ALL-type therapy without local radiotherapy provides a 90% event-free survival for children with T-cell lymphoblastic lymphoma: a BFM group report. *Blood* 2000; **95**: 416–421.

13 Mora J, Filippa DA, Qin J, Wollner N. Lymphoblastic lymphoma of childhood and the LSA2-L2 protocol: the 30-year experience at Memorial Sloan–Kettering Cancer Center. *Cancer* 2003; **98**: 1283–1291.

14 Laver JH, Mahmoud H, Pick TE *et al.* Results of a randomised phase III trial in children and adolescents with advanced stage diffuse large cell non-Hodgkin's lymphoma: a Pediatric Oncology Group study. *Leuk Lymphoma* 2001; **42**: 399–405.

15 Brugieres L, Deley MC, Pacquement H *et al*. CD30(+) anaplastic large-cell lymphoma in children: analysis of 82 patients enrolled in two consecutive studies of the French Society of Pediatric Oncology. *Blood* 1998; **92**: 3591–3598.

16 Seidemann K, Tiemann M, Schrappe M *et al*. Short-pulse B-non-Hodgkin lymphoma-type chemotherapy is efficacious treatment for pediatric anaplastic large cell lymphoma: a report of the Berlin-Frankfurt-Munster Group Trial NHL-BFM 90. *Blood* 2001; **97**: 3699–3706.

17 Williams DM, Hobson R, Imeson J. Anaplastic large cell lymphoma in childhood: analysis of 72 patients treated on the United Kingdom Children's Cancer Study Group chemotherapy regimen. *Br J Haematol* 2002; **117**: 812–820.

18 le Deley MC, Reiter A, Williams D *et al*. Prognostic factors in childhood anaplastic large cell lymphoma: result of the European Intergroup Study. In: *Proceedings of the Seventh International Conference on Malignant Lymphoma* 1998.

19 Brugieres L, Quartier P, Le Deley MC *et al*. 2000. Relapses of childhood anaplastic large-cell lymphoma: treatment results in a series of 41 children – a report from the French Society of Pediatric Oncology. *Ann Oncol* 2000; **11**: 53–58.

20 Reiter A, Schrappe M, Parwaresch R *et al*. Non-Hodgkin's lymphomas of childhood and adolescence: results of a treatment stratified for biologic subtypes and stages. A report of the Berlin-Frankfurt-Munster Group. *J Clin Oncol* 1995; **13**: 359–372.

21 Reiter A, Schrappe M, Tiemann M *et al*. Improved treatment results in childhood B-cell neoplasms with tailored intensification of therapy: a report of the Berlin-Frankfurt-Munster Group Trial NHL-BFM 90. *Blood* 1999; **94**: 3294–3306.

22 Patte C, Auperin A, Michon J *et al*. The Societe Francaise d'Oncologie Pediatrique LMB89 protocol: highly effective multiagent chemotherapy tailored to the tumor burden and initial response in 561 unselected children with B-cell lymphomas and L3 leukemia. *Blood* 2001; **97**: 3370–3379.

23 Patte C, Philip T, Rodary C *et al*. Improved survival rate in children with stage III and IV B cell non-Hodgkin's lymphoma and leukemia using multi-agent chemotherapy: results of a study of 114 children from the French Paediatric Oncology Society. *J Clin Oncol* 1986; **4**: 1219–1226.

24 Patte C, Philip T, Rodary C *et al*. High survival rate in advanced stage B cell lymphoma and leukemias without CNS involvement with a short intensive polychemotherapy: results from the French Paediatric Oncology Society of a randomized trial of 216 children. *J Clin Oncol* 1991; **9**: 123–132.

25 Atra A, Gerrard M, Hobson R *et al*. Improved cure rate in children with B-cell acute lymphoblastic leukaemia (B-ALL) and stage IV B-cell non-Hodgkin's lymphoma (B-NHL) – results of the UKCCSG 9003 protocol. *Br J Cancer* 1998; **77**: 2281–2285.

26 Cairo MS, Sposto R, Perkins SL *et al*. Burkitt's and Burkitt-like lymphoma in children and adolescents: a review of the Children's Cancer Group experience. *Br J Haematol* 2003; **120**: 660–670.

27 Gerrard M, Cairo MS, Weston C *et al*. Results of the FAB LMB 96 international study in children and adolescents (C+A) with localised, resected B cell lymphoma (large cell [LCL], Burkitt's [BL] and Burkitt-like [BLL]). France. *Proc Am Soc Clin Oncol* 2003: 795.

28 Patte C, Gerrard M, Auperin A *et al*. Results of the randomised international trial FAB LMB 96 for the 'intermediate risk' childhood and adolescent B-cell lymphoma: reduced therapy is efficacious. *Proc Am Soc Clin Oncol* 2003: 796.

29 Cairo MS, Gerrard M, Sposto R *et al*. Results of a randomized FAB LMB96 international study in children and adolescents (C+A) with advanced (bone marrow

[BM] [B-ALL] and/or CNS) B-NHL (large cell [LCL], Burkitt's [BL] and Burkitt-like [BLL]): Pts with L3 leukemia/CNS- have an excellent prognosis. *Proc Am Soc Clin Oncol* 2003: 796.

30 Zebrack BJ, Zeltzer LK, Whitton J *et al.* Psychological outcomes in long-term survivors of childhood leukemia, Hodgkin's disease, and non-Hodgkin's lymphoma: a report from the Childhood Cancer Survivor Study. *Pediatrics* 2002; **110**: 42–52.

31 Silber JH, Cnaan A, Clark BJ *et al.* Enalapril to prevent cardiac function decline in long-term survivors of pediatric cancer exposed to anthracyclines. *J Clin Oncol* 2004; **22**: 820–828.

32 Leung W, Sandlund JT, Hudson MM *et al.* Second malignancy after treatment of childhood non-Hodgkin lymphoma. *Cancer* 2001; **92**: 1959–1966.

CHAPTER 8

Hodgkin's disease and adolescents: the lost tribe?

K. P. Windebank

Introduction

In 1832 Thomas Hodgkin presented a paper to the Medical Chirurgical Society in London entitled 'On some morbid appearances of the absorbent glands and spleen'. The report was based on cases he had seen since his appointment in 1825 as the first curator of Guy's Hospital Medical School Museum. The paper was forgotten and his name is associated with the disease only because Sir Samuel Wilks, when he described the disease more accurately 30 years later, insisted on giving Hodgkin the credit. Some 172 years on, although the disease is well characterized in children and adults, adolescents are only just beginning to be recognized as a distinct subgroup with Hodgkin's disease.

One of the axioms of child health is that children are not miniature adults. Few would dispute this, but where does that leave adolescents? Given their behaviour, ought we to treat them as big children or should they be thought of physiologically as the real miniature adults? While in some areas of the life and health of adolescents this is irrelevant, in the case of significant illness and consequent major treatment interventions, dealing with these questions may be crucial to ensuring optimal care and concordance. This is no more relevant to anyone than to the adolescent diagnosed with Hodgkin's disease.

At first consideration, it seems reasonably straightforward to begin by defining adolescence. It is the phase of human development between the onset of puberty and the achievement of adult maturity. Unfortunately, neither puberty nor maturity is determined by age, immediately confounding the standard models whereby medical care is delivered. Depending on the configuration of local health-care services, adolescents are treated in a children's hospital (upper age 16 years), an adult hospital (lower age 16 years) or a general hospital (potentially 10–25 years).[1] Not surprisingly, the age of 16 falls exactly midway through the teenage years, neatly (if artificially) cutting the adolescent group in two and thereby causing a multitude of problems.

Apart from the evident psychosocial need, is there a separate need to identify any potential curative advantage to be gained by targeting an adolescent group with Hodgkin's disease? In effect, definition and need are complementary. If a group can be separated out on disease criteria, then it is a group that almost certainly would benefit from closer scrutiny. So, is it possible to set apart a unique adolescent cohort by examining the features of the disease occurring across this age range?

Incidence

Certainly the incidence pattern of a particular cancer can help select a discrete patient population. Osteogenic sarcoma and Ewing's tumour are commonest in the 10- to 24-year-old group, peaking in 15- to 19-year-olds (Fig. 8.1a). This supports a compelling argument for these tumours to be treated regionally

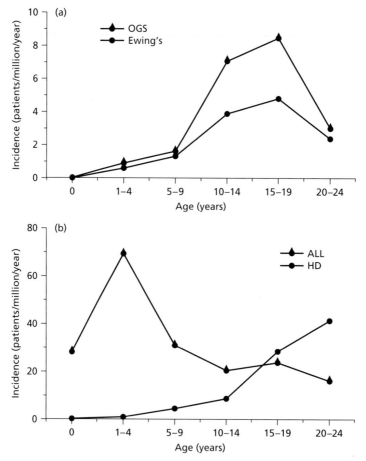

Fig. 8.1 Incidence of osteogenic sarcoma (OGS) and Ewing's tumour (a) and acute lymphoblastic leukaemia (ALL) and Hodgkin's disease (HD) (b) by age group. (Reproduced with kind permission from the Northern Region Children's and Young Persons' Malignant Disease Registries.)

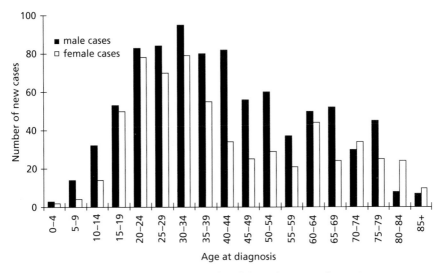

Fig. 8.2 Number of new cases diagnosed of Hodgkin's disease in the UK in 2000 according to sex (modified from http://www.cancerresearchuk.org/aboutcancer/statistics/statstables/hodgkinsdisease).

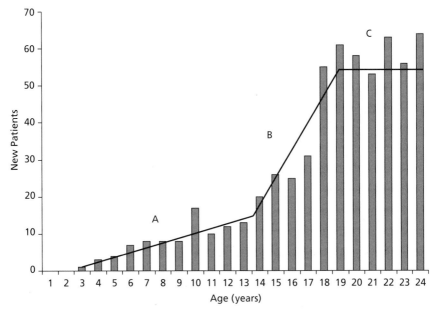

Fig. 8.3 Age of patients diagnosed with Hodgkin's disease in the Northern Region of England 1968–2000. (Reproduced with kind permission from the Northern Region Children's and Young Persons' Malignant Disease Registries.)

under a single multidisciplinary team. In an analogous way, acute lymphoblastic leukaemia is clearly a disease of young children and, not unexpectedly, the expertise for treatment of this condition lies within the boundaries of paediatrics (Fig. 8.1b). Following the same logic, it could be argued from Fig. 8.1b that, as Hodgkin's disease is rare in children and younger adolescents, patients should be looked after most appropriately by adult-oriented multidisciplinary teams, who see the vast majority of cases.

Hodgkin's disease has a bimodal lifetime incidence with peaks in early and late adulthood (Fig. 8.2). The disease is rare in children in industrialized societies and then the incidence rises steeply to the young adult plateau that covers the third decade of life. Focusing on this changing incidence through childhood to the young adult peak, a pattern emerges (Fig. 8.3). There is a minimally increasing incidence during childhood (A), followed by a very steep rise in teenagers (B) and reaching a plateau in the early twenties (C). This could just reflect developmental variation in biological susceptibility to a single disease entity at different ages. Alternatively, it could reflect something different about the pathogenesis of the type of disease in children compared with young adults, with both occurring in a mixed picture during the transition period of adolescence.

Epidemiology

Socio-economic status and exposure to infections are important factors influencing the prevalence of the disease.[2] Children with Hodgkin's disease tend to come from lower socio-economic groups with larger family sizes and consequently wider exposure to infections at a younger age. Conversely, the risk factors for developing Hodgkin's disease in the young adult plateau are associated with higher social classes.

Complementing these general observations, and further suggesting a difference in aetiology between children and young adults, are the specific findings relating to the causal association between the Epstein–Barr virus (EBV) and Hodgkin's disease. Based on serological evidence, it has been known for some time that Hodgkin's disease is often EBV-associated, with a higher rate of association among children compared with young adults.[3,4] More recently, using EBV-encoded RNA *in situ* hybridization techniques on biopsy tissue, it has become apparent that the young adult peak is indeed driven largely by EBV-negative cases, the changeover occurring during the teenage years.[5] Notwithstanding that, there are still considerable numbers of EBV-associated cases in early compared with mid-adulthood.

Data are emerging to suggest that EBV-associated disease has a separately definable prognosis, which may be worse in children and older adults than in younger adults.[6] This component of the aetiology may soon begin to influence treatment intensity decisions. With the advent of more specifically directed anti-EBV immunological modalities, it will also change whole therapeutic strategies.

These observations suggest that the adolescent group merits individual consideration, insofar as it encompasses a changeover period in the aetiology of the disease. Some adolescents have children's Hodgkin's disease and others have the young adult type of disease.

Pathology

The malignant Hodgkin's cell is of B-cell lineage, but unlike most types of B-cell non-Hodgkin's lymphoma (NHL), in which there are sheets of malignant cells, as few as 1 in 100 cells may be neoplastic in a node infiltrated by Hodgkin's disease. The rest of the cells are inflammatory migrants, which explains why Hodgkin's disease nodes can wax and wane over months. Teenagers prone to self-medication with over-the-counter analgesics may notice this phenomenon particularly.

Depending on the pattern of the accompanying inflammatory response, four subtypes of Hodgkin's disease are currently recognized: nodular sclerosing, grade I and II (NSI and NSII); mixed cellularity (MC); lymphocyte-depleted; and classical lymphocyte-rich. Nodular lymphocyte-predominant Hodgkin's disease has been reclassified as a low-grade NHL. The prognostic significance of the subtypes has been debated for years, but there is some evidence that, of the two commonest, MC has a poorer prognosis than NSI.[7]

In children, while NSI predominates (60% of diagnoses), up to 30% of cases of Hodgkin's disease may be MC.[8] In contrast, MC Hodgkin's disease becomes much rarer in the young adult peak and has been observed in as few as 4% (7 out of 180) of centrally reviewed 17- to 20-year-olds entered into the CCG 5942 clinical trial (J. Nachman, personal communication). Interestingly, MC Hodgkin's disease in general is associated preferentially with EBV positivity.[6]

These findings lend further credence to the likelihood that adolescence reflects a complex period in the pathology of Hodgkin's disease with the declining incidence of prognostically possibly less favourable MC disease, with or without the presence of the EBV genome.

Presentation, diagnosis and staging

In common with other age groups, in adolescence the usual presentation of low-stage disease is painless, enlarging cervical lymphadenopathy. The later-stage presentations in teenagers are associated often with primary intra-abdominal disease or, in young women, with mediastinal disease that has progressed significantly to chest wall involvement before they seek medical advice.

The clinical history should document the presence or absence of 'B' symptoms, suggestive of widespread disease (recurrent fever, night sweats or unexplained weight loss of more than 10% in the preceding 6 months). Interestingly, vasculitic rashes and pruritus do not constitute B symptoms and may be seen occasionally in early-stage disease. The initial interview and physical examination of the younger adolescent should include documentation of pubertal status and the initial assessment of competence to give informed consent relevant to impending therapeutic decisions and issues about the preservation of fertility.

To make the diagnosis, nodal or other involved tissue should be obtained, as the subtype can be determined accurately only against the background of overall cellular architecture. Owing to the rarity of carcinoma in the first two decades of life, this is almost always the initial approach adopted to suspicious lymphadenopathy in children. However, some young adults will go along the carcinoma diagnostic route and have a fine needle aspiration that reveals Hodgkin's cells. With this result they should proceed to excisional node biopsy to ensure allocation to the correct subtype.

Unlike NHL, in Hodgkin's disease the pattern of dissemination is by contiguous lymphatic spread. The disease begins in one nodal group and then gradually spreads out to involve the surrounding groups, as defined in Fig. 8.4.[9] This is reflected in the original 1971 Ann Arbor staging system (Stage I, single group; Stage II, two groups or more on same side of diaphragm; Stage III, two groups or more on opposite sides of diaphragm; and Stage IV, extralymphatic spread) and its subsequent modifications applied to patients with Hodgkin's disease. Initial staging must provide accurate information on the extent of the disease in order to guide the intensity of therapy required to cure with the least adverse effects.

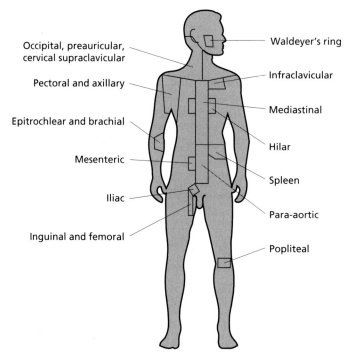

Fig. 8.4 Lymph node groups used in assigning the stage of Hodgkin's disease. (After Kaplan.)[9]

Peripheral lymphadenopathy can be assessed generally by clinical examination, but intrathoracic and intra-abdominal disease need more sophisticated approaches. This was particularly important in the pre-chemotherapy era, when radiotherapy was the main therapeutic modality. Areas of disease not identified, and therefore excluded from the radiation field, would declare themselves subsequently as a 'relapse'.

In the past, chest X-ray alone was used to exclude or confirm mediastinal disease and intra-abdominal staging was accomplished by lymphangiography, to look at the retroperitoneum, and surgical staging was performed by laparotomy with splenectomy. With the advent of effective chemotherapy and computerised tomography (CT), the continued need for such invasive procedures and their subsequent complications was debated during the 1980s.[10] By the end of that decade surgical staging had been largely abandoned.

Whilst in children CT visualization of retroperitoneal nodal tissue is poor due to a relative paucity of fat, in adolescents it is usually adequate and staging is accomplished reliably by CT in the majority of teenagers. Recently, positron emission tomography (PET) scanning has been advocated as a more sensitive technique for identifying tissue involved with Hodgkin's disease at diagnosis, and has been proposed to be of particular benefit in assessment of remission when a residual mass remains in an area of original bulky disease.[11] Using small amounts of radioactive substrate, commonly fluorodeoxyglucose (FDG), tissue that is highly metabolically active can be visualized. As tumour cells are proliferating, they take up the tagged substrate preferentially. However, normal white cells responding to any tissue insult are also metabolically very active, so that areas of inflammation or infection may appear positive.

The studies on PET scanning have centred predominantly on adult populations and should be interpreted with care when attempts are made to extrapolate to Hodgkin's disease in children and teenagers.[12] Extreme caution must be exercised always in transposing interpretations based on adult physiology to growing children and hormonally maturing adolescents. For initial diagnostic evaluation, it is important to establish what is normal before pronouncing with confidence what constitutes an abnormal area of uptake. In addition, as mentioned above, as few as 1 in 100 cells in tissue effaced by Hodgkin's disease are actually malignant, the rest being inflammatory. At the end of treatment a positive scan could represent bystander inflammatory tissue, whereas a negative result may be missing significant numbers of viable tumour cells scattered through a metabolically inactive background of fibrosis. Rigorous evaluation of this technique in longitudinal studies beginning at diagnosis should be considered mandatory before its widespread application to childhood and adolescent Hodgkin's disease can be justified.

In the presence of B symptoms or suspicious peripheral blood findings, bilateral bone marrow aspirates and trephine biopsies should be performed. On occasion, when localized bone pain is prominent, a radionuclide bone scan is indicated. Other haematological and biochemical parameters should be documented and, where available, incorporated into the calculation of a prognostic index, which may be useful in deciding the intensity or duration of therapy. Such scoring systems have been validated in adults and can include older teenagers.[13] It has been suggested that five pretreatment factors may predict the prognosis in children and teenagers: male sex; Stage IIB, IIIB or IV; bulky mediastinal disease; white blood cell count greater than 13.5×10^9/litre; and haemoglobin concentration less than 11 g/dl.[14] Interestingly, age above or below 14 years did not reach significance even on univariate analysis.

Preparation and planning for treatment

Adolescents are in the crucial phase of coming to terms with who they are and what they want to be. The impact of a diagnosis of cancer cannot be underestimated in psychological and practical terms. Ideally, access to an independent confidant should be established before treatment is started. This may be a psychologist, social worker or specifically trained nurse counsellor. The aim is to provide a contact who will prevent the young person developing a feeling of isolation and encourage them to explore and understand their feelings of anger, frustration, guilt and rebellion.

Resentment at losing recently hard-fought-for independence can be a powerful force in generating non-concordance. This is particularly hazardous in terms of ensuring the meticulous taking of oral chemotherapy and reporting the early onset of symptoms that potentially warn of septicaemia during periods of febrile neutropenia. It is helpful to emphasize this eventuality by going over potentially extreme scenarios. For example, 'You're about to go out to your girlfriend's 18th birthday party and you feel a bit dizzy and hot. What do you do? You don't ignore it, you check your temperature and discuss it with your family.' Or 'It's 4.00 a.m. in the morning, you wake up feeling hot and ill, but you know you've got an appointment at the clinic at 10.00 a.m. What do you do? You don't roll over and go back to sleep.' This may seem to be overstating the case, but most young people with Hodgkin's disease are treated in an outpatient setting and will not necessarily appreciate the dangers of delaying antibiotic therapy in this situation.

Concerns relating to the preservation of fertility of adolescents are labyrinthine in their complexity and in Hodgkin's disease they are complicated further by the fact that many patients, especially those with advanced disease, are subfertile at diagnosis. Although they are discussed in detail elsewhere in these proceedings, there are particularly important issues in Hodgkin's disease. Probably the most significant is that the vast majority of adolescents will survive their disease with few external signs of therapeutic sequelae. While the move from therapy based on alkylating agents to less gonadotoxic therapy has led to a significant reduction in infertility in Hodgkin's disease survivors, it should be remembered that, in aiming to give the minimum effective chemotherapy, some patients will relapse. Given this possibility of return to more therapy and the variance in normal baseline fertility, it is prudent to store appropriate samples even for those patients whose proposed definitive therapy is not felt to be sterilizing.

In educational terms, this period in a young person's life is critical, and careful consideration must be given to minimizing disruption of schooling and other training. Liaison with the patient's school or college should include the practical side of allowing the student the freedom to come and go as they feel well enough to do, and the academic side of encouraging work at home and appropriate input to examination boards to prevent double jeopardy.

Most first-line Hodgkin's disease chemotherapy can be given in the clinic, but the after-effects often put the patient in bed at home for a few days. Our practice is to give chemotherapy on Friday, leaving the weekend for the teenager to recover enough to get back to school or college, and parents to get to work, on Monday. Needless to say, this is sometimes more popular with the other members of the family than with the patient.

Some of the drugs used are highly emetogenic and it is important to plan how appropriate changes will be made if nausea is a persistent problem. Adolescents are notoriously prone to anticipatory vomiting and getting in the car to come to clinic can herald the start of severe vomiting that can end as dramatically as it started, if chemotherapy is delayed because of low counts. Simple antiemetics such as metoclopramide, ondansetron, cyclizine and haloperidol should be used initially. Anxiolytics such as lorazepam can be helpful, and in resistant cases nabilone, with its dual relaxant and antiemetic action, can produce spectacular relief. Nabilone therapy should be instituted with caution as its effects may be unpredictable, especially in younger teenagers.

Children are usually offered the convenience of an indwelling central venous catheter (CVC) that may be totally implanted or externalized to suit parental competencies, the child's lifestyle and the intensity of chemotherapy. Adults are frequently offered repeated peripheral cannulation as their lone option. Adolescents, with their changing body imagery and their frequently chaotic lifestyle, deserve careful individual consideration, rather than being made to fit in with the practice of the centre where they are receiving treatment. Matters have been helped by the rise of interventional radiology leading to the resolution of many of the issues relating to the surgical ownership of adolescents between paediatric and general surgery. They should be offered the most appropriate CVC for their own perceived comfort, their maturity and their lifestyle and family circumstances.

Treatment and side-effects

Surgery has little role in Hodgkin's disease, apart from at diagnosis and the insertion of indwelling CVCs except in nodular lymphocyte-predominant Hodgkin's disease, now reclassified among NHL, in which there is evidence accruing that when a small number of nodes is involved and these are excised completely, cure may be expected without additional therapy.[15,16]

Not surprisingly, younger adolescents have tended to receive the same chemotherapy as children, whereas older adolescents have been looked after by adult-based multidisciplinary teams. While numerous regimens used in adult practice have proved to be very effective in children, the high survival rates have been gained at the cost of significant morbidity. This has been revealed clearly in long-term follow-up studies in children.[17] In particular, regimens based on alkylating agents, such as the original MOPP (mustard, oncovin, procarbazine and prednisolone) pose the risks of infertility and secondary cancers, whereas the introduction of ABVD (adriamycin, bleomycin, vinblastine and dacarbazine) came with its alternative long-term effects on cardiac muscle and lung parenchyma.

Various strategies have been invoked using these drugs, or closely related ones, with and without the addition of etoposide and radiotherapy.[18,19] Alternating the MOPP and ABVD regimens on a monthly basis is effective in earlier stages of disease, with a reduction in individual cumulative doses of drugs and consequent side-effects. The length of treatment with these regimens has been related to both the initial stage and the speed of response. In more advanced cases, all these drugs can be given in a dose-intensive fashion in a 1-month hybrid rather than spread over 2 months. Such hybrid regimens can be used alone or in combination with stem-cell rescue procedures.[20] There are also numerous combinations of drugs used in second- and third-line therapies. Allogeneic bone marrow transplantation has not been of major value, owing to the heavy pretreatment received by relapsing Hodgkin's disease patients. Recently, however, the reduced conditioning required for so-called mini transplants has enabled the salvage of multiply relapsed patients.[21,22] A degree of alopecia is universal and relates to the intensity of therapy. Surprisingly, it is often not as big an issue for the patient as expected by the rest of the family. Fortunately, today the teenage years are recognized as a time for experimentation, making any hair fashion acceptable.

Radiotherapy is used in a variety of situations. In early-stage, localized disease in children, it has been used to cure 70% of cases without resorting to systemic chemotherapy.[23] This is normally in cervical disease and, apart from some muscle wasting, the main side-effect is thyroid failure that requires life-long replacement therapy with thyroxine. At the other end of the spectrum, and commonly seen in adults, is advanced disease, with bulky, often mediastinal masses that respond but do not disappear after chemotherapy. This leaves potential residual disease among fibrotic reactive nodal tissue, and radiotherapy is used as consolidation. The main side-effect of mediastinal radiotherapy is the recently increasingly documented complication of breast cancer.[24] This is a very significant risk in adolescent females who have had breast tissue included in the radiation field. There is such concern over this that national trial organizations have instituted regular screening programmes for patients in this group. In the meantime, improved equipment and planning have resulted in much smaller doses being given to areas involving breast tissue.

Combined modality therapy, employing chemotherapy and then targeted radiotherapy, has the potential advantage of using lower doses of both modalities, thereby reducing side-effects. Perhaps the most difficult question under intensive current investigation is where the balance should lie between radiotherapy and chemotherapy in low- and intermediate-risk cases.[19,25] It is likely that the answers may be different for growing children and maturing adolescents compared with adults. It has been advocated that PET scanning may be a useful guide to whether radiotherapy should be used to treat areas of original or residual bulk disease. As discussed above, this would need careful evaluation before being incorporated into trials of adolescent Hodgkin's disease.

Immunotherapy has exciting potential in Hodgkin's disease, in which, it seems, malfunction of the patient's immune system may be playing a major role in oncogenic transformation. The efficacy of anti-CD20 antibody in resistant cases of Hodgkin's disease has been reported.[26] The potential for using antiviral therapy is widening in EBV-associated Hodgkin's disease, either with antibodies or EBV-specific cytolytic T cells cloned *in vitro* and HLA matched to the patient's tissue type.

Looking at the therapeutic questions to be asked and given the heterogeneity of Hodgkin's disease in adolescents, the ultimate aim should be to develop clinical trials that are targeted specifically at this group of older children and younger adults.

Conclusions

Adolescents are unique. They are immersed in a distinct phase of human development in which they are neither an end-stage child nor a nascent adult. As evolution dictates, their logic, values and sense of immortality strive relentlessly to make strangers of their family. To put all this on hold with a diagnosis of cancer, and the news that if they do not do exactly as they are told from now on they will die, is not the best way to begin a complex course of medical treatment. Clearly, the need for psychosocial support and an appropriate therapeutic environment should not be underestimated if optimal therapy is to be accomplished.

Hodgkin's disease in adolescents is almost certainly not a single disease. To achieve cure at least cost, the patients who need less treatment must be teased out as soon as possible from those who need the most intensive combined-modality therapy. As well as haematological and biochemical factors, EBV status and pathological subtype may be important predictors of outcome in adolescents. A slow response to chemotherapy, perhaps monitored by PET scanning, is also likely to identify those with more resistant disease.

It may seem that the obvious answer is also the simplest. Adolescents with Hodgkin's disease should be treated according to specifically designed pro-tocols, in adolescent units by adolescent multidisciplinary teams with full and appropriate psychosocial support. While we are striving for this ideal, what are the priorities? The most important is the need to design further comprehensive, randomized adolescent studies to answer the questions relating to the balance of chemotherapy and radiotherapy in early stages and the best intensive therapy in advanced cases. Such protocols would need to be agreed by and accessed by those currently looking after adolescents, namely paediatricians and adult physicians. This will take time.

In the meantime, in this age of rapidly expanding information technology, are there any other approaches worth considering? In the UK, under the auspices of the National Cancer Network, a web-based registration project is currently being rolled out to all physicians looking at another cohort of Hodgkin's disease patients – the over 60-year age group (www.shieldstudy.co.uk). The study aims to collect information on all patients in this age range, irrespective of whether they are treated according to a suggested protocol or with other treatment. Having this study already in place offers an excellent opportunity to follow on with a study registering and collecting data on a nationally defined population of adolescents. The lost tribe would become the unique cohort.

References

1 Windebank K, Morgan S. Starting an adolescent cancer unit: why does it take so long? *Pediatr Blood Cancer* 2004; **42**: 241–248.

2 Mueller NE. Epidemiology – Hodgkin's disease. In: Hancock BW, Selby PJ, MacLennan K, Armitage JO, eds. *Malignant Lymphoma*. London: Arnold, 2000: Chapter 13, 161–167.

3 Evans AS, Gutensohn NM. A population-based case-control study of EBV and other viral antibodies among persons with Hodgkin's disease and their siblings. *Int J Cancer* 1984; **34**: 149–157.

4 Armstrong AA, Alexander FE, Paes RP *et al.* Association of Epstein–Barr virus with pediatric Hodgkin's disease. *Am J Pathol* 1993; **142**: 1683–1688.

5 Jarrett RF, Krajewski AS, Angus B *et al.* The Scotland and Newcastle epidemiological study of Hodgkin's disease: impact of histopathological review and EBV status on incidence estimates. *J Clin Pathol* 2003; **56**: 811–816.

6 Young LS, Murray PG. Epstein–Barr virus and oncogenesis: from latent genes to tumours. *Oncogene* 2003; **22**: 5108–5121.

7 MacLennan KA, Vaughan Hudson B, Vaughan Hudson G. Histopathology – Hodgkin's disease. In: Hancock BW, Selby PJ, MacLennan K, Armitage JO, eds. *Malignant Lymphoma*. London: Arnold, 2000: Chapter 2, 9–19.

8 Schwartz CL. The management of Hodgkin disease in the young child. *Curr Opin Pediatr* 2003; **15**: 10–16.

9 Kaplan HS. *Hodgkin's Disease*, 2nd edn. Cambridge (MA): Harvard University Press, 1980.

10 Windebank KP, Gilchrist GS. Hodgkin's disease. *Pediatr Ann* 1988; **17**: 204–223.

11 Weirauch MR, Re D, Scheidhauer K *et al.* Thoracic positron emission tomography using 18F-flurodeoxyglucose for the evaluation of residual mediastinal Hodgkin disease. *Blood* 2001; **98**: 2930–2934.

12 Hudson MM, Krasin MJ, Kaste SC. PET imaging in pediatric Hodgkin's lymphoma. *Pediatr Radiol* 2004; **34**: 190–198.

13 Proctor SJ, Taylor P, Donnan P *et al.* A numerical prognostic index for clinical use in identification of poor risk patients with Hodgkin's disease at diagnosis. *Eur J Cancer* 1991; **27**: 624–629.

14 Smith RS, Chen Q, Hudson MM, *et al.* Prognostic factors for children with Hodgkin's disease treated with combined-modality therapy. *J Clin Oncol* 2003; **21**: 2026–2033.

15 Pellegrino B, Terrier-Lacombe MJ, Oberlin O *et al.* Lymphocyte-predominant Hodgkin's lymphoma in children: therapeutic abstention after initial lymph node resection – a study of the French Society of Pediatric Oncology. *J Clin Oncol* 2003; **21**: 2948–2952.

16 Murphy SB, Morgan ER, Katzenstein HM, Kletzel M. Results of little or no treatment for lymphocyte-predominant Hodgkin disease in children and adolescents. *J Pediatr Hematol Oncol* 2003; **25**: 684–687.

17 Bhatia S, Yasui Y, Robison LL *et al.* High risk of subsequent neoplasms continues with extended follow-up of childhood Hodgkin's disease: report from the Late Effects Study Group. *J Clin Oncol* 2003; **21**: 4386–4394.

18 Thomson AB, Wallace WH. Treatment of paediatric Hodgkin's disease: a balance of risks. *Eur J Cancer* 2002; **38**: 468–477.

19 Diehl V. Chemotherapy or combined modality treatment: the optimal treatment for Hodgkin's disease. *J Clin Oncol* 2004; **22**: 15–18.

20 Proctor SJ, Mackie M, Dawson A *et al.* A population-based study of intensive multi-agent chemotherapy with or without autotransplant for the highest risk Hodgkin's disease patients identified by the Scotland and Newcastle Lymphoma Group (SNLG) prognostic index. A Scotland and Newcastle Lymphoma Group study (SNLG HD III). *Eur J Cancer* 2002; **38**: 795–806.

21 Carella AM, Cavaliere M, Lerma E *et al.* Autografting followed by nonmyeloablative immunosuppressive chemotherapy and allogenic peripheral-blood hematopoietic stem-cell transplantation as treatment of resistant Hodgkin's disease and non-Hodgkin's lymphoma. *J Clin Oncol* 2000; **18**: 3918–3924.

22 Anderlini P, Giralt S, Andersson B *et al.* Allogeneic stem cell transplantation with fludarabine-based, less intensive conditioning regimens as adoptive immunotherapy in advanced Hodgkin's disease. *Bone Marrow Transplant* 2000; **26**: 615–620.

23 Shankar AG, Ashley S, Radford M *et al.* Does histology influence outcome in childhood Hodgkin's disease? Results from the United Kingdom Children's Cancer Group. *J Clin Oncol* 1997; **15**: 2622–2630.

24 Wahner-Roedler DL, Nelson DF, Croghan IT *et al.* Risk of breast cancer and breast cancer characteristics in women treated with supradiaphragmatic radiation for Hodgkin's lymphoma: The Mayo Clinic experience. *Mayo Clin Proc* 2003; **78**: 708–715.

25 Nachman JB, Sposto R, Herzog P *et al.* Randomized comparison of low-dose involved-field radiotherapy and no radiotherapy for children with Hodgkin's disease who achieve a complete response to chemotherapy. *J Clin Oncol* 2002; **20**: 3765–3771.

26 Rehwald U, Schulz H, Reiser M *et al.* Treatment of relapsed CD20+ Hodgkin lymphoma with the monoclonal antibody rituximab is effective and well tolerated: results of a phase 2 trial of the German Hodgkin Lymphoma Study Group. *Blood* 2003; **101**: 420–424.

CHAPTER 9

Adolescent CNS tumours: my brain has damaged my life

D. A. Walker

Introduction

The age incidence of CNS tumours has two peaks: one in childhood and early adolescence and a second peak is preceded by a gradual rise in incidence towards the end of a natural lifespan (Fig. 9.1).[1] The peak in early life suggests a different aetiology from tumours occurring later in life, which is presumably related to ageing. This early peak in tumour formation may be linked to the processes of brain growth and neurodevelopment, which occur rapidly in the first 3 years of life and then episodically throughout the rest of childhood and adolescence, when a wide variety of different processes occur at different times, linked to brain maturation, myelinization, neuronal arborization and synapse formation.

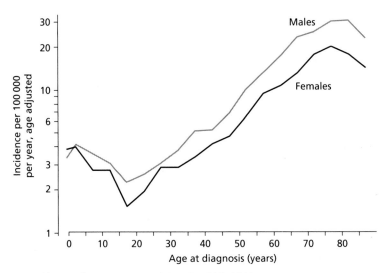

Fig. 9.1 Incidence of CNS tumors, US SEER, 1997–2001.

In childhood, the commonest group of CNS tumours are low-grade astrocytomas, followed by malignant medulloblastoma, ependymoma, other gliomas, the embryonic malformation of craniopharyngioma, pineal region tumours and a variety of other very rare tumours. In teenagers and young adults, astrocytomas predominate; low-grade tumours change from a pilocytic grade 1 morphology to a grade 2 morphology and high-grade tumours increase in incidence during this period. Intracranial germ cell tumours have a peak in adolescence and are consequently thought to be driven by endogenous pubertal hormones. The embryonic tumours, such as medulloblastoma and ependymoma, become rare.

Survival Eurocare

Over the past 10 years, survival rates in CNS tumours of childhood have risen from 55% to 72% in the UK overall. Data from teenagers and young adults is harder to come by, the most recent European data shows 5-year survival rates at 66% in the early 1990s based on the Eurocare study (Table 9.1).[2,3] Internationally, there are wide confidence intervals for survival rates in PNET, the most malignant tumour of childhood. Cure in this tumour relies upon excellent multimodal treatment, and the wide range of outcomes indicates a considerable range of availability of effective radiotherapy and chemotherapy in countries contributing to this study. Note the lack of data for ependymoma and PNET in the older age range, indicating their rarity at this stage in life.

Diagnostic imaging, anatomy and function

From the clinical perspective, symptomatology at the time of presentation is dictated by the anatomical location of the tumour as the brain is regionally organized from the functional standpoint. The anatomical location of the tumour therefore determines not only the symptoms but also the decisions regarding biopsy, resectability, histological interpretation, radiation treatments and their toxicity, risks of acquired disability and their potential for recovery. Modern imaging provides exceptionally clear definition of anatomical

Table 9.1 Eurocare study CNS tumour survival rates, 1990–1994 (19 countries)

| Tumour type (ICCC) | 0–14 years | | | 15–24 years | | |
	n	5-year survival (95% CI)	Inter-country range	n	5-year survival (95% CI)	Inter-country range
Ependymoma (IIIa)	453	55% (49–62%)	36–73%	NA	NA	NA
Astrocytoma (IIIb)	2241	79% (74–83%)	63–89%	738	66% (62–69%)	33–88%
PNET (IIIc)	1156	50% (46–55%)	11–100%	NA	NA	NA

CI, confidence intervals; ICCC, International Childhood Cancer Classification. NA, not applicable.

Table 9.2 Healthcare professionals involved in comprehensive care of children and young people with brain and spinal tumours

Primary and secondary health-care team
General practitioner
District nurse
Health visitor
School nurse
Educational psychologist
Paediatrician working in hospital and community
Paediatric nursing teams working in hospital and community
Audiometrist
Speech and language therapist
Dietician
Paediatric radiographers (diagnostic)

Tertiary health-care team
Paediatric oncologist
Paediatric neurosurgeon
Paediatric radiotherapist supported by radiotherapy team skilled in the care of children and young people and their families
Neuropathologist
Neuroradiologist
Paediatric neurosurgical and oncology nursing team
Specialist liaison nurses
Specialized chemotherapy pharmacy support
Specialist play therapist
Specialist rehabilitation team (paediatric physiotherapists and occupational therapists)
Specialist social worker
Educational liaison worker
Paediatric endocrinologist
Paediatric neurologist
Paediatric ophthalmologist
Neurophysiologist
Paediatric surgeon
Paediatric surgical specialists in ENT, orthopaedics, maxillofacial and plastic surgery
Child psychiatrist
Clinical psychologist

location, and is providing increasingly valuable information about tumour biology, metastatic disease, and can direct surgical interventions aimed at biopsy and the relief of intracranial pressure through cyst aspiration or endoscopic ventriculostomy.

Once the anatomical and staging pathological processes are complete, the pathway of care commences. This combines the efforts of a huge range of clinical specialists, who make up multiprofessional, multidisciplinary teams in hospital, in the community, in education and local communities, but most importantly of all within the family (Table 9.2). For teenagers and young adults facing a life-threatening diagnosis of brain tumour, this array of individuals committed to their well-being, working in different institutions and organizations, poses a unique challenge of communication if these individuals are not only going to help the young person recover physically but are also going to help them to return the point in their life trajectory where they can move forward with their personal development, their career and their education or training with a view to achieving independence in all senses of the word. This is not always achievable, and residual disability that may affect up to 60% has inevitable long-term consequences for the young person, the family, the health services and society. This is further compounded by the risk of recurrent or second tumours and further need for life-saving or palliating interventions at intervals after completion of the initial treatment programme.

Workshop

During the Third International Conference on Cancer and the Adolescent, sponsored by the Teenage Cancer Trust the audience was asked to take part in a workshop that aimed to identify, from the young person's perspective:
- the information they require for decision-making about treatment
- the qualities of a rehabilitation service
- service arrangements for support for ongoing education and vocational training
- support for families of the young person with a brain or spinal tumour.

The prioritized responses, derived from the audience's contributions, are shown in Tables 9.3–9.6.

Table 9.3 Information – prioritized information required by teenagers and young adults to support decision-making about treatment

1 Clear facts about disease, treatment, complications of treatment and likely outcomes
2 Access to written information prepared in age-appropriate format, in paper, computerized or video formats – the more interactive the better
3 Time for in-depth individualized counselling with professional support, keeping the young person informed, giving them time to reflect upon the impact of the information upon their lives as their treatment and rehabilitation progress
4 Access to and communication with professionals offering advocacy support, providing honest information and providing continuity of contact. These interactions should be non-judgemental
5 With time and access to others with similar problems for discussion, i.e. peers, friends and family from home and school
6 Access to specialist psychology support
7 Access to information about fertility risks
8 Access to social work support

Table 9.4 Rehabilitation – prioritized qualities of a rehabilitation service for a teenager or young adult

1. Ease of access to multiprofessional rehabilitation team including physiotherapy, occupational therapy, speech therapy, with clear objectives and specific arrangements for liaison between the hospital and community-based services. This may include access to a specialist rehabilitation unit with age-appropriate facilities
2. Flexibility and individualization of timetabling and appointments
3. Specific arrangements for liaison with school, college and work, if appropriate, to facilitate re-integration
4. Selection of rehabilitation staff who are sensitive to the needs of teenagers and young adults who are familiar with the pathways of rehabilitation and cancer treatments for this young age group
5. Therapy sessions including others from similar age groups
6. Opportunity to meet with other young people and families facing similar problems
7. An age-appropriate therapy environment which should be stimulating and contemporary, with the help of specialist equipment, such as computer and state-of-the-art gymnastic equipment
8. Information about the impact of any disabilities upon education, quality of life and activities of daily living
9. The opportunity for individualized rehabilitation sessions as well as family involvement in rehabilitation sessions
10. The opportunity for long-term planning of rehabilitation, in liaison with therapists in adult services
11. Access to careers advice, individualized and specialized
12. Access to a nutritional team for advice
13. Emphasis on maintaining hope for the future
14. Communication and liaison with primary care team
15. Rehabilitation team involvement in treatment planning throughout
16. Training of rehabilitation team for communication techniques in adolescence and young adulthood

Table 9.5 Education-prioritized service arrangements for support for ongoing education and vocational training

1. Special arrangements for liaison between the clinical environment and the educational environment through the special educational needs coordinators, mentors, tutors and educational welfare officers
2. Health service and educational funding for special educational needs in schools, colleges and universities
3. Access to Connexions services, educational counselling and careers counselling
4. Access to distance learning, resources, tutors and special arrangements for examinations linked to disability, particularly cognitive disability
5. Access to educational or neuropyschological assessment
6. Strong links between schools, colleges and universities and the rehabilitation team, particularly with an emphasis on occupational therapy
7. Links between community nursing, schools and GP aimed at promoting flexibility and individualization of arrangements
8. Access to transport for health and educational attendances. Arrangements for adaptation of existing vehicles and support of applications for personal specialist transport
9. Access to an activity coordinator or youth worker within the clinical team and in the local environment
10. Access to social work support
11. Access to individual and family counselling or therapy where appropriate

Table 9.6 Family – prioritized support required for families of the young person with a brain and spinal tumour

---

1 Opportunity for families to link in with networks of other families in similar situations and access to specific facilities for family support
2 Access to educational support
3 Access to psychotherapy and psychology support
4 Access to social work and Sibling Support
5 Access to dietetic and therapy advice
6 Access to disease information
7 Access to financial support, particularly for transport
8 Access to respite care and palliative care
9 Access to the outreach nurse specialist
10 Access to youth worker and activity coordinator
11 Specific arrangements to involve the extended family in support
12 Time for counselling with regard to emotional difficulties
13 The philosophy where needs are individualized rather than standardized
14 Emphasis upon maintaining peer support with friends at home but also identifying peers in the health system for sharing of experiences
15 Access to specialist equipment for maintaining family life and access to support spiritual needs

---

Conclusion

The wide range and complex nature of rehabilitation support that is needed for a young person and his or her family when facing up to disability and when the cancer is a brain tumour is bewildering. There are defined neuro-oncology teams for children in the UK and teams for adults have also been developed. However, to our knowledge, none have been arranged to meet the special needs of teenagers and young adults. The opportunity is there for this sort of team-working to develop, drawing experience from both the younger and the older age groups, creating an age-specific philosophy of care, and identifying resources that will meet the unique needs of teenagers and young adults with central nervous system tumours.

References

1 Ries LAG, Eisner MP, Kosary CL *et al.*, eds. *SEER Cancer Statistics Review, 1975–2001.* Bethesda (MD): National Cancer Institute. http://seer.cancer.gov/csr/1975_2001/, 2004.
2 Gatta G, Corazziari I, Magnani C *et al.*; EUROCARE Working Group. Childhood cancer survival in Europe. *Ann Oncol* 2003; **14** (Suppl. 5): v119–v127.
3. Gatta G, Capocaccia R, De Angelis R, Stiller C, Coebergh JW; EUROCARE Working Group. Cancer survival in European adolescents and young adults. *Eur J Cancer* 2003; **39**: 2600–2610.

CHAPTER 10

Ewing's sarcoma

A. Craft

Introduction

In 1918 a 14-year-old girl was referred to Dr James Ewing in New York because she had what appeared to be a pathological fracture of her left forearm. It was thought that this was probably an osteogenic sarcoma as this was the only bone tumour of young people known about at the time. Radiation therapy was just beginning to emerge as a possible way of treating cancer and Ewing took the opportunity to try this out. He applied a radium pack and repeated this twice at 2-week intervals. Not expecting much response, he was surprised when the application of the radium pack resulted in almost complete resolution of the swelling. The girl remained well for 17 months but then developed a local recurrence and distant metastases from which she died.

Ewing recognized this as an unusual clinical situation and in addition the microscopic appearance of the tumour, obtained at local relapse, was completely different from that of osteosarcoma. He therefore called it a diffuse endothelioma of bone or endothelial myeloma. Ewing was an eminent pathologist and clinician and by the time of the fourth edition of his book *Neoplastic Diseases*, written in 1940, the tumour that he described was well established, although modestly he did not call it Ewing's tumour.[1] As regards treatment, he wrote:

Treatment – When the diagnosis of endothelial myeloma is suspected the writer believes that the first indication is for treatment by radiation in full doses, and over considerable periods. This recommendation is based on the reported cure of certain cases in the Registry by radiation alone, and on the clinical disappearance of the disease for variable periods in many more cases. The response to radiation also confirms the diagnosis. The danger of metastases occurring while this treatment is in progress is probably negligible, since the tumour tissue generally undergoes rapid liquefaction and necrosis.

The difficulties of wisely managing the case after the primary regression under radiation remain, however, quite formidable. Recurrence is the rule, and unless one continues the treatment long after all signs of the disease have disappeared, a sudden recurrence may completely alter the outlook. The safest method would seem to call for amputation or local excision to prevent recurrence. Until a larger series of 5-year cures from radiation are secured with inaccessible tumours, operative measures cannot safely be dispensed with. In young children, secondary tumours occur so uniformly after amputation, and so early, that there seems little to be gained by amputation. The older the subject, the better is the prognosis from amputation. There are four reports of cures by radiation and excision.

For many years radiotherapy and surgery were the only forms of treatment available and the survival rate was at best 5%. Death was usually due to lung and bone or bone marrow metastases, suggesting that in the vast majority of cases this is a disseminated disease at diagnosis. It was not until the advent of chemotherapy that the outlook began to improve. Progress was made first in the USA, where in the early 1970s Mark Nesbit formed the Intergroup Ewing's Sarcoma Study (IESS) Group. They undertook an important three-armed randomized study which concluded that doxorubicin was an essential drug in this disease, but that similar survival could be seen if lung irradiation was substituted. This study established that vincristine, cyclophosphamide, doxorubicin and actinomycin D were the most effective drugs.[2] Interestingly, since then, ifosfamide and etoposide are the only two additional drugs which have found their way into common practice.

The importance of local control was also identified by the IESS group, as it had been by Ewing. Their other main contribution was the recognition that the site of tumour was an important prognostic factor, limb tumours faring better than axial sites.

Most treatment protocols being used around the world now use a combination of these six drugs. Survival rates have improved as can be seen from

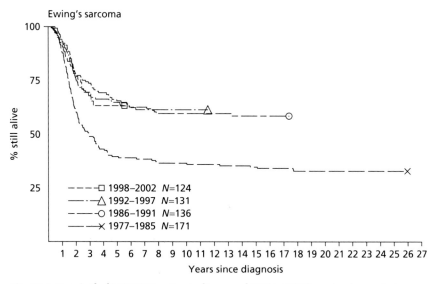

Fig. 10.1 Survival of UKCCSG patients diagnosed 1977–2002 by calendar period.

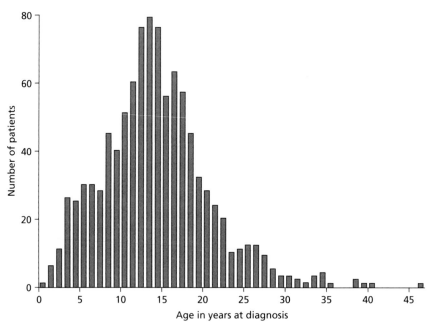

Fig. 10.2 Age incidence of 975 Ewing's sarcoma patients in UK and German studies.

Fig. 10.1, which shows the progress over four successive quinquennia. These figures are taken from the United Kingdom Children's Cancer Study Group (UKCCSG) Registry and include only those under 15 years of age. Ewing's sarcoma, however, is not just a childhood disease, as can be seen from Fig. 10.2, which shows the age distribution of 946 cases treated by the UK and German/Austrian (CESS) group.[3]

As can be seen from Fig. 10.1, there has been little improvement in outcome over the past few years. However, there has been much research not only into treatment but also into epidemiology and, more importantly, into a basic understanding of the biology of this fascinating disease. This chapter reviews this recent research activity.

Epidemiology

Ewing's sarcoma is uncommon, affecting annually 0.6 per million population. It can occur in babies and in adults up to the age of 40 years or more. The peak is clearly in the adolescent years. In his 1940 textbook, Ewing recognized that there might be physical differences with those who develop osteogenic sarcoma. He said 'Contrary to the rule with osteosarcoma, the subjects of endothelial myeloma are usually of delicate build and have suffered from nutritional disorders of childhood'. There has long been controversy about the stature of those who develop bone tumours. Cotterill and colleagues[4] have recently reviewed the stature of 720 young people with malignant bone tumours entered into clinical trials in the UK. Those with osteosarcoma were significantly taller than the general population, and this was especially marked for those with a femur primary. Those patients with Ewing's sarcoma who presented before the age of 16 years were also significantly tall, but those presenting later were not. For both types of tumour the mean age at diagnosis was significantly earlier for females than males, reflecting their earlier growth spurt.

Osteosarcoma occurs in all racial groups but Ewing's sarcoma is extremely rare in black populations. The reason for this racial difference is unknown.

Ewing thought that trauma was a factor in the aetiology of the tumour. Like osteosarcoma, it is likely that trauma reveals the presence of the tumour rather than being a causative element. A number of case–control studies have been performed, none of which have identified any major factor that could be conclusively implicated as a causal factor. Exposure to an agricultural way of life and possibly, therefore, to chemical exposure has been suggested in two studies.[5,6] A strong association with inguinal hernia, and its repair, was found in the Australian study. There is no obvious explanation for this.

Molecular diagnosis

For many years diagnosis has relied on the histological appearance of the tumour, using immunohistochemistry and, where available, electron micro-scopy. The discovery of a characteristic chromosomal translocation, t(11:22), has led many to suggest that without this the diagnosis cannot be made. The early years of cytogenetic investigation have not been easy as the number of 'unsatisfactory' samples and preparations was substantial. However, now that new techniques such as FISH and RT-PCR are available it is possible to be more dogmatic about the need to identify the translocation before a diagnosis can be confidently made. Helman and his colleagues at the National Institutes of Health[7] have suggested that 'in apparently translocation negative samples, close attention should be given to the possibility of an alternative diagnosis'.

Whilst the initial diagnosis is important, an equally valuable use of the new molecular diagnostic techniques is likely to be the identification of individual tumour cells in blood and bone marrow. This would allow better staging at diagnosis and also provide evidence of the speed of response to therapy and the presence of minimal residual disease. A study by the Société Française d'Oncologie Pediatrique (SFOP) has recently reported results in 172 patients at diagnosis using an RT-PCR targeting the two common gene transcripts, EWS-FL1-1 and EWS-ERG. RT-PCR positivity of the bone marrow was signific-antly correlated with adverse outcome ($P = 0.007$). Although molecularly diagnosed metastases were more common in large tumours known to have a poor prognosis, they were also significantly associated with poor outcome in tumours with an otherwise good prognosis.[8] The current Euro-Ewing's EE99 study is investigating the importance of molecularly detectable disease at diagnosis and follow-up in a large randomized study (see below).

Pathobiology

Although the major chromosomal aberrations and the common gene transcripts are now well known, it is not clear how they are actually involved in the genesis of the sarcoma. An understanding of how the various factors interact within the cell could lead to possible therapeutic targets. The stunning success of imatinib mesylate (Gleevec®) (ST1-571) in chronic myeloid leukaemia has led to a search for other tumours in which tyrosine kinase inhibition might be of potential therapeutic value. Expression of c-*kit* appears to be a prerequisite for the possible activity of imatinib, and when approximately 30% of Ewing's sarcomas were shown to express c-*kit* there was optimism. However, there was no correlation between the expression of c-*kit* and outcome. Very high levels of imatinib were needed to cause some inhibition of growth of Ewing's sarcoma cell lines *in vitro*. It is unlikely that imatinib will be effective on its own in the clinical situation.[9]

The p53 tumour suppressor gene has been studied as a possible prognostic marker. Overexpression has been reported to be associated with a worse outcome, as has the cell proliferation nuclear antigen Ki-67. The proto-oncogene HER2/neu was not expressed.[10] An intriguing association between telomerase activity and outcome in Ewing's sarcoma has also been reported.[11]

Kovar and his colleagues in Vienna have been searching for the function of the RNA-binding protein which is encoded by *EWS*. They have shown that it is dispensable for growth of Ewing's sarcoma.[12] More recently they have shown that an interaction between the *EWS* NH$_2$ terminus and *BARD1* links the Ewing's sarcoma gene to a common tumour suppression pathway.[13]

Treatment

Protocols of treatment for Ewing's sarcoma over the past few years have evolved from those that originated in the IESS studies in the 1970s. In the UK the UKCSSG/MRC studied a regimen similar to that studied by IESS with the four known active drugs. The ETI protocol[14] demonstrated a 5-year overall survival of 39% whilst at the same time in Germany, Austria and the Netherlands the co-operative Ewing's Sarcoma Study group (CESS) was formed and undertook a very similar study. In the CESS 81 study they demonstrated a clear association between tumour volume and outcome.[15] The UK moved on to ET-2, which substituted ifosfamide for cyclophosphamide but treated all patients with the same protocol. The overall 5-year survival improved to 62%. In the CESS 86 study ifosfamide was used only for those with large tumours with poorer prognosis. Ifosfamide was concluded to be superior to cyclophosphamide and has been subsumed into all subsequent studies.[16,17] Neither group was large enough to undertake randomized studies so in 1989 the European Intergroup Co-operative Ewing's Sarcoma Study (EI-CESS) group was formed. The EICESS 92 study stratified patients into those with good and bad prognosis on the basis of tumour volume. Those in the high-risk group were randomized to receive or not receive etoposide in addition to the four known active drugs. The definitive analysis will be undertaken in 2004 but preliminary results suggest that the addition of etoposide may confer a marginal but so far non-significant advantage. It is certainly no worse even allowing for possible increased morbidity of the additional drug.[18]

In the USA a similar approach was adopted in which addition of ifosfamide and etoposide to standard chemotherapy was randomized.[19] In patients with metastatic disease there was no benefit from the two extra drugs, but for those with non-metastatic disease survival was 11% better (72 versus 61%), similar to that seen when comparing ET-1 with ET-2. Very similar results have been obtained by groups in Scandinavia[20] and Italy,[21] although the French found no benefit from the addition of ifosfamide alone.[22]

Prognostic factors

Several large groups have reviewed their databases to determine prognostic factors. Although any prognostic factor is clearly dependent on the treatment given, most treatments are similar so it is likely that prognostic factors across different groups will be valid.[23,24] The two most prognostic factors in multivariate analyses are metastatic disease at diagnosis and the response to initial chemotherapy. Many other factors, important on their own, such as tumour site and size and raised levels of lactose dehydrogenase (LDH), are of lesser importance when multiple factors are taken into account. Prognostic factors allow us to target potential improvements in treatment to those who might benefit most.

Possible improvements in therapy

Dose intensification

Survival rates have improved over the last 30 years yet we are still using the same basic drugs. Ifosfamide has largely been substituted for cyclophosphamide and this has probably been responsible for 10% of the improvement. The rest is likely to be due to the use of more intensive chemotherapy with increased doses. This has been made possible by better supportive care and the use of growth factors such as granulocyte colony stimulating factor (GCSF). Marina and colleagues[24] reported that considerable dose intensification was feasible but had serious side-effects and did not improve disease-free survival. A similar study by Womer and colleagues[25] using GCSF to allow interval compression of therapy was a pilot for a randomized study which is now under way in the USA.

Megatherapy

The use of high-dose chemotherapy with or without total body irradiation as consolidation treatment has been considered and indeed used over the last 25 years.

Chemotherapy has consisted of various combinations of busulfan, melphalan and thiotepa with either bone marrow or peripheral blood stem cell rescue. These various strategies were reviewed by Pinkerton and colleagues.[26] They concluded that using increased doses of alkylating agents could improve survival to 30–40% in some series for those with bad prognostic disease, with better outcomes seen in those with lung metastases. Meyers and colleagues[27] were disappointed with survival in their series of high-risk Ewing's sarcoma patients. They reported that, in all three patients in whom analysis of peripheral blood stem cell collections for Ewing's cells by RT-PCR was possible, tumour cells were found.

Other topical issues

Survival after relapse

Several studies have shown that the outcome is poor for patients who relapse with metastatic disease after modern intensive therapy. Relapse within 2 years of completion of therapy is usually fatal. However, there are some long-term survivors of those who relapse after 2 years.[28] Weston and colleagues have recently used a new statistical technique to identify 'cure'. They conclude that survival for 5 years is likely to be synonymous with cure.[29]

Response to chemotherapy

For many tumours, especially sarcomas, the histological response to initial chemotherapy is one of the most important prognostic factors, but is of no value in stratifying initial chemotherapy as it can only be determined once the tumour has been surgically removed. Abudo and colleagues[30] reviewed tumour volume as measured by CT and/or MRI and found a reduction in size to be strongly correlated with tumour necrosis. Dyke and his colleagues[31] found that dynamic contrast-enhanced MRI correlated with the histological appearance of necrosis. However, these findings are too preliminary to be of reliable value in determining initial treatment.

New agents

Topotecan and irinotecan have been investigated in Phase I/II settings and have both been shown to have potential activity against Ewing's sarcoma.[32,33]

Second malignancies

It has long been known that one of the late side-effects of the use of local irradiation is the subsequent development of secondary tumours, usually sarcomas, in the irradiated site.[34] More recently the use of epipodophyllotoxin inhibitors, such as etoposide, has caused concern because of their potential to initiate myelodysplasia and acute myelogenous leukaemia. The risk appears to be less than when these drugs are used in other situations.[35]

Long-term functional outcome

In both the USA and in the UK there are long-term cancer survivor studies.[36] In addition, the European Bone Tumour Outcome Study (EBTOS) is evaluating survivors of bone tumours. Overall health and social outcome seems to be good and, at least in one study, no significant differences were reported between amputees and those treated in other ways.[36]

The current Euro-Ewing Study: EE 99

The EICESS group was expanded in 1999 to include the French (SFOP), the Swiss (SIAK) and the pan-European, largely adult, European Organization for the Research and Treatment of Cancer (EORTC). This new Euro-Ewing intergroup has the potential for rapid accrual of patients and the ability to answer important randomized questions. At the inception it was decided that the most important question to be asked was whether or not high-dose consolidation therapy after maximally tolerable chemotherapy would improve survival in those of moderate to high risk of relapse. The study design is shown in Fig. 10.3. Patients are allocated to the three regimes R1, R2 and R3 after six courses of intensive chemotherapy using VIDE (vincristine, ifosfamide, doxorubicin and etoposide; Table 10.1). This induction therapy was piloted in London and a report of the first 30 patients has been published.[37]

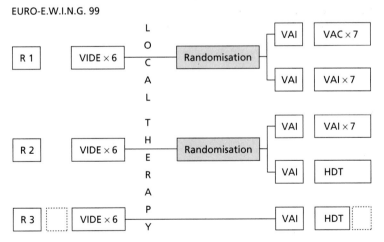

Fig. 10.3 Schema for EE 99 study.

Table 10.1 Chemotherapy for EE 99 using VIDE (vincristine, ifosfamide, doxorubicin and etoposide)

Vincristine	1.5 mg/m^2	Day 1
Ifosfamide	3000 mg/m^2	Days 1, 2, 3
Doxorubicin	20 mg/m^2	
Etoposide	150 mg/m^2	

Conclusion

Ewing's sarcoma is one of the more common tumours in adolescents and young people. Improvements in survival have occurred over the last 30 years, but the rate of progress is now slow. This tumour does have a characteristic chromosomal translocation and a search is on to find the gene product. The hope is that the next few years will lead us to better and more targeted therapy, for which major multinational trials will be necessary. We are moving towards this with the current Euro-Ewing's collaboration, in which the US Children's Oncology Group has recently become a partner.

James Ewing would have been amazed at the progress that has been made. Perhaps our goal should be 95% cure with minimal morbidity by the centenary of the diagnosis of Ewing's first patients. If so, we have 13 years in which to achieve it.

References

1 Ewing J. *Neoplastic Diseases. A Treatise on Tumours*, 4th edn. Philadelphia: Saunders, 1940: 370.
2 Nesbit MEJ, Gehan EH, Burgert EOJ *et al.* Multimodel therapy for management of primary, non metastatic Ewing's sarcoma of bone: a long term follow up of the first Intergroup Study. *J Clin Oncol* 1990; **8**: 1664–1674.
3 Cotterill SJ, Ahrens S, Paulussen M *et al.* Prognostic factors in Ewing's tumour of bone: an analysis of 975 patients from the European Intergroup Co-operative Ewing's Sarcoma Study Group. *J Clin Oncol* 2000; **18**: 3108–3114.
4 Cotterill SJ, Wright CM, Pearce MS, Craft AW. Stature of young people with malignant tumours. *Pediatr Blood Cancer* 2004; **42**: 59–63.
5 Valery PC, McWhirter W, Selight A *et al.* A national case control study of Ewing's sarcoma family of tumours in Australia. *Int J Cancer* 2003: **105**: 825–830.
6 Valery PC, McWhirter W, Sleigh A *et al.* Farm exposures, parental occupation and risk of Ewing's sarcoma in Australia. *Cancer Causes Control* 2002; **13**: 263–270.
7 Dagher R, Pham TA, Sorbara L *et al.* Molecular confirmation of Ewing sarcoma. *J Ped Hematol Oncol* 2001; **23**: 221–224.
8 Schleiermacher C, Peter M, Oberlin *et al.* for Société Française d'Oncologie Pediatrique. Increased risk of systemic relapses associated with bone marrow micrometastasis and circulating tumor cells in localized Ewing tumour. *J Clin Oncol* 2003; **21**: 85–91.
9 Scotlandi K, Manara MC, Stramiello R *et al.* c-kit Receptor expression in Ewing's sarcoma: lack of prognostic value but therapeutic targeting opportunities in appropriate conditions. *J Clin Oncol* 2003; **21**: 1952–1960.
10 Amir G, Issakov J, Meller I *et al.* Expression of p53 gene product and cell proliferation marker Ki-67 in Ewing's sarcoma: correlation with clinical outcome. *Human Pathol* 2002; **33**: 170–174.
11 Ohali A, Avigad S, Cohen IJ *et al.* Association between telomerase activity and outcome in patients with nonmetastatic Ewing family of tumours. *J Clin Oncol* 2003; **21**: 3836–3843.
12 Kovar H, Jug G, Hattinger C *et al.* The EWS protein is dispensable for Ewing tumour growth. *Cancer Res* 2001; **61**: 5992–5997.

13 Spahn L, Petermann R, Silligan C *et al.* Interaction of the EWS NH2 terminus with BARD 1 links the Ewing's sarcoma gene to a common tumour suppressor pathway. *Cancer Res* 2002: **62**: 4583–4587.

14 Craft AW, Cotterill SJ, Bullimore JA *et al.* Long term results from the first UKCCSG Ewing's Tumour Study (ET-1). *Eur J Cancer* 1997; **33**: 1061–1069.

15 Jurgens H, Exner J, Gadner H *et al.* Multidisciplinary treatment of primary Ewing's sarcoma of bone. A 6 year experience of a European co-operative trial. *Cancer* 1988; **61**: 23–32.

16 Craft AW, Cotterill SJ, Malcolm AJ *et al.* Ifosfamide containing chemotherapy in Ewing's sarcoma. The second UKCCSG/MRC Ewing's tumour study (ET-2). *J Clin Oncol* 1998; **16**: 3628–3633.

17 Paulussen M, Ahrens S, Dunst J *et al.* Localized Ewing tumour of bone: final results of the Co-operative Ewing's Sarcoma Study CESS 86. *J Clin Oncol* 2001; **19**: 1818–1829.

18 Paulussen M, Craft AW, Lewis I *et al.* Ewing tumour of bone – updated report of the European Intergroup Co-operative Ewing's Sarcoma Study EICESS 92. *ASCO Proc* 2002: A1568.

19 Grier HE, Krailo MD, Garbell NJ *et al.* Addition of ifosfamide and etoposide to standard chemotherapy for Ewing's sarcoma and primitive neuroectodermal tumour of bone. *N Engl J Med* 2003; **348**: 694–701.

20 Elomaa I, Blomqvist CP, Saeter G *et al.* Five year results in Ewing's sarcoma. The Scandinavian Sarcoma Group experience with the SSG IX protocol. *Eur J Cancer* 2000; **36**: 875–880.

21 Bacci G, Ferrari S, Bertoni F *et al.* Neoadjuvant chemotherapy for peripheral malignant neuroectodermal tumour of bone: Recent experience at the Instituto Rizzoli. *J Clin Oncol* 2000; **18**: 885–892.

22 Oberlin O, Habrand JL, Zucker JM *et al.* No benefit of ifosfamide in Ewing's sarcoma: a randomised study of the French Society of Pediatric Oncology. *J Clin Oncol* 1992; **10**: 1407–1412.

23 Ahrens S, Hoffmann C, Jabar S *et al.* Evaluation of prognostic factors in a tumour volume-adapted treatment strategy for localized Ewing sarcoma of bone: the CESS 86 experience. *Med Paediatr Oncol* 1999; **32**: 186–195.

24 Marina NM, Pappo AS, Parham DM *et al.* Chemotherapy dose-intensification for pediatric patients with Ewing's family of tumours and desmoplastic small round-cell tumours: a feasibility study at St. Jude Children's Research Hospital. *J Clin Oncol* 1999; **17**: 180–190.

25 Womer RB, Daller RT, Fenton JG, Miser JS. Granulocyte colony stimulating factor permits dose intensification by interval compression in the treatment of Ewing's sarcomas and soft tissue sarcomas in children. *Eur J Cancer* 2000; **36**: 87–94.

26 Pinkerton CR, Bataillard A, Guillo S *et al.* Treatment strategies for metastatic Ewing's sarcoma. *Eur J Cancer* 2001; **37**: 1338–1344.

27 Meyers PA, Krailo MD, Ladany M *et al.* High-dose melphalan, etoposide, total-body irradiation and autologous stem-cell reconstitution as consolidation therapy for high risk Ewing's sarcoma does not improve prognosis. *J Clin Oncol* 2001; **19**: 2812–2820.

28 Rodrigues-Galindo C, Billups C, Kun LE *et al.* Survival after recurrence of Ewing tumours. The St. Jude Children's Hospital Experience 1979–1999. *Cancer* 2002; **94**: 561–569.

29 Weston CL, Douglas C, Craft AW *et al.* Establishing long term survival and cure in young patients with Ewing's sarcoma. *Br J Cancer* 2004; **91**: 225–232.

30 Abudu A, Davies AM, Pynsent PB *et al.* Tumour volume as a predictor of necrosis after chemotherapy in Ewing's sarcoma. *J Bone Joint Surg* 1999; **81**: 317–322.

31 Dyke JP, Panicek DM, Healey JH *et al.* Osteogenic and Ewing sarcomas: estimation of necrotic fraction during induction chemotherapy with dynamic contrast-enhanced MR imaging. *Radiology* 2003; **228**: 271–278.

32 Cosetti M, Wexler LH, Calleja E *et al.* Irinotecan for paediatric solid tumours: the Memorial Sloan-Kettering experience. *J Pediatr Hematol/Oncol* 2002; **24**: 1001–1005.

33 Saylors RL, Stine KC, Sullivan J *et al.* for the Pediatric Oncology Group. Cyclophosphamide plus topotecan in children with recurrent or refractory solid tumours: a Pediatric Oncology Group Phase II Study. *J Clin Oncol* 2001; **19**: 3463–3469.

34 Paulussen M, Ahrens S, Lehnert M *et al.* Second malignancies after Ewing tumour treatment in 690 patients from a cooperative German/Austrian/Dutch study. *Ann Oncol* 2001; **12**: 1619–1630.

35 Numata A, Shioda K, Gondo H *et al.* Therapy related chronic myelogenous leukaemia following autologous stem cell transplantation for Ewing's sarcoma. *Br J Haematol* 2002; **117**: 613–616.

36 Nagarajan R, Neglia JP, Clohisy DR *et al.* Education, employment insurance and marital status among 694 survivors of pediatric lower extremity bone tumours. A report from the childhood cancer survivor study. *Cancer* 2003; **97**: 2554–2564.

37 Strauss SJ, McTiernan A, Driver D *et al.* Single center experience of a new intensive induction therapy for Ewing's family of tumours: feasibility, toxicity and stem cell mobilization properties. *J Clin Oncol* 2003; **21**: 2974–2981.

CHAPTER 11

Advances in osteosarcoma

J. Whelan

Introduction

Among the several cancers that affect teenagers, osteosarcoma comes nearest to being a characteristic cancer of adolescence. Extremely uncommon before 5 years of age and infrequent up to the age of 10 years, the extraordinary peak of incidence occurring in the early teenage years is quickly followed by as rapid a decline, so that osteosarcoma in those aged over 25 once again becomes a very uncommon cancer. While a second peak is described in the elderly, this accounts for a relatively small number of cases and the aetiological factors are generally different.[1]

Although osteosarcoma and the other common bone sarcoma in this age group, Ewing's tumour, constitute the fourth commonest group of malignancies affecting teenagers and young adults, they are the second commonest cause of death after brain tumours. Improvements in survival for this disease were rapid in the 1970s and 1980s but have changed little over the past 20 years. Understanding of the biology of osteosarcoma has certainly improved in recent years but there is as yet little promise of therapeutic benefit from the insights provided by the molecular biology revolution, as is increasingly being seen in other cancers.

The diagnosis of cancer in a teenager is always traumatic and acutely disrupting to normal development. Treatment, too, is an ordeal. Achieving cure from osteosarcoma is only possible after chemotherapy and surgery. But the chemotherapy for osteosarcoma is among the most toxic given for any solid tumour. After a couple of months of systemic treatment, major surgery is undertaken, often with an accompanying fear of limb loss and always to be followed by gruelling rehabilitation at the same time as continuing chemotherapy. This treatment carries lifelong functional costs for most patients and ongoing orthopaedic problems are common. Sadly, survival is unsatisfactory – perhaps no more than two-thirds of patients have a realistic chance of cure.

The new guard of cancer treatments provide exciting prospects for an ever-closer future, headed by rationally designed drugs and novel approaches, such as gene therapy, perhaps soon to be backed up by the individualization of treatment promised by pharmacogenomics. Simpler measures would be welcomed first by many of those diagnosed with osteosarcoma. Many patients would immediately benefit from changes in attitude that lead both to earlier recognition of the disease and a readiness to refer to specialist oncologists. Teenagers and young adults often find their symptoms of a bone tumour dismissed in primary care, and even when an X-ray is carried out subsequent referral can be slow. This contrasts with the referral pathway that a teenager with acute leukaemia may experience after the first abnormal blood test.

How 'good' is treatment for osteosarcoma?

Most osteosarcomas arise in the extremity, around the knee or shoulder girdle. After staging with an isotope bone scan and computed tomography of the chest, most are found to be localized. In these circumstances cure is sometimes achieved with complete surgical resection and combination chemotherapy based around cisplatin, doxorubicin, methotrexate and sometimes ifosfamide. Most clinical research has focused on localized disease and the outcome of first-line therapy. Tumours that arise in other sites, particularly the pelvis and spine, or when metastatic, are less well studied although universally acknowledged to be associated with inferior outcome. In order to advise patients, how do we determine the effectiveness of current treatments for osteosarcoma, or indeed which is the best treatment?

Population and registry studies

Data derived from population and cancer registries have several advantages, in particular the potential to include all patients with osteosarcoma rather than subpopulations selected for a clinical trial or referred to a specialist centre. These sources can also allow comparison between countries and detect shifts in survival trends over time. In contrast, case inclusion and verification by registries is variable and explanations for differences and changes may be obscure or speculative. Finally, registry data may not reflect more recent treatment innovations.

There are only a few published registry reports of osteosarcoma to aid comparisons, both over time and between countries where different treatment philosophies or health-care systems may prevail.

The recently published EUROCARE study of mortality from cancer in 15- to 24-year-olds analysed data from over 15,000 cases diagnosed between 1990 and 1994. Five-year survival from osteosarcoma was 58%. This was significantly lower than survival from all cancers in this age group, which was 76%. Survival was poorer in 15- to 19-year-olds than in 20- to 24-year-olds and both groups fared worse than the 10- to 14-year group. There were also considerable variations in survival between countries. However, there were only 370 cases of osteosarcoma recorded, which indicates marked underrepresentation of the total number of cases that one would expect from the participating countries.[2] Registry data on mortality from all bone cancers have recently provided evidence of improvement in survival since 1965 but the improvement is less evident in Eastern Europe compared with Western Europe,

Japan and the USA. In the latter three areas, the trend in improvement appears to be less evident since 1990.[3]

What do clinical trials tell us?

The importance of clinical trials of cancer treatment is repeatedly and rightly emphasized. The quality of information about effectiveness of treatment for osteosarcoma that can be derived from clinical trials will reflect the quality of the trial itself and in particular the selection of patients for inclusion in that trial. Thus caution is essential when making comparisons between the results of different clinical trials. When seeking information about the efficacy of different treatments, data from large, well-conducted, randomized trials is the most reliable. As osteosarcoma is a rare disease requiring complex management that is often undertaken in relatively few specialist centres, such studies have not been commonly undertaken.

The European Osteosarcoma Intergroup (EOI) has undertaken three consecutive randomized trials in localized extremity osteosarcoma. These have addressed the value of different chemotherapy regimens, each using a combination of doxorubicin and cisplatin as the standard arm. The first trial suggested that this regimen was of equal efficacy to a similar schedule of these two drugs plus methotrexate.[4] The second study compared the two-drug schedule with a more complex prolonged multidrug regimen similar to the T10 regimen devised in the USA, which had been reported to be associated with outstanding outcomes.[5] In the EOI study there was no difference in survival between the two schedules.[6] Furthermore, the results of the T10-like regimen were notably inferior to that originally reported and, indeed, to results from other groups using T10 as a standard treatment in single-arm studies.

Early reporting is one cause of overoptimistic trial outcomes. The pooled data from the 570 subjects randomized in these trials now allows analysis to be made at a time when 94% have been followed beyond 5 years or to death, and demonstrate an overall survival of 56% with progression-free survival of 44%, both at 5 years.[7] These data are an accurate reflection of outcomes for extremity osteosarcoma treated with neo-adjuvant chemotherapy in multiple institutions participating in well-conducted randomized studies. However, these trials were conducted between 1983 and 1992 so may not reflect more recent improvements in treatment and supportive care.

The third trial, for which accrual of 504 subjects was completed in 2003, asked whether increasing the dose intensity of this two-drug schedule was beneficial. The interval between courses was reduced from 3 to 2 weeks by the use of granulocyte colony stimulating factor. Preliminary results have now been analysed and presented.[8] At a median follow-up of 4.2 years, estimated progression-free survival for the 504 patients was 43% and overall survival 55%, similar to figures from the previous studies. Despite an increase in dose intensity of 25%, no survival advantage was demonstrated for the dose-intensive schedule.

There are several limitations to these data which restrict their applicability in osteosarcoma. We know little about the reasons for non-inclusion of potentially eligible subjects, who are, for example, estimated to be as many as 50% of UK patients. We learn nothing about those tumours that arise elsewhere in the skeleton or have metastases at diagnosis. Above all, survival from osteosarcoma described by these studies is poor, particularly when compared with outcomes from other cancers of children and young people, and the accrual time for clinical trials (10 years for the third EOI study) is simply too long when answers to questions about improving treatments are needed as soon as possible.

The EOI studies have been described here as an example, but have other trials groups achieved better results? The largest randomized study completed in localized extremity osteosarcoma was conducted in the USA by the Pediatric Oncology Group and Children's Cancer Group.[9] Intergroup 0133 recruited 693 subjects between 1993 and 1997 in order to answer (i) whether the addition of ifosfamide to cisplatin, doxorubicin and methotrexate improved event-free survival, and (ii) whether the addition of muramyl tripeptide to chemotherapy improved event-free survival. Disappointingly, the trial failed to give clear answers to either question, possibly because of an unexpected interaction between two arms of this 2×2 factorial study. However, the overall results are informative. The event-free survival for the whole group is 69% at 3 years, which would appear to be far superior to that recorded in the EOI study taking place over the same period.

There are few major differences in approach between other groups striving to improve the treatment of osteosarcoma, as the number of active chemotherapy agents is limited and new agents have not been identified. Thus, whether from single institutions, other randomized studies or study groups, results similar to the above are reported.[10–12] It is unsafe to construct firm conclusions about the value of individual treatments by direct comparisons between trials, but in general we see that little improvement has occurred in the treatment of osteosarcoma in the past 20 years; that whether chemotherapy regimens are based on two, three or four drugs, overall survival for reported patients lies somewhere between 55 and 70%; and that no one treatment schedule is obviously preferable with regard to either survival or toxicity. Randomized trials remain the best source of information regarding treatment efficacy but are limited by the prolonged accrual time and the lack of new approaches that can be tested.

One way forward for clinical research in osteosarcoma

In acknowledgement of the problems outlined above, which are common to all osteosarcoma clinical investigators, an international dialogue began between several study groups in 2001 with the aim of seeking common ground to form the basis for cooperative research. As a result, the EURAMOS Group (European and American Osteosarcoma Study Group) has been formed, comprising representatives from four major groups, the EOI (representing affiliated centres in the UK, the Netherlands and Belgium), the Co-operative Osteosarcoma Study Group (centres in Germany, Austria, Switzerland and Hungary), the Scandinavian Sarcoma Group (centres in Sweden, Norway, Finland, Denmark and Iceland) and the Children's Oncology Group (centres in the USA, Canada and Australia).

The aim of the EURAMOS collaboration is to improve survival from osteosarcoma by (i) carrying out large international randomized trials, (ii) facilitating biological research, (iii) seeking new therapeutic approaches, and (iv) developing common understanding and methodologies for staging, pathology and other aspects of osteosarcoma. It is anticipated that by working together these groups will be able to recruit 1400 patients to a randomized study in less than 4 years.

The first randomized study, EURAMOS 1, is in the advanced stages of planning and is anticipated to open later in 2004 (Fig. 11.1). The study addresses two questions in the treatment of resectable osteosarcoma: (i) whether changing chemotherapy on the basis of histological response improves event-free survival, and (ii) whether the addition of pegylated α-interferon as maintenance treatment after completion of chemotherapy improves event-free survival for those who have had a good histological response to preoperative chemotherapy. The standard chemotherapy arm chosen for this trial is based on the standard arm of the US randomized study discussed above, Intergroup 0133, and comprises cisplatin, doxorubicin and methotrexate. Randomization will take place after surgery according to whether more than 90% necrosis is recorded in the resection specimen. Those subjects whose response exceeds 90% will complete standard three-drug chemotherapy and will either be treated with interferon for a total treatment time of 2 years or be observed. Those with an inferior response will be randomized to receive more intensive chemotherapy by the addition of ifosfamide and etoposide to the three-drug backbone. The study will also evaluate overall survival, short- and long-term toxicity and quality of life, and will have parallel biological correlative studies.

A further objective is to test the feasibility of this international collaboration for the development of clinical research in osteosarcoma. Very important obstacles and delays can be identified in the realization of this trial that have wider implications for research in other rare cancers. Certainly, the initial challenge was finding clinical consensus from which trial questions could be formed; bearing in mind the different and indeed strong pedigrees of the four groups, this might have been predicted to be unachievable. In fact, the common goal and objectives outlined above have been a powerful cohesive force to aid in tackling a shared problem.

A significant limitation of the design of a first trial was the relatively small number of questions that could feasibly be addressed by a large study. A far greater problem has been the regulatory bureaucracy that applies to clinical trials. Different regulatory systems operate in the USA and Europe and the processes for joining these up are unwieldy. The development of EURAMOS 1

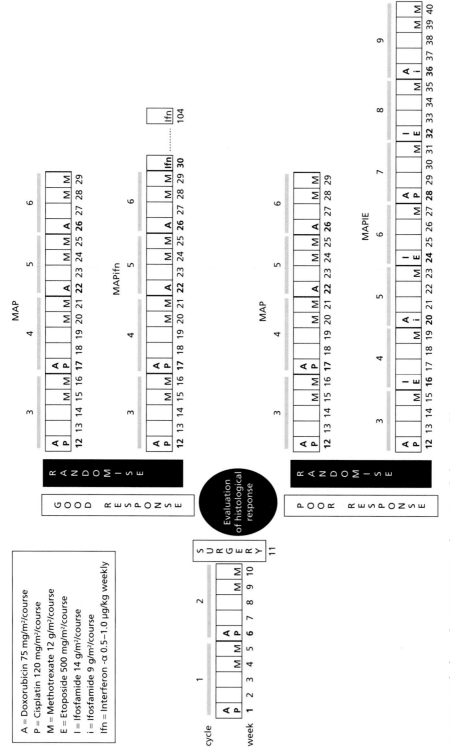

Fig. 11.1 Trial schema for EURAMOS I phase III study for resectable osteosarcoma.

has coincided with the introduction of complex new legislation in the European Union which challenges every aspect of trial development and operation. Facilitation through these new minefields has been insufficient, and has produced frustration amongst clinical investigators and delay in opening of the study, ultimately to the cost of patients with osteosarcoma. In addition, funding sources for a study such as this are extremely limited, again contributing to the time lost.

Conclusion

Improvements in every aspect of understanding and treatment of osteosarcoma are needed. These should begin with early referral to specialist care that can be undertaken in an appropriately experienced and resourced centre. Much greater support is needed for clinical research and new collaborations are required in order to gain information from clinical trials more quickly. Basic research must yield new therapeutic opportunities if major improvements in survival from osteosarcoma are to be seen. Clinical investigators must be ready to adapt traditional methodologies to properly evaluate new agents as they become available, in recognition that their effects may differ from those of conventional cytotoxic agents.

References

1 Whelan JS, Cannon SR. Osteosarcoma. In: Souhami RL, Tannock I, Hohenberger P, Horiot J-C, eds. *Oxford Textbook of Oncology*, 2nd edn. Oxford: Oxford University Press, 2001: 2553–2570.

2 Gatta G, Capocaccia R, De Angelis R, Stiller C, Coebergh JW. Cancer survival in European adolescents and young adults. *Eur J Cancer* 2003; **39**: 2600–2610.

3 Levi F, Lucchini F, Negri E, La Vecchia C. Trends in cancer mortality at age 15 to 24 years in Europe. *Eur J Cancer* 2003; **39**: 2611–2621.

4 Bramwell VH, Burgers M, Sneath R *et al*. A comparison of two short intensive adjuvant chemotherapy regimens in operable osteosarcoma of limbs in children and young adults: the first study of the European Osteosarcoma Intergroup. *J Clin Oncol* 1992; **10**: 1579–1591.

5 Rosen G, Nirenberg A. Neoadjuvant chemotherapy for osteogenic sarcoma: a five year follow-up (T-10) and preliminary report of new studies (T-12). *Prog Clin Biol Res* 1985; **201**: 39–51.

6 Souhami RL, Craft AW, Van der Eijken JW *et al*. Randomised trial of two regimens of chemotherapy in operable osteosarcoma: a study of the European Osteosarcoma Intergroup. *Lancet* 1997; **350**: 911–917.

7 Whelan JS, Weeden S, Uscinska B *et al*. for the European Osteosarcoma Intergroup. Localised extremity osteosarcoma: mature survival data from two European Osteosarcoma Intergroup randomised clinical trials. *Proc ASCO* 2000; **19**: 552.

8 Lewis IJ, Nooij M. Chemotherapy at standard or increased dose intensity in patients with operable osteosarcoma of the extremity: a randomised controlled trial conducted by the European Osteosarcoma Intergroup (ISRCTN 86294690). *Proc ASCO* 2003; **22**: 3281.

9 Meyers P, Schwartz CL, Bernstein M *et al.* Addition of ifosfamide and muramyl tripeptide to cisplatin, doxorubicin, and high-dose methotrexate improves event-free survival (EFS) in localised osteosarcoma (OS). *Proc ASCO* 2001; **20**: 1483a.

10 Bacci G, Ferrari S, Mercuri M *et al.* Neoadjuvant chemotherapy for extremity osteosarcoma – preliminary results of the Rizzoli's 4th study. *Acta Oncol* 1998; **37**: 41–48.

11 Bielack S, Kempf-Bielack B, Schwenzer D *et al.* [Neoadjuvant therapy for localized osteosarcoma of extremities. Results from the cooperative osteosarcoma study group COSS of 925 patients]. [In German]. *Klin Padiatr* 1999; **211**: 260–270.

12 Smeland S, Muller C, Alvegard TA *et al.* Scandinavian Sarcoma Group Osteosarcoma Study SSG VIII: prognostic factors for outcome and the role of replacement salvage chemotherapy for poor histological responders. *Eur J Cancer* 2003; **39**: 488–494.

CHAPTER 12

Osteosarcoma and surgery

R. J. Grimer

Introduction

Osteosarcomas are primary malignancies of bone that peak in incidence during adolescent years. The most common age to develop osteosarcoma is 16 years and almost 50% of patients developing an osteosarcoma will be teenagers. The cause of the vast majority of osteosarcomas is unknown. In many cases there will be a history of trauma that initiated the symptoms but there is no evidence that trauma actually causes osteosarcoma. The most common site for osteosarcoma to develop is around the knee and almost half of all tumours will be in the distal femur; the next most common site is the proximal tibia, followed by the proximal humerus. At all ages above 10 years the tumour is more common in males than females, by an average ratio of 1.3:1. Before age 10, girls are as likely as boys to develop osteosarcoma. The vast majority of patients with an osteosarcoma will have had a considerable duration of symptoms prior to diagnosis, and in retrospect many will admit to vague and non-specific symptoms that were present for up to 4 months or more prior to diagnosis. The tumours are not infrequently misdiagnosed as athletic injuries.[1]

Diagnosis

Guidelines for the early diagnosis of all bone and soft tissue tumours are available to all doctors and have been widely publicized.[2] There is as yet no evidence that this is leading to earlier diagnosis of primary sarcomas. The average size of bone tumour at presentation is 11 centimetres. The key features that should suggest the possible presence of a malignant bone tumour are:
- non-mechanical pain (pain not related to activity or that may wake the patient at night)
- bony swelling or tenderness.

The radiological features that should alert the clinician include (Fig. 12.1):
- bone destruction
- new bone formation
- soft tissue swelling
- periosteal elevation.

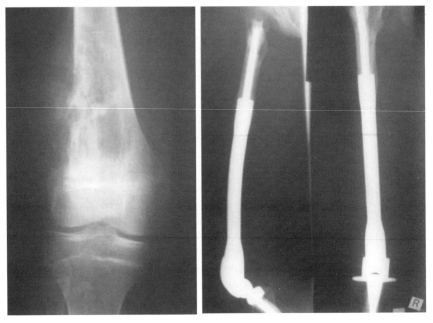

Fig. 12.1 A typical osteosarcoma of the distal femur and its subsequent resection and replacement with a metal endoprosthesis.

The presence of one or more of these should alert the clinician to the possibility of a bone tumour but the differential diagnosis of these features remains wide. Further investigation is clearly warranted, however.

Management

The management of osteosarcoma has changed little in the past 25 years. Since chemotherapy has been shown to dramatically improve survival, it has become essential in the management of all high-grade osteosarcomas. Unfortunately, there has been little improvement in survival since chemotherapy was first introduced and a series of MRC trials in the UK have consistently shown an overall survival rate of 54% at 5 years.[3–5]

Although chemotherapy is undoubtedly the thing that is likely to cure the greatest proportion of patients, surgery remains an essential part of the management programme of all patients with osteosarcoma. In the absence of effective chemotherapy, surgery offers the only possible chance of cure. Even with effective chemotherapy, osteosarcoma is rarely cured without surgical resection.[6]

Surgery

The aim of surgical management of osteosarcoma is to completely resect the tumour to produce the minimum risk of local recurrence and the maximum chance of overall survival. The secondary role of surgery is to reconstruct the patient's limb after resection of the tumour in order to try to restore maximum function to the individual. In some situations the only safe way of carrying out surgery will be with an amputation, but in most cases limb salvage surgery will be possible. The risks and benefits of each do, however, need highlighting to the individual and the options for limb salvage need explaining.

Amputation used to be the surgical treatment of choice for osteosarcoma. Because most tumours arise around the knee joint, this meant that the amputation was usually high above the knee or sometimes a disarticulation of the hip. Limb salvage surgery and, in particular, the use of endoprosthetic replacements has dramatically altered the surgical possibilities available to the patient – but not without complications.

There are some situations in which amputation is still the only safe option and these constitute approximately 15% of cases. The main indication for amputation is where a tumour has not responded to chemotherapy and in which there is an extensive soft tissue component involving the neurovascular bundle. Relative indications for amputation include those patients with a modest soft tissue extension of tumour in whom resection margins are likely to be very close, and patients in whom for some other reason complete resection of tumour cannot be achieved. Tumour growth into the adjacent joint is not an absolute contraindication to limb salvage as extra-articular resection can be carried out. In some situations amputation remains the treatment of choice. This is particularly the case for those osteosarcomas involving the distal part of the skeleton such as the digits, foot and ankle. In most other situations patients prefer limb salvage even though the procedure is associated with increased risks.

What are the advantages of limb salvage surgery? In theory, the advantage is that the patient retains the limb and should thus have improved function. Their limb should look more normal and this should have psychological benefit. The disadvantages of limb salvage surgery are that it is complicated and has to be carried out in specialist centres. It is, certainly initially, expensive and the surgeon may be tempted to try to carry out limb salvage surgery when it may not be completely safe to do so. This remains one of the most controversial areas of the surgery of osteosarcoma.

Proving that limb salvage surgery is safe has been quite a challenge but most authors now accept that limb salvage surgery, if carried out properly, does not decrease the chance of survival.[7] Surprisingly, this lack of difference in survival is not matched by the risk of local recurrence, which is consistently greater in patients with limb salvage.[8] In one study, centre A had an 85% limb salvage rate whilst centre B, using the same chemotherapy, had a 50% limb salvage rate. The local recurrence rate at centre A was over 10% whilst at centre B it was 2%. Despite this apparent difference in local tumour control, the overall survival of the patients at the two centres was identical.[9]

Some studies have shown that there are significant functional benefits for limb salvage,[10] and other studies have shown that limb salvage surgery is in fact cost-effective simply because the cost of replacing artificial limbs on a regular basis in a fit and active population is far greater than the cost of servicing and replacing the endoprosthetic replacements used in limb salvage surgery.[11]

The question of the safety of limb salvage surgery is principally one of identifying the price of local recurrence and then trying to work out what effect this has on the patient's survival. It has been shown by numerous authors that the risk of local recurrence is related to two factors: the margins of excision and the effectiveness of neoadjuvant chemotherapy. If a wide surgical margin can be achieved (a good layer of tissue between the surgeon and the tumour) and there is greater than 90% necrosis of the tumour following chemotherapy, the risk of local recurrence will be extremely low – about 2%. If however there is less than 90% necrosis but wide margins then the risk is increased to approximately 11%, a risk similar to that with a very close margin of resection in the presence of a good response to chemotherapy. If, however, the surgeon carries out a resection extending very close to the margins of the tumour, through what is known as the 'reactive layer', and there is a poor response to chemotherapy, the risk of local recurrence may be 30% or higher. The number of patients likely to be at risk of local recurrence depends on the effectiveness of chemotherapy. The chemotherapy used in the UK has consistently produced only 28% of patients with a so-called good response to chemotherapy, whilst series from Italy have shown up to 70% with a good response.[6] The closest margin of resection is usually adjacent to the neurovascular bundle and removal and replacement of this is not usually feasible; thus, marginal surgery in the presence of poor necrosis may arise in one-quarter of the patients.

In order to be able to assess how this risk of local recurrence translates into subsequent events, the significance of local recurrence should be known. Approximately one-third of patients with a local recurrence already have metastatic disease by the time they present and in these cases the prognosis is very poor, few surviving beyond 2 years. Of the patients who do not have metastases at the time of development of local recurrence, approximately two-thirds will subsequently develop metastatic disease, and in them the prognosis is also very poor. However, one-third will not have metastases and these patients can thus be cured simply by treatment of the local recurrence alone. Some authors consider local recurrence as having such a poor prognosis that it is to be avoided at all costs. In this situation, they often recommend that a patient with close or involved margins and a poor response to chemotherapy should undergo immediate amputation.[6] There is no proof that this doctrine produces improved survival. Local recurrence is clearly a significant risk factor for subsequent survival but it has not convincingly been shown to be an independent risk factor compared with the effects of chemotherapy.

Prognostic factors

The prognosis for survival in osteosarcoma is related to a number of factors:[12]
- site (proximal sites do worse than distal; truncal sites are worse than extremities)
- elevated blood alkaline phosphatase at diagnosis
- percentage necrosis after preoperative chemotherapy (response to chemotherapy)
- sex (in some series females do better)
- size (bigger tumours do worse).

Patients having an amputation as opposed to limb salvage do worse but this is almost certainly because they have large tumours that often do not respond to chemotherapy. Interestingly, the duration of symptoms has not been shown to be a risk factor and in some series a short duration of symptoms had a better prognosis than a long duration, as these are more likely to be aggressive, rapidly growing tumours responsive to chemotherapy.

Limb salvage options

The types of limb salvage surgery available have increased dramatically as the ingenuity of surgeons has increased and as biotechnology has advanced. The options available for limb salvage include:
- resection of tumour without replacement
- endoprosthetic replacement
- rotationplasty
- allografts
- autografts.

Resection of the tumour alone without reconstruction is clearly the most attractive option but unfortunately it is only available in some sites. The fibula, clavicle and rib are the most obvious expendable bones, but osteosarcoma rarely arises in these sites.

The most common limb salvage surgery practised over the past 20 years in the UK has undoubtedly been endoprosthetic replacements.[13] Considerable experience has been gained in their use and in their limitations. Endoprosthetic replacements are made of metal, usually titanium, and are used to replace joints and long lengths of bone. Endoprostheses can be used to replace all or part of the humerus, radius, pelvis, femur or tibia. The success of the various implants varies from site to site and depends very much upon the amount of normal soft tissue that can be retained to provide function. In general, if no functioning soft tissues can be retained at the time of surgery then an endoprosthetic replacement is not likely to be of much value, except in the upper humerus, and amputation should be considered. The main advantages of endoprosthetic replacements are that they are readily available, they are predictable and they provide immediate and secure fixation, allowing the individual to get up and walk as soon as the soft tissues have healed. The disadvantages are that they do impose restrictions on the individual's lifestyle; in particular, contact and other active sports are to be discouraged as they can produce dramatic failure of the implants. Most of the endoprosthetic replacements will be fixed to the skeleton with cement, often augmented with hydroxyapatite. In the earlier designs of prosthesis, mechanical loosening was common but this is now increasingly rare and prostheses will have failed due to the wear of the high-density polyethylene used in the joints, to fatigue failure or to infection.[14] The risk of infection in these endoprostheses is significant and infection can develop at any time. The risk of infection is somewhere between 6 and 10% over a 10-year period. Infection can be very difficult to treat and sometimes requires amputation.[15] Overall, however, endoprosthetic replacements have a failure rate, in terms of major revision surgery, of about 3% per year, based on historical series. Modern implants should do better but patients do need to be aware that almost inevitably their prostheses will require revision at some stage in the future, resulting in significant further hospitalization and an increased risk of complications, etc.

Rotationplasty is a most interesting concept. The principle is that the whole segment of the limb bearing the tumour is removed and the healthy limb below is attached to the healthy limb above (i.e. a segment of lower thigh may be removed and the upper tibia joined to the upper femur). The only structure left linking the two following removal of the tumour will be the sciatic nerve, and the blood vessels are anastomosed. The procedure is called rotationplasty because as the distal part is connected to the upper leg, it is rotated through 180°. This will result in a very short limb with the ankle and foot facing backwards. The advantage of this is that the ankle will now act like a knee joint and will be fitted with an artificial limb much like a below-knee amputation, something which gives a huge functional advantage compared with an above-knee amputation. The operation has enjoyed great popularity in Europe and in Canada but is being done less frequently as the perceived advantages of endoprosthetic replacement become known. The main advantage of a rotationplasty is that it provides very good function with little need for further surgical intervention.[16] The disadvantages are the need for regular replacement of artificial limbs (which is costly) and the individual's perception of their abnormal appearance. The vast majority of children cope well with this; adults find it more difficult to cope with. Long-term series, however, suggest that patients accept the procedure well and continue to function at a high level. There is no evidence as yet that the ankle develops arthritis due to its unusual role as a knee joint.[17]

Allografts were also very popular in North America. The advantage of an allograft is that it is a biological as opposed to a mechanical reconstruction. Allografts are obtained from tissue donors, usually patients who have died and given permission for the kidneys, heart, liver and other organs to be transplanted. The bone is harvested under strict sterile precautions and is stored at −80°C. When a bone is required, a suitable one can be obtained from the bone bank. The service is not currently widely available in the UK but allografts can be obtained from tissue banks in North America or Europe. The bone is dead and acts merely as a scaffolding. Studies have shown that when an allograft is used, the junction with the normal bone heals like a fracture but the remainder of the bone does not revascularize. The bones are weaker than normal and there is a significant risk of non-union at the bone–allograft junction, infection and fractures. It is generally accepted that the best use of allografts is following diaphyseal resection of bone rather than in situations where joints need replacing.[18] There are, however, notable long-term successes even in this situation.[19] The theoretical advantage that soft tissues can be attached to the allograft better than to endoprostheses has not been substantiated, particularly in the upper limb, where it was hoped that improved function around the shoulder would result from the use of allografts. This has not been proved to be the case.[20] The disadvantages of an allograft include the high risk of infection, non-union and graft failure. Allografts are cheaper than endoprosthetic replacements but do not allow weight-bearing until the bone allograft junction has united, something which often takes many months. There is evidence that allografts used in patients on chemotherapy have a higher rate of complications than in those not requiring such treatment.[21]

Autografts are another attractive option. In this situation, an expendable bone is moved from elsewhere in the patient to replace the diseased one that is being resected. In reality, there are only three bones which can be moved with ease: the fibula, the iliac crest of the pelvis and the rib. The latter two are too small and too weak to be used in most situations and hence it is only bones that can be replaced by the fibula that are likely to be suitable for the use of autografting. The most obvious situation is in the mid-tibia, where the fibula can be swung across and used to replace the diseased portion of tibia. The advantages of this are that the bone that is moved is the patient's own bone and there is usually a rapid rate of union. However, there is then a significant delay until the bone hypertrophies sufficiently to allow weight-bearing, and during this time the patient will have to remain non-weight-bearing or partially weight-bearing. Once the bone has hypertrophied, however, it becomes as thick and as strong as the normal host bone. In the femur, one fibula is not likely to be sufficient to take the patient's weight for a very long time and consequently this type of autograft is rarely used.

Another interesting and attractive option is to use the individual's own bone, removing it, sterilizing it and reimplanting it![22] The tumour-bearing bone can be sterilized using high-dose radiotherapy (90 Gy), autoclaving, pasteurization and microwaving. All these techniques are effective in killing the tumour (and bone) DNA. Tumour is removed from the bone macroscopically and then, after sterilization, the bone, which will of course fit perfectly, is replaced, just like an allograft. In some situations this technique has been used to replace joints and in others it has simply been used as a method of replacing part of the bone along with other supplementary fixation. It is likely that this type of reconstruction will become more common, particularly in situations where endoprosthetic replacements or other options are not readily available, such as in the pelvis.[23]

Decision-making

Deciding what is best for an individual patient is thus very difficult. There is a whole range of issues to be confronted and the decision as to how much in-depth discussion an individual can cope with in making this decision has to be made. The surgeon will usually meet the patient for the first time when a biopsy is carried out. At that time the patient will not know whether or not a tumour is present and is confronted with the possibility that his/her whole life is likely to be changed by the diagnosis of cancer. Few individuals, let alone adolescents, will be able to cope with the complexities of whether they should have an amputation or limb salvage, and if so what sort of limb salvage.

In an ideal world, the patient commences on chemotherapy and, having adjusted to the idea of this, will have further consultation to discuss all the relevant challenges ahead. They need to be aware of the risks and benefits of each of the procedures and the likely impact on their life. What we do know, however, is that most survivors of childhood cancer cope remarkably well. They seem to adapt and accept their situation and accept any failures of the type of surgery they have undergone. Most patients, whether they have amputation or limb salvage, will accept what they have had done.

Adolescents are notorious risk-takers. This attitude leads to the dilemma of patients who are unwilling to have an amputation because the tumour is too large or because it has not responded to chemotherapy. Amputation holds fears of the unknown and even attending an artificial limb centre or meeting other individuals with an amputation will rarely abate this. For these patients, the thought of losing their limb may be so dreadful that they could not contemplate life without it. Yet the fact that they adapt so remarkably when they do have an amputation is a testament to how the human can adapt. Patients will, however, accept a significant increase in the risk to their life in order to avoid amputation. This concept of accepting risk in order to achieve a perceived gain is not new but to quantify it has always proved difficult. The challenge that the surgeon and other care providers must meet is to estimate risks and to confront these openly and honestly with our patients.

References

1 Muscolo DL, Ayerza MA, Makino A, Costa-Paz M, Aponte-Tinao LA. Tumors about the knee misdiagnosed as athletic injuries. *J Bone Joint Surg* 2003; **85A**: 1209–1214.
2 Department of Health. Guidelines for early diagnosis of cancer. Department of Health. http://www.doh.gov.uk/pub/docs/doh/guidelines.pdf.
3 Bramwell VHC, Burgers M, Sneath RS *et al*. A comparison of two short intensive adjuvant chemotherapy rgimens in operable osteosarcoma of limbs in children and young adults: the first study of the European Osteosarcoma Intergroup. *J Clin Oncol* 1992; **10**: 1579–1591.
4 Souhami RL, Craft AW, Van der Eijken JW *et al*. Randomised trial of two regimes of chemotherapy in operable osteosarcoma: a study of the European Osteosarcoma Intergroup. *Lancet* 1997; **350**: 911–917.

5 Lewis IJ, Weeden S, Machin D, Stark D, Craft AW. Received dose and dose-intensity of chemotherapy and outcome in nonmetastatic extremity osteosarcoma. *J Clin Oncol* 2000; **18**: 4028–4037.

6 Jaffe N, Carrasco H, Raymond K, Ayala A, Eftekhari F. Can cure in patients with osteosarcoma be achieved exclusively with chemotherapy and abrogation of surgery? *Cancer* 2003; **95**: 2202–2210.

7 Bacci G, Ferrari S, Lari S *et al*. Osteosarcoma of the limb. *J Bone Joint Surg* 2002; **84B**: 88–92.

8 Rougraff BT, Simon MA, Kneisl JS, Greenberg DG, Mankin HJ. Limb salvage compared with amputation for osteosarcoma of the distal end of the femur. A longterm oncological, functional and quality of life study. *J Bone Joint Surg* 1994; **76A**: 649–656.

9 Grimer RJ, Taminiau AM, Cannon SR. Surgical outcomes in osteosarcoma. *J Bone Joint Surg* 2003; **84B**: 395–400.

10 Postma A, Kingma A, De Ruiter JH *et al*. Quality of life in bone tumour patients comparing limb salvage and amputation of the lower extremity. *J Surg Oncol* 1992; **51**: 47–51.

11 Grimer RJ, Carter SR, Pynsent PB. The cost-effectiveness of limb salvage surgery for bone tumours. *J Bone Joint Surg* 1997; **79B**: 558–561.

12 Davis AM, Bell RS, Goodwin PJ. Prognostic factors in osteosarcoma: a critical review. *J Clin Oncol* 1994; **12**: 423–431.

13 Cannon SR. Massive prostheses for malignant bone tumours of the limbs. *J Bone Joint Surg* 1997; **79**: 497–506.

14 Unwin PS, Cannon SR, Grimer RJ, Kemp HB, Sneath RS, Walker PS. Aseptic loosening in cemented custom-made prosthetic replacements for bone tumours of the lower limb. *J Bone Joint Surg* 1996; **78**: 5–13.

15 Grimer RJ, Belthur N, Chadrasekar C, Carter SR, Tillman RM. Two-stage revisions for infected endoprostheses used in tumor surgery. *Clin Orthop* 2002; **395**: 193–203.

16 Hillmann A, Hoffmann C, Gosheger G, Krakau H, Winkelmann W. Malignant tumour of the distal part of the femur or proximal tibia: endoprosthetic replacement or rotationplasty. Functional outcome and quality of life measurements. *J Bone Joint Surg* 1999; **81A**: 462–468.

17 Rodl RW, Pohlmann U, Gosheger G, Lindner NJ, Winkelmann W. Rotationplasty – quality of life after 10 years in 22 adults. *Acta Orthop Scand* 2002; **73**: 85–88.

18 Mankin HJ, Gebhardt MC, Jennings LC, Springfield DS, Tomford WW. Long-term results of allograft replacement in the management of bone tumours. *Clin Orthop* 1996; **324**: 86–97.

19 Muscolo DL, Ayerza MA, Aponte-Tinao LA. Survivorship and radiographic analysis of knee osteoarticular allografts. *Clin Orthop* 2000; **373**: 73–79.

20 Gebhardt MC, Roth YF, Mankin HJ. Osteoarticular allografts for reconstruction of the proximal part of the humerus after excision of a musculoskeletal tumour. *J Bone Joint Surg* 1990; **72**: 334–345.

21 Hazan EJ, Hornicek FJ, Tomford W, Gebhardt MC, Mankin HJ. The effect of adjuvant chemotherapy on osteoarticular allografts. *Clin Orthop* 2001; **385**: 176–181.

22 Uyttendaele D, De Schryver A, Claessens H *et al*. Limb conservation in primary bone tumours by resection, extracorporeal irradiation and re-implantation. *J Bone Joint Surg* 1988; **70**: 348–353.

23 Hong A, Stevens G, Stalley P *et al*. Extracorporeal irradiation for malignant bone tumours. *Int J Radiat Oncol Biol Phys* 2001; **50**: 441–447.

Part three
Survivorship

CHAPTER 13

Subfertility in adolescents with cancer: who is at risk and what can be done?

W. H. B. Wallace and M. F. H. Brougham

Introduction

Cancer affects approximately 1 in 5000 adolescents aged 15–19 years.[1] Recent advances in both available treatments and supportive care have resulted in markedly improved survival rates (Fig. 13.1), such that now around 75–80% of patients with the most common malignancies in the age group achieve long-term survival.[2,3]

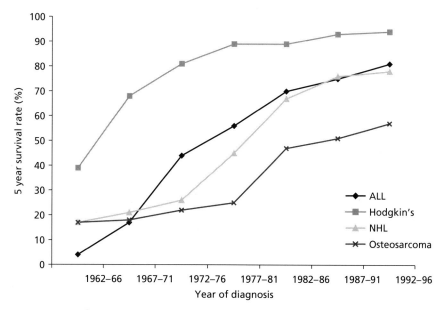

Fig. 13.1 Trends in 5-year survival rates (%) in selected childhood and adolescent cancers from 1962 to 1996. (Source: National Registry of Childhood Tumours.) ALL, acute lymphoblastic leukaemia. NHL, non-Hodgkin's lymphoma.

There are, therefore, increasing numbers of young adults who have survived cancer but who must live with the consequences of curative treatment. It has been estimated that by the year 2010 about one in 715 of the adult population will be a long-term survivor of childhood and adolescent cancer.[4] Attention must therefore be directed to minimizing the impact of the late effects of treatment, in order to improve the quality of life for this patient group. Adverse effects of cancer therapy are diverse and include disorders of the endocrine system, cardiac and pulmonary dysfunction, renal and hepatic impairment, secondary malignancies and psychosocial difficulties.

Many treatments for cancer, both in childhood and in later life, can affect future fertility.[5,6] Adolescence represents the start of reproductive life, and issues of sexuality, including fertility, are of particular importance at this time. Thus treatment received during this period that affects future fertility can have a devastating impact, both at the time with regard to the acceptance of treatment, and in later life, when the patient may wish to start a family.[7] It is therefore imperative to consider, at an early stage, strategies that may protect or restore fertility in later life.

This article will discuss the aetiology of subfertility following treatment for cancer in adolescence, and in particular which patient groups are likely to be at increased risk. Strategies to protect or restore fertility will then be discussed, including consent and ethical issues.

Gonadal toxicity following cancer treatment in the adolescent

Gonadal damage in adolescents treated for cancer can result from either systemic chemotherapy or radiotherapy delivered to fields involving the craniospinal or pelvic regions of the body.

In males normal testicular function is dependent on a complex interplay between the Sertoli, Leydig and germ cells. Sertoli cells are responsible for nurturing developing germ cells, whereas the most important function of Leydig cells is testosterone production. Cytotoxic treatment, by its nature, targets rapidly dividing cells and therefore spermatogenesis may be impaired following such treatment. The exact mechanism of this damage is uncertain but appears to involve depletion of the proliferating germ cell pool.[8–10] The adult testis is continually producing mature spermatozoa and is therefore not surprisingly very susceptible to cytotoxic damage. However, it is clear that gonadotoxic treatment received at any age can lead to subsequent infertility,[11,12] and there is increasing evidence that the testis demonstrates significant cellular activity before puberty and that this activity is essential for normal adult testicular function.[13] Thus, the timing of the gonadotoxic insult in relation to puberty is of less importance than the nature of the insult itself.

In contrast, the female is born with her full complement of eggs, which thereafter declines in an exponential fashion to the menopause, at an average age of 51 years. Indeed, this decline actually begins before birth (Fig. 13.2).

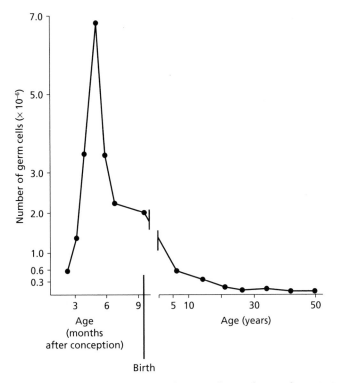

Fig. 13.2 Exponential decline in oocyte population with age (from Baker, 1968; Block, 1952).

Both chemotherapy and radiotherapy may accelerate oocyte depletion, leading to truncated fecundity and premature menopause.[14,15]

The effects of radiotherapy

The gonads are sensitive to irradiation and the resulting damage depends on the field of treatment, total dose and fractionation schedule and the age of the patient.[15–17,19]

Males

In males, radiation doses as low as 0.1–1.2 Gy can result in detectable effects on spermatogenesis, with doses over 4 Gy causing a more permanent detrimental effect.[16–18] The somatic cells of the testis are more resistant to radiotherapy-induced damage than the germ cells. Indeed, Leydig cell dysfunction is not observed until doses of around 20 Gy in prepubertal boys and 30 Gy in sexually mature males.[19] Therefore, many patients will produce testosterone and develop normal secondary sexual characteristics, despite severe impairment of spermatogenesis.

Within the adolescent age group, radiation-induced testicular damage is most often encountered following direct irradiation of the testes for leukaemic infiltration. Radiation doses of 24 Gy are used, and this invariably results in permanent azoospermia.[20] Total body irradiation, given as conditioning treatment before bone marrow transplantation (BMT) at doses of 14.4 Gy, is also sterilizing, although Leydig cell function may be preserved.[21]

Females

In female patients, total body, abdominal or pelvic irradiation not only causes ovarian damage but may also affect uterine function. As with males, the degree of impairment depends on the radiation dose, field, fractionation schedule and age at the time of treatment.[15,22–24] In healthy women the oocyte pool declines with age in an exponential manner.[25] Depletion of primordial follicles secondary to radiotherapy is proportional to the size of the existing oocyte pool and therefore, for a given dose of radiation, the younger the patient at the time of radiotherapy the later the onset of a premature menopause. The human oocyte is very sensitive to radiation, and we have estimated the LD_{50} (the lethal dose required to kill 50% of the total oocytes) to be less than 2 Gy.[26] Indeed, premature ovarian failure has been reported following total body irradiation (14.4 Gy) received during adolescence.[24]

Irradiation involving the uterus in childhood and adolescence is associated with an increased incidence of nulliparity, spontaneous miscarriage and intrauterine growth retardation.[23,24,27] The mechanisms underlying these problems remain unclear, but may be secondary to reduced elasticity of the uterine musculature and uterine vascular damage.[24,27] Patients who have received radiation involving the pelvis should be counselled appropriately, and good communication with the obstetrician is essential.

Tumours of the central nervous system are the second commonest solid malignancy in adolescence.[1] Cranial irradiation is frequently used as a therapeutic modality in this patient group. Whilst not harming the gonads directly, fertility can be impaired by disruption to the hypothalamic–pituitary–gonadal axis. Indeed, patients receiving radiation doses of 35–45 Gy have demonstrated subsequent deficiencies in plasma gonadotrophins.[28] If severe enough, this may result in a significant reduction in circulating sex hormone levels and delayed puberty. Hypogonadism following cranial irradiation has been demonstrated to be secondary to hypothalamic GnRH deficiency.[29] Thus, exogenous GnRH can be used as replacement therapy in order to restore gonadal function and fertility.

The effects of chemotherapy

Cytotoxic chemotherapy can cause gonadal damage, and the nature and extent of this damage is dependent upon the agent administered, the dose received and the age and sex of the patient.[11,30–32] Although a number of agents have been identified as being gonadotoxic (Table 13.1), including procarbazine, cisplatin and the alkylating agents, such as cyclophosphamide, melphalan and chlorambucil, it is important to note that not all chemotherapeutic agents

Table 13.1 Gonadotoxic chemotherapy agents

Alkylating agents
Cyclophosphamide
Ifosfamide
Nitrosoureas, e.g. carmustine, lamustine
Chlorambucil
Melphalan
Busulphan
Vinca-alkaloids
Vinblastine
Anti-metabolites
Cytarabine
Others
Cisplatin
Procarbazine

cause permanent gonadal damage. In addition, the relative contribution of each individual drug can be difficult to determine as most treatments are administered in multi-agent regimens.

Males

As with radiotherapy, the testicular seminiferous epithelium, which supports spermatogenesis, is very sensitive to the detrimental effects of chemotherapy irrespective of pubertal status at the time of treatment. Therefore, after receiving gonadotoxic agents, patients may be rendered oligospermic or azoospermic but testosterone production by the Leydig cell is usually unaffected, and thus secondary sexual characteristics develop normally.[33,34] Following higher cumulative doses of gonadotoxic chemotherapy, Leydig cell dysfunction may also become apparent.[35]

Hodgkin's disease is the commonest solid malignancy seen in the adolescent age group.[1] Treatment of this lymphoma has involved the use of procarbazine together with alkylating agents such as chlorambucil, mustine and cyclophosphamide. Whilst these drug combinations have resulted in excellent survival rates, the majority of male patients have subsequently developed permanent azoospermia.[33] Mackie and colleagues[30] studied patients with a mean age at diagnosis of 12.2 years and who were treated with ChlVPP, a regimen containing both chlorambucil and procarbazine. On follow-up, 89% of these patients demonstrated severe damage to the seminiferous epithelium up to 10 years after therapy. Because of this, treatment for Hodgkin's disease has been modified in an attempt to reduce the gonadotoxicity whilst maintaining long-term survival.[36] Treatment with the ABVD regimen (adriamycin, bleomycin, vinblastine and dacarbazine), which contains no alkylating agents or procarbazine, results in significantly less gonadotoxicity, with no patients demonstrating permanent azoospermia.[37] However, the anthracycline agent in this regimen renders it potentially cardiotoxic.

Current treatment of Hodgkin's disease for adolescents in the UK involves combination chemotherapy that alternates courses of ChlVPP and ABVD. Although this exposes patients to both alkylating agents and anthracyclines, both are delivered at reduced total cumulative dosage, with the goal of maintaining excellent survival rates with minimal long-term adverse effects. This regimen has been shown to result in significantly less gonadotoxicity than does therapy based on alkylating agents and procarbazine alone,[38,39] with approximately half of all male patients preserving their fertility.

Females

In contrast to the effects of radiotherapy, females are, in general, less susceptible to the gonadotoxic effects of the chemotherapeutic agents discussed above. However, ovarian dysfunction following chemotherapy has been described.[40] As with male patients, procarbazine and alkylating agents, as used for the treatment of Hodgkin's disease, are particularly gonadotoxic. Mackie and colleagues[30] demonstrated that more than half of the female patients studied had evidence of ovarian dysfunction after ChlVPP chemotherapy. As with the male patients, alternating cycles of ChlVPP and ABVD are being tested to reduce gonadotoxicity in female patients.

As with radiotherapy, the degree of ovarian damage following chemotherapy is dependent on the age of the patient, older females being more susceptible to the development of premature ovarian failure.[14] The larger reserve of surviving primordial follicles available after treatment probably explains the relative protection afforded to younger females, particularly prepubertally but also within adolescence.

Long-term follow-up is essential for these patients, as premature ovarian failure will result in an early menopause. Byrne and colleagues[41] followed up women treated for cancer before the age of 20 and found that 42% of women treated with radiotherapy and alkylating agent-based chemotherapy had reached menopause by the age of 31, compared with 5% of controls. Patients who are at risk must be counselled appropriately, not only because their fertile window is substantially reduced but also with regard to the additional implications of premature menopause, such as reduced bone mineral density and osteoporosis.

The effects of disease

Although many aspects of cancer treatment may affect fertility, it is important to note that the disease itself may contribute to gonadal dysfunction. Indeed, it has been demonstrated that up to 70% of male patients with Hodgkin's disease assessed before commencing treatment have impaired semen quality.[42] This may also be observed in patients with other malignancies prior to treatment,[43] although perhaps to a lesser extent. In addition to the disease itself, other non-specific conditions commonly observed at presentation, such as fever and cachexia, can impair semen quality.[44]

Similarly, oocytes harvested from female patients before cancer therapy are of impaired quality and exhibit an impaired fertilization rate compared with those from control females.[45]

These findings will have implications when considering fertility preservation strategies before the commencement of gonadotoxic therapy.

Fertility potential and assessment following cancer treatment

Due to the varied nature of the gonadal insult following chemotherapy or radiotherapy, it can often be very difficult to predict whether an adolescent undergoing cancer treatment will subsequently have impaired fertility. The risk of subfertility can be categorized according to the type of malignancy and its associated treatment (Table 13.2). As can be seen, treatment for Hodgkin's disease with alkylating agent-based therapy is profoundly gonadotoxic, as discussed above. Conditioning prior to bone marrow transplantation with

Table 13.2 Best assessment of risk of subfertility following current treatment for childhood and adolescent cancer by disease

Risk of subfertility	Disease/treatment
Low	Acute lymphoblastic leukaemia
	Wilms' tumour
	Soft tissue sarcoma: stage 1
	Germ cell tumours (with gonadal preservation and no radiotherapy)
	Retinoblastoma
	Brain tumour
	Surgery only
	Cranial irradiation <24 Gy
Medium	Acute myeloblastic leukaemia
	Hepatoblastoma
	Osteosarcoma
	Ewing's sarcoma
	Soft tissue sarcoma
	Neuroblastoma
	Non-Hodgkin's lymphoma
	Hodgkin's disease: 'alternating therapy'
	Brain tumour
	Craniospinal radiotherapy
	Cranial irradiation >24 Gy
High	Total body irradiation
	Localized radiotherapy: pelvic/testicular
	Chemotherapy conditioning for bone marrow transplant
	Hodgkin's disease: alkylating agent-based therapy
	Soft tissue sarcoma: metastatic

high-dose chemotherapy and total body irradiation also carries a substantial risk of gonadotoxicity, as do most treatments of metastatic sarcoma. However, current therapies for acute lymphoblastic leukaemia, the commonest malignancy in childhood and adolescence, and for many other common paediatric cancers (Table 13.2) constitute a relatively low risk of gonadotoxicity.

It is important to note that treatment protocols for malignant disease are continually evolving in order to improve survival and reduce adverse effects. Whereas treatment for acute lymphoblastic leukaemia has intensified over the past decade, the management of non-Hodgkin's lymphoma, for example, has tended to become less intensive. In addition, as more is known about the biology of malignant disease, there is an increasing trend to stratify treatments according to the risk of relapse. Therefore, this assessment of risk represents a guide, which needs to be continually reviewed in the light of ongoing research. To complicate matters further, there are reports of patients having received sterilizing treatment who have subsequently demonstrated recovery of spermatogenesis or ovarian function.[46,47] In view of these uncertainties, counselling adolescents and their families is difficult. Long-term follow-up of these patients must include appropriate discussion and assessment of fertility.

The assessment of gonadal function currently involves regular clinical assessment of pubertal progression, biochemical assessment of plasma gonadotrophins and sex steroids, semen analysis in males and menstrual history in females.

Testicular enlargement is the initial sign of puberty in boys, followed by penis enlargement and the development of pubic hair.[48] As discussed earlier, after gonadotoxic therapy many male patients will have preserved Leydig cell function and will therefore develop normal secondary sexual characteristics. Their testes, however, will be small and atrophied, with a loss of tubular space (Fig. 13.3), suggestive of reduced sperm production.[49] On clinical examination, using the Prader orchidometer, a testicular volume of 12 ml or less in a postpubertal male is likely to be associated with azoospermia.

In females puberty commences with development of the breast bud and menarche occurs around 2 years later.[48] As in males, ovarian volume can be indicative of gonadal function and is reduced in patients treated for cancer.[50]

Biochemical analysis of patients who have impaired fertility following treatment will usually demonstrate a raised follicle stimulating hormone, and reduced oestradiol in females. In males follicle stimulating hormone is increased but Leydig cell function may be normal, characterized by normal plasma testosterone and only marginally elevated luteinizing hormone.

Assessment of fertility, clinically and biochemically, is not possible before and during puberty. A potential marker is inhibin B,[51] a glycoprotein, secreted predominantly from Sertoli cells in males and developing antral follicles in females,[52,53] that plays an important role in spermatogenesis and folliculogenesis in adult males and females respectively. There is evidence to suggest that gonadotoxic chemotherapy is associated with a reduction in inhibin B levels in adult males,[54] presumably indicating reduced sperm production.[52] However, this relationship has not been clearly demonstrated in childhood and

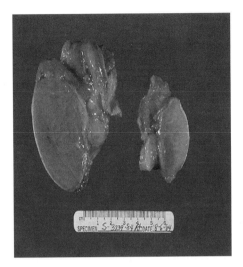

Fig. 13.3 Testicular atrophy following gonadotoxic therapy. Normal testis on left, atrophied testis on right.

adolescence,[51] and it remains to be seen whether inhibin B will become a useful tool in the fertility assessment of these patients in the future.

In female patients there is also much interest in anti-Mullerian hormone (AMH) as a potential marker of ovarian reserve. AMH is a glycoprotein that is predominantly expressed in the fetal testis, causing regression of the Mullerian ducts.[55] However, in females it is produced by the granulosa cells of preantral and small antral follicles, and serum levels of AMH correlate with ovarian follicular reserve.[56] Indeed, AMH levels are lower in female cancer survivors[50] and may therefore contribute to the assessment of gonadal function in this patient group.

Options for fertility preservation

Preservation of fertility is dictated by sexual maturity, and currently the only established options are cryopreservation of spermatozoa in the male and of oocytes in the female, or of embryos in those with a partner.

Male patients

Semen cryopreservation is particularly problematic in the adolescent population. Sperm banking is not universally practised in paediatric oncology centres, and there are very few suitable 'adolescent-friendly' facilities. Following confirmation of a diagnosis of malignancy, cancer therapy is usually required to commence as soon as possible. After having received such devastating news regarding the diagnosis, it can often be very difficult for teenagers to then discuss fertility and their thoughts about having children and subsequently produce a semen specimen. Discussions must therefore be handled with sensitivity, using appropriate language which the patient understands. On the positive side, however, many patients and their families derive benefit from open discussion regarding fertility, particularly as this places emphasis on looking to the future and provides reassurance that curative treatment is the aim.[57]

Semen specimens are usually produced by masturbation. However, should this not be possible, sperm may be retrieved following testicular or epididymal aspiration. Rectal electrostimulation techniques under anaesthetic can also be used.

The semen specimens produced in adolescence are frequently of poor quality.[58] Many patients will have only recently commenced spermarche, which may partially explain this, but many other factors contribute. The disease itself may impair semen quality, as discussed above. Psychological stress, nearly always present after a diagnosis of cancer, can also impair spermatogenesis.[59] The freeze–thawing process used for cryopreservation can then cause further damage, resulting in impaired sperm motility[60] and damage to chromatin structure and sperm morphology.[61]

Following cryopreservation, stored spermatozoa are subsequently used to produce offspring via *in vitro* fertilization (IVF). With advances in assisted reproduction techniques, particularly intracytoplasmic sperm injection (ICSI), which involves the injection of a single spermatozoon directly into an oocyte, the problems of low sperm numbers and poor motility may be circumvented.[62,63]

All male patients who are able to produce semen should have the opportunity of sperm banking prior to the commencement of cancer treatment. If the production of semen is not possible, alternative methods of sperm retrieval should be considered if the likelihood of infertility is significant and the patient is sufficiently mature, both physically (testicular volume greater than 10 ml) and emotionally, with a demonstrable understanding of what is involved and why cryopreservation is being offered.

For patients who have not yet commenced puberty, the options for fertility preservation remain entirely experimental at present. However, with ongoing research efforts, there is optimism for these patients in the future.

Although the prepubertal testis does not produce mature spermatozoa, it does contain the diploid stem germ cells from which haploid spermatozoa will ultimately be derived. Therefore, in theory, testicular tissue could be harvested prior to gonadotoxic cancer therapy and cryopreserved. Following cure and on entering adulthood, this tissue could be thawed and used in one of two ways in order to produce offspring. Firstly, the stored germ cells could be reimplanted into the patient's own testes in order to restore natural fertility, a procedure known as germ cell transplantation.[64] Alternatively, the stored cells could be matured *in vitro* until they are able to achieve fertilization using ICSI.

Whilst these techniques have enormous potential, they are associated with a number of problems that must be addressed before their clinical application. Optimal techniques for obtaining the tissue and the subsequent cryopreservation process are uncertain at present. In addition, the procedure for returning the germ cells to the testis for germ cell transplantation has yet to be established.

However, one of the most important issues to be addressed with auto-transplantation is that it requires tissue that was removed from a patient with cancer before treatment to be returned to the patient following cure. There is, therefore, a risk of reintroducing malignant cells, with potentially fatal consequences. This is unlikely to occur with malignancies such as Hodgkin's disease, which is often localized at presentation, but the risk would be substantial with haematological malignancies,[65] in which the testes can act as sanctuary sites for leukaemic cells. In principle, any theoretical risk of returning cancer cells following treatment, however small, is not acceptable.

The technique of maturing stem germ cells *in vitro* would circumvent this risk. However, although the restoration of fertility following *in vitro* spermatogenesis has been reported,[66] this process involved maturation from the later stages of spermatogenesis rather than from stem cells. Indeed, it appears unlikely that *in vitro* maturation of diploid stem cells into haploid spermatozoa will be technically possible in the near future.

An alternative to these techniques in the prepubertal patient is hormonal manipulation. Because cytotoxic treatment acts principally on rapidly dividing cells, it has been postulated that by rendering the testes quiescent with hormonal treatments, the germ cells will be less susceptible to the cytotoxic effects. Although this technique, based on suppression of the hypothalamic–pituitary–gonadal axis, has been successful in rodent models treated with chemotherapy and radiotherapy,[67,68] clinical trials have thus far failed to demonstrate any benefit.[69,70] There may be a number of reasons for the lack of protection afforded to humans, but recent evidence suggests that the proliferation of germ cells in prepubertal primates is actually gonadotrophin-independent.[71] Therefore, hormonal manipulation based on suppression of this axis is unlikely to be protective in patients receiving gonadotoxic therapy. Studies are currently in progress in order to identify what factors do regulate spermatogonial proliferation, with the hope that these may offer novel targets of gonadal protection during cytotoxic therapy.

Female patients

At present there are only two established practices of fertility preservation in female patients receiving gonadotoxic cancer therapy.

Firstly, young women who are due to receive pelvic irradiation may have their ovaries shielded, or indeed removed from the radiation field, a procedure known as oophoropexy. This can be performed laparoscopically,[72] with the ovaries placed behind the uterus or into the paracolic gutters, or can involve transfer to a distant site within the body.[73] However, although ovarian function may be preserved with such techniques in carefully selected patients, radiation-induced uterine damage may reduce the chances of carrying a successful pregnancy.

Secondly, fertility may be preserved by collection of mature oocytes before gonadotoxic therapy for IVF and subsequent embryo cryopreservation. This method is only applicable to sexually mature females, and requires a partner or donor sperm for fertilization. For women without a partner, cryopreservation of mature oocytes is an alternative option, but subsequent pregnancy rates are significantly lower as these cells sustain more damage during the freeze–thaw process than do embryos.[74] These techniques, however, are not suitable for the majority of cancer patients as they require a period of ovarian hyperstimulation for several weeks, which will inevitably delay the commencement of treatment. In addition, this method is inappropriate for adolescent and prepubertal patients, in whom all fertility preservation strategies remain experimental at present.

Although mature oocytes cannot be harvested from this group of patients, ovarian tissue containing germ cells could be removed and stored prior to gonadotoxic therapy. Following cure this tissue could either be returned to the patient by autotransplantation or matured *in vitro* to produce offspring by IVF, in a manner similar to that proposed in male patients at this age.

Ovarian tissue can be removed by either taking multiple biopsies from the ovary or by performing an oophorectomy. However, perhaps the most promising technique is the harvesting of ovarian cortical strips. This can be done laparoscopically, and this tissue is rich in primordial follicles. Poirot and colleagues[75] have reported their experience of cryopreservation of ovarian tissue in women exposed to gonadotoxic treatments. Ovarian tissue was cryopreserved in 31 of 51 patients assessed. The patients were aged from 2.7 to 34 years and 16 of them were under 18 years old. In 24 cases a whole ovary was harvested by laparoscopy or laparotomy and in seven approximately half the ovary was removed. Ovarian cortex histology was performed for all patients. In patients under 7 years old the mean number of primordial and primary follicles was $20.36/mm^2$ ($n = 6$). This decreased to $4.13/mm^2$ for patients aged between 10 and 15 years ($n = 8$) and to $1.63/mm^2$ for those over 15 years ($n = 17$). Only nine of the 31 patients had not received previous chemotherapy and no data on long-term ovarian function are presented. The authors conclude that cryopreservation of ovarian tissue may be offered to women at risk of ovarian damage, and that younger patients should be given priority.

Autologous transplantation of this tissue would aim to both restore natural fertility and maintain sex steroid production. Cortical strips are ideal for this purpose as the tissue survives cryopreservation and undergoes revascularization on return.[76] The feasibility of this process has been demonstrated in sheep,[77] with both the return of ovarian hormonal activity and the subsequent production of offspring. The success of such techniques in animal models has led to similar procedures being attempted in adult females.

The first attempt at reimplantation of ovarian cortical strips into a patient following gonadotoxic therapy did result in a return of ovarian function, but this was only temporary and did not result in the restoration of fertility.[78] Although further experimentation in sheep has suggested that ovarian function may be maintained long term after autotransplantation,[79] it seems likely that ovarian grafts will have a limited life span.

Oktay and colleagues[80] have since demonstrated the return of sex steroid production following heterotopic transplantation. Ovarian cortical strips, removed following oophorectomy in two patients, either as part of treatment or before gonadotoxic therapy, were reimplanted into the forearm. Transplantation into this site allows percutaneous aspiration of ovarian follicles, and indeed a metaphase I oocyte was obtained in this manner. The recent reports by Oktay and colleagues,[81] of human embryo development after heterotopic transplantation of cryopreserved ovarian tissue, and of Donnez and colleagues,[82] of a live birth after orthotopic transplantation of cryopreserved ovarian tissue, are important advances in demonstrating that it may be realistic to preserve ovarian function after sterilizing treatment.

Although these reports are extremely encouraging, and offer significant hope to adolescent cancer patients, a number of issues remain to be clarified before the widespread clinical application of these techniques. Perhaps the greatest concern, as with male patients in whom germ cell transplantation may be considered, is the potential to return malignant cells back to the patient following cure. This is of particular importance in patients with haematological malignancies,[83] but any theoretical risk, however small, is unlikely to be acceptable.

Oocyte maturation *in vitro*, followed by assisted reproduction, would eliminate this risk. Techniques to artificially mature oocytes, even from early stages of development, have yielded some success in murine models.[84,85] However, the clinical application of this procedure would be most beneficial in adolescent cancer patients if it were possible to artificially mature primordial follicles, as these are abundant within the ovarian cortical strips. At present little is known about the support required for this process to occur using human tissue,[86] and the clinical potential of this technique may therefore take some time to be fully realized.

Opportunities for preserving fertility in these patients must be grasped, even though the potential of these strategies is yet to be fully realized. However, it is equally essential to work within acceptable guidelines, and a working party from the Royal College of Obstetricians and Gynaecologists (RCOG) has published a comprehensive document[87] outlining standards of best practice regarding the collection and future use of such tissue. It would be inappropriate to recommend ovarian tissue harvesting for all girls and young women who require cytotoxic treatment, and thus suitable patients should be carefully selected. Suggested criteria for this selection process, based on the RCOG working group report, are outlined in Table 13.3.[81,82]

Table 13.3 Edinburgh criteria for selection of patients for cryopreservation of ovarian cortical tissue

Age ≤30 years
No previous chemotherapy/radiotherapy (if aged <15 years consider if previous 'low-risk' chemotherapy)
A realistic chance of long-term survival
A high risk of treatment-induced immediate ovarian failure (estimated at >50%)
Informed consent (from patient or, in the case of an incompetent child, from the parents)
Negative HIV and hepatitis serology
No existing children

It is emphasized that these criteria are based on multidisciplinary discussion and the RCOG working group report. They are for guidance only, with each patient assessed individually, and should be updated in the light of emerging evidence and experience.

As in male patients, an alternative strategy to protect the gonads from cytotoxic damage has been attempted by suppression of ovarian activity, using GnRH analogues to suppress the hypothalamic–pituitary–ovarian axis. Gonadal protection from alkylating agents has been demonstrated in both primate models and clinical studies using this technique,[88,89] and thus the coadministration of GnRH analogues in patients receiving these agents may be beneficial. However, primordial follicles are not under the influence of gonadotrophins and therefore a decline in their numbers will not be affected by such strategies. Indeed, this technique offers no protection against radiation-induced damage.[90]

The decline in follicle numbers is by apoptosis and therefore inhibition of this process may preserve ovarian function. Murine studies have demonstrated that disruption of the gene encoding acid sphingomyelinase, or treatment with sphingosine-1-phosphate, attenuates apoptotic destruction of primordial fetal oocytes, causing an increase in numbers of primordial follicles at birth.[91] These oocytes demonstrated resistance to both chemotherapy- and radiotherapy-induced apoptosis. Although this approach is potentially interesting, inhibiting apoptosis in such patients may be associated with serious adverse effects, and thus further studies in animal models are required.

Offspring of cancer survivors

Whilst these strategies offer real hope of improved fertility prospects for patients, consideration must be given to the offspring subsequently produced. Concerns have been raised that the mutagenic potential of cancer therapy could predispose children of patients who receive such treatment to congenital abnormalities, or even to cancer themselves. A large epidemiological study has failed to demonstrate any such link,[92] except in those with familial malignances. However, these offspring resulted from natural conception and it remains to be seen if problems may arise from the use of assisted reproduction techniques, whereby the natural selection processes of normal sexual reproduction are circumvented. Long-term surveillance of future offspring is therefore essential.

Many of the experimental strategies discussed above will use ICSI as a fertilization technique. As nuclear material from a sperm is injected directly into an oocyte, natural mechanisms that prevent either sperm or oocytes with defective DNA from being involved in fertilization are bypassed. Indeed, offspring born using ICSI do have a higher incidence of chromosomal abnormalities, particularly of the sex chromosomes.[93] However, rather than the technique itself predisposing to these abnormalities, the increased incidence is felt to reflect the higher rate of constitutional chromosomal abnormalities observed in infertile couples using ICSI. These problems may therefore be less likely in cancer survivors as their infertility is secondary to gonadotoxic treatment. Indeed, a recent study has demonstrated that sperm from men previously treated for childhood cancer do not carry a greater burden of damaged DNA compared with sperm from age-matched controls.[34] This provides some reassurance with regard to the use of spermatozoa from oligospermic men following cancer therapy.

Offspring born using ICSI are at an increased risk of congenital malformations[94] and low birth weight.[95] Although this can be partially explained by associated factors, such as maternal age and multiple births, it emphasizes the need for ongoing follow-up studies of children born after the use of assisted reproduction technology.

Ethical and legal issues

Harvesting gonadal tissue for future use, and indeed the other techniques discussed above to improve future fertility, are exciting prospects that provide hope for adolescents with cancer. Although there are still many scientific and technical issues to resolve, this technology also raises a number of important ethical and legal issues, which must be addressed before these procedures are used in a clinical setting.

Of prime importance, when considering options for future fertility following cancer treatment, must be that any decision is taken in the patient's best interests. Thus, the advantages of any intervention, or of an active decision not to intervene, must outweigh any disadvantages, both in the short and the long term. Attempts to preserve fertility must not raise unrealistic expectations and must not have undue adverse effects in either the patient or any subsequent offspring.

Comparing potential benefits with long-term risks is particularly problematic in this situation. The effectiveness of therapeutic intervention is still unknown at present, and it will be many years until expertise has improved sufficiently to assess it realistically. However, unless these techniques are considered and appropriate methods offered now, the opportunity of fertility preservation will be missed. Deleterious effects will also take many years to fully evaluate, particularly with respect to future progeny. Thus, fertility preservation must be considered in the context of clinical benefit within the management of adolescent cancer, and also in the context of ongoing research. Valid consent to perform these procedures is therefore both a legal and an ethical requirement.

For consent to be valid it must be informed, obtained voluntarily and given by a competent person. Legal competence to consent requires that the individual giving it is able to understand the information given, believes it applies to them, retains it, and uses it to make an informed choice. In view of the complexity of the issues surrounding fertility preservation, the anxieties of both patients and their families at the time of diagnosis, and the limited time for discussion due to the urgency of commencing treatment, the validity of such consent may be compromised.

The issue of valid consent is further complicated by the age of the patient involved and their degree of understanding of the issues being discussed. Young persons over the age of 16 years in Scotland and 18 years in England and Wales may consent to treatment under the Family Law Reform Act (1969). Otherwise consent is obtained by proxy, from a parent or legal guardian. Younger patients may give valid consent if they demonstrate sufficient understanding and intelligence to enable them to make an informed decision – so-called Gillick competence.[96] However, with respect to the storage and future use of gametes, consent by proxy is specifically excluded by the Human Fertilisation and Embryology Act (HFEA).[97] Thus, parents, or legal guardians, cannot give consent on behalf of the child. However, immature germ cells, which include both those from prepubertal males and primordial follicles from ovarian cortical strips, are not within the HFEA definition of a gamete as they are unable to take part in fertilization. Therefore these cells could be harvested with parental consent, if the procedure were in the patient's best interests. If this immature material were subsequently matured to produce gametes this tissue would then fall under the jurisdiction of the HFEA and the patient's informed consent would be required.

Consent in situations such as this should be viewed as a dynamic, continual process that is adapted as new information becomes available. Indeed, obtaining consent in different stages may alleviate many of the difficulties discussed above.[98] The first stage of consent would be for the harvest and storage of the gonadal tissue. The second stage, at a later date, would involve consent for the use of stored germ cell material for both fertilization and research. In addition, it is important to obtain consent at the time of collection for what should happen to gonadal tissue in the event of the patient's death. Whilst some would advocate destruction of the tissue in this situation, others have suggested allowing the parents to give consent for the tissue to be used for research purposes.[99] Ownership of the gonadal tissue in this situation should not be transferred to the patient's relatives.

These issues must be addressed in order that new techniques are adequately regulated. Following extensive, collaborative discussion within a multidisciplinary setting, a number of recommendations have been suggested.[99,100] These include ongoing, structured research with centralization of data and rapid dissemination of results, a rigorous review of procedures and development of the process of obtaining informed consent. This will ensure that adolescents with cancer have a realistic and safe prospect for fertility in the future.

Conclusions

Whilst many adolescents diagnosed with cancer can now realistically hope for long-term survival, they must often live with the consequences of achieving cure. Infertility is one of the most devastating adverse effects of cancer treatment in this patient group, and it is therefore imperative to consider methods of protecting or restoring fertility at an early stage.

Both chemotherapy and radiotherapy can impair future fertility, and treatments for certain cancers can be sterilizing. Although the prediction of future fertility following treatment is extremely difficult, there is currently much interest in potential markers of gonadal damage that may, in the future, be of use in adolescence.

Although strategies exist for fertility preservation in sexually mature patients, there is very little to offer younger patients who are at risk of infertility following treatment. However, a number of potential therapeutic interventions are the focus of much research attention, and although many scientific, technical, legal and ethical issues need to be addressed, there is genuine hope for adolescent cancer survivors in the future.[101]

References

1 Stiller C. Epidemiology of cancer in adolescents. *Med Pediatr Oncol* 2002; **39**: 149–155.

2 Mertens AC, Yasui Y, Neglia JP *et al*. Late mortality experience in five-year survivors of childhood and adolescent cancer: the Childhood Cancer Survivor Study. *J Clin Oncol* 2001; **19**: 3163–3172.

3 Campbell J, Wallace WHB, Bhatti LA *et al*. Childhood cancer in Scotland: trends in incidence, mortality and survival 1975–1999. Edinburgh: NHS Scotland Information and Statistics Division, 2004.

4 Scottish Intercollegiate Guidelines Network. Guideline 76: Long term follow up care of survivors of childhood cancer. Scottish Intercollegiate Guidelines Network, 2004.

5 Waring AB, Wallace WHB. Subfertility following treatment for childhood cancer. *Hosp Med* 2000; **61**: 550–557.

6 Barber HR. The effect of cancer and its therapy upon fertility. *Int J Fertil* 1981; **26**: 250–259.

7 Green T. Having a brain tumour: a journey through life. *Med Pediatr Oncol* 2002; **39**: 195–197.

8 Meistrich ML, Finch M, da Cunha MF, Hacker U, Au WW. Damaging effects of fourteen chemotherapeutic drugs on mouse testis cells. *Cancer Res* 1982; **42**: 122–131.

9 Bucci LR, Meistrich ML. Effects of busulfan on murine spermatogenesis: cytotoxicity, sterility, sperm abnormalities, and dominant lethal mutations. *Mutat Res* 1987; **176**: 259–268.

10 Kangasniemi M, Huhtaniemi I, Meistrich ML. Failure of spermatogenesis to recover despite the presence of A spermatogonia in the irradiated $LBNF_1$ rat. *Biol Reprod* 1996; **54**: 1200–1208.

11 Whitehead E, Shalet SM, Jones PH, Beardwell CG, Deakin DP. Gonadal function after combination chemotherapy for Hodgkin's disease in childhood. *Arch Dis Child* 1982; **57**: 287–291.

12 Relander T, Cavallin-Stahl E, Garwicz S, Olsson AM, Willen M. Gonadal and sexual function in men treated for childhood cancer. *Med Pediatr Oncol* 2000; **35**: 52–63.

13 Chemes HE. Infancy is not a quiescent period of testicular development. *Int J Androl* 2001; **24**: 2–7.

14 Whitehead E, Shalet SM, Blackledge G *et al.* The effect of combination chemotherapy on ovarian function in women treated for Hodgkin's disease. *Cancer* 1983; **52**: 988–993.

15 Wallace WH, Shalet SM, Crowne EC, Morris-Jones PH, Gattamaneni HR. Ovarian failure following abdominal irradiation in childhood: natural history and prognosis. *Clin Oncol (R Coll Radiol)* 1989; **1**: 75–79.

16 Speiser B, Rubin P, Casarett G. Aspermia following lower truncal irradiation in Hodgkin's disease. *Cancer* 1973; **32**: 692–698.

17 Clifton DK, Bremner WJ. The effect of testicular x-irradiation on spermatogenesis in man. A comparison with the mouse. *J Androl* 1983; **4**: 387–392.

18 Centola GM, Keller JW, Henzler M, Rubin P. Effect of low-dose testicular irradiation on sperm count and fertility in patients with testicular seminoma. *J Androl* 1994; **15**: 608–613.

19 Shalet SM, Tsatsoulis A, Whitehead E, Read G. Vulnerability of the human Leydig cell to radiation damage is dependent upon age. *J Endocrinol* 1989; **120**: 161–165.

20 Castillo LA, Craft AW, Kernahan J, Evans RG, Aynsley-Green A. Gonadal function after 12-Gy testicular irradiation in childhood acute lymphoblastic leukaemia. *Med Pediatr Oncol* 1990; **18**: 185–189.

21 Leiper AD, Stanhope R, Lau T. The effect of total body irradiation and bone marrow transplantation during childhood and adolescence on growth and endocrine function. *Br J Haematol* 1987; **67**: 419–426.

22 Wallace WH, Shalet SM, Hendry JH, Morris-Jones PH, Gattamaneni HR. Ovarian failure following abdominal irradiation in childhood: the radiosensitivity of the human oocyte. *Br J Radiol* 1989; **62**: 995–998.

23 Sanders JE, Hawley J, Levy W. Pregnancies following high-dose cyclophosphamide with or without high-dose busulfan or total-body irradiation and bone marrow transplantation. *Blood* 1996; **87**: 3045–3052.

24 Bath LE, Critchley HO, Chambers SE *et al.* Ovarian and uterine characteristics after total body irradiation in childhood and adolescence: response to sex steroid replacement. *Br J Obstet Gynaecol* 1999; **106**: 1265–1272.

25 Faddy MJ, Gosden RG. A model conforming the decline in follicle numbers to the age of menopause in women. *Hum Reprod* 1996; **11**: 1484–1486.

26 Wallace WHB, Thomson AB, Kelsey TW. The radiosensitivity of the human oocyte. *Hum Reprod* 2003; **18**: 117–121.

27 Critchley HO, Wallace WH, Shalet SM *et al.* Abdominal irradiation in childhood: the potential for pregnancy. *Br J Obstet Gynaecol* 1992; **99**: 392–394.

28 Littley MD, Shalet SM, Beardwell CG, Robinson EL, Sutton ML. Radiation-induced hypopituitarism is dose-dependent. *Clin Endocrinol* 1989; **31**: 363–373.

29 Hall JE, Martin KA, Whitney HA, Landy H, Crowley WF Jr. Potential for fertility with replacement of hypothalamic gonadotrophin-releasing hormone in long term female survivors of cranial tumors. *J Clin Endocrinol Metab* 1994; **79**: 1166–1172.

30 Mackie EJ, Radford M, Shalet SM. Gonadal function following chemotherapy for childhood Hodgkin's disease. *Med Pediatr Oncol* 1996; **27**: 74–78.

31 Wallace WH, Shalet SM, Lendon M, Morris-Jones PH. Male fertility in long-term survivors of childhood acute lymphoblastic leukaemia. *Int J Androl* 1991; **14**: 312–319.

32 Wallace WH, Shalet SM, Crowne EC, Morris-Jones PH, Gattamaneni HR, Price DA. Gonadal dysfunction due to cis-platinum. *Med Pediatr Oncol* 1989; **17**: 409–413.

33 Kreuser ED, Xiros N, Hetzel WD, Heimpel H. Reproductive and endocrine gonadal capacity in patients treated with COPP chemotherapy for Hodgkin's disease. *J Cancer Res Clin Oncol* 1987; **113**: 260–266.

34 Thomson AB, Campbell AJ, Irvine DS *et al.* Semen quality and spermatozoal DNA integrity in survivors of childhood cancer: a case-control study. *Lancet* 2002; **360**: 361–367.

35 Gerl A, Muhlbayer D, Hansmann G, Mraz W, Hiddemann W. The impact of chemotherapy on Leydig cell function in long term survivors of germ cell tumors. *Cancer* 2001; **91**: 1297–1303.

36 Thomson AB, Wallace WH. Treatment of paediatric Hodgkin's disease: a balance of risks. *Eur J Cancer* 2002; **38**: 468–477.

37 Viviani S, Santoro A, Ragni G, Bonfante V, Bestetti O, Bonadonna G. Gonadal toxicity after combination chemotherapy for Hodgkin's disease. Comparative results of MOPP vs ABVD. *Eur J Cancer Clin Oncol* 1985; **21**: 601–605.

38 Anselmo AP, Cartoni C, Bellantuono P *et al.* Risk of infertility in patients with Hodgkin's disease treated with ABVD vs. MOPP vs. ABVD/MOPP. *Haematologica* 1990; **75**: 155–158.

39 Longo DL, Glatstein E, Duffey PL. Alternating MOPP and ABVD chemotherapy plus mantle-field radiation therapy in patients with massive mediastinal Hodgkin's disease. *J Clin Oncol* 1997; **15**: 3338–3346.

40 Chiarelli AM, Marrett LD, Darlington G. Early menopause and infertility in females after treatment for childhood cancer diagnosed in 1964–1988 in Ontario, Canada. *Am J Epidemiol* 1999; **150**: 245–254.

41 Bryne J, Fears TR, Gail MH. Early menopause in long-term survivors of cancer during adolescence. *Am J Obstet Gynecol* 1992; **166**: 788–793.

42 Rueffer U, Breuer K, Josting A. Male gonadal dysfunction in patients with Hodgkin's disease prior to treatment. *Ann Oncol* 2001; **12**: 1307–1311.

43 Hallak J, Mahran A, Chae J, Agarwal A. The effects of cryopreservation on semen from men with sarcoma or carcinoma. *J Assist Reprod Genet* 2000; **17**: 218–221.

44 Agarwal A, Shekarriz M, Sidhu RK, Thomas AJ Jr. Value of clinical diagnosis in predicting the quality of cryopreserved sperm from cancer patients. *J Urol* 1996; **155**: 934–938.

45 Pal L, Leykin L, Schifren JL. Malignancy may adversely influence the quality and behaviour of oocytes. *Hum Reprod* 1998; **13**: 1837–1840.

46 Marmor D, Duyck F. Male reproductive potential after MOPP therapy for Hodgkin's disease: a long-term survey. *Andrologia* 1995; **27**: 99–106.

47 Nasir J, Walton C, Lindow SW, Masson EA. Spontaneous recovery of chemotherapy-induced primary ovarian failure: implications for management. *Clin Endocrinol* 1997; **46**: 217–219.

48 Tanner JM. *Growth at Adolescence*, 2nd edn. Oxford: Blackwell Science, 1962.

49 Siimes MA, Rautonen J. Small testicles with impaired production of sperm in adult male survivors of childhood malignancies. *Cancer* 1990; **65**: 1303–1306.

50 Bath LE, Wallace WH, Shaw MP, Fitzpatrick C, Anderson RA. Depletion of ovarian reserve in young women after treatment for cancer in childhood: detection by anti-Mullerian hormone, inhibin B and ovarian ultrasound. *Hum Reprod* 2003; **18**: 2368–2374.

51 Crofton PM, Thomson AB, Evans AEM. Is inhibin B a potential marker of gonado-toxicity in prepubertal children treated for cancer? *Clin Endocrinol* 2003; **58**: 296–301.

52 Anderson RA, Sharpe RM. Regulation of inhibin production in the human male and its clinical applications. *Int J Androl* 2000; **23**: 136–144.

53 Roberts VJ, Barth S, el-Roeiy A, Yen SS. Expression of inhibin/activin subunits and follistatin messenger ribonucleic acids and proteins in ovarian follicles and the corpus luteum during the human menstrual cycle. *J Clin Endocrinol Metab* 1993; **77**: 1402–1410.

54 Wallace EM, Groome NP, Riley SC, Parker AC, Wu FC. Effects of chemotherapy-induced testicular damage on inhibin, gonadotrophin, and testosterone secretion: a prospective longitudinal study. *J Clin Endocrinol Metab* 1997; **82**: 3111–3115.

55 Lee MM, Donahoe PK. Mullerian inhibiting substance: a gonadal hormone with multiple functions. *Endocr Rev* 1993; **14**: 152–164.

56 van Rooij IA, Broekmans FJ, te Velde ER. Serum anti-Mullerian hormone levels: a novel measure of ovarian reserve. *Hum Reprod* 2002; **17**: 3065–3071.

57 Wallace WHB, Thomson AB. Preservation of fertility in children treated for cancer. *Arch Dis Child* 2003; **88**: 493–496.

58 Postovsky S, Lightman A, Aminpour D *et al.* Sperm cryopreservation in adolescents with newly diagnosed cancer. *Med Pediatr Oncol* 2003; **40**: 355–359.

59 Clarke RN, Klock SC, Geoghegan A, Travassos DE. Relationship between psychological stress and semen quality among in-vitro fertilization patients. *Hum Reprod* 1999; **14**: 753–758.

60 Alvarez JG, Storey BT. Evidence for increased lipid peroxidative damage and loss of superoxide dismutase activity as a mode of sublethal cryodamage to human sperm during cryopreservation. *J Androl* 1992; **13**: 232–241.

61 Hammadeh ME, Askari AS, Georg T, Rosenbaum P, Schmidt W. Effect of freeze-thawing procedure on chromatin stability, morphological alteration and membrane integrity of human spermatozoa in fertile and subfertile men. *Int J Androl* 1999; **22**: 155–162.

62 Chen SU, Ho HN, Chen HF *et al.* Pregnancy achieved by intracytoplasmic sperm injection using cryopreserved semen from a man with testicular cancer. *Hum Reprod* 1996; **11**: 2645–2647.

63 Rosenlund B, Sjoblom P, Tornblom M, Hultling C, Hillensjo T. In-vitro fertilization and intracytoplasmic sperm injection in the treatment of infertility after testicular cancer. *Hum Reprod* 1998; **13**: 414–418.

64 Brinster RL, Zimmermann JW. Spermatogenesis following male germ-cell transplantation. *Proc Natl Acad Sci USA* 1994; **91**: 11298–11302.

65 Jahnukainen K, Hou M, Petersen C, Setchell B, Soder O. Intratesticular transplantation of testicular cells from leukemic rats causes transmission of leukemia. *Cancer Res* 2001; **61**: 706–710.

66 Tesarik J, Bahceci M, Ozcan C, Greco E, Mendoza C. Restoration of fertility by in-vitro spermatogenesis. *Lancet* 1999; **353**: 555–556.

67 Ward JA, Robinson J, Furr BJ, Shalet SM, Morris ID. Protection of spermatogenesis in rats from the cytotoxic procarbazine by the depot formulation of Zoladex, a gonadotropin-releasing hormone agonist. *Cancer Res* 1990; **50**: 568–574.

68 Kurdoglu B, Wilson G, Parchuri N, Ye WS, Meistrich ML. Protection from radiation-induced damage to spermatogenesis by hormone treatment. *Radiat Res* 1994; **139**: 97–102.

69 Waxman JH, Ahmed R, Smith D. Failure to preserve fertility in patients with Hodgkin's disease. *Cancer Chemother Pharmacol* 1987; **19**: 159–162.

70 Thomson AB, Anderson RA, Irvine DS *et al.* Investigation of suppression of the hypothalamic-pituitary-gonadal axis to restore spermatogenesis in azoospermic men treated for childhood cancer. *Hum Reprod* 2002; **17**: 1715–1723.

71 Kelnar CJ, McKinnell C, Walker M. Testicular changes during infantile 'quiescence' in the marmoset and their gonadotrophin dependence: a model for investigating susceptibility of the prepubertal human testis to cancer therapy? *Hum Reprod* 2002; **17**: 1367–1378.

72 Williams RS, Littell RD, Mendenhall NP. Laparoscopic oophoropexy and ovarian function in the treatment of Hodgkin disease. *Cancer* 1999; **86**: 2138–2142.

73 Leporrier M, von Theobald P, Roffe JL, Muller G. A new technique to protect ovarian function before pelvic irradiation. Heterotopic ovarian autotransplantation. *Cancer* 1987; **60**: 2201–2204.

74 Salha O, Picton H, Balen A, Rutherford A. Human oocyte cryopreservation. *Hosp Med* 2001; **62**: 18–24.

75 Poirot C, Vacher-Lavenu MC, Helardot P *et al.* Human ovarian tissue cryopreservation: indications and feasibility. *Hum Reprod* 2002; **17**: 1447–1452.

76 Gosden RG, Boulton MI, Grant K, Webb R. Follicular development from ovarian xenografts in SCID mice. *J Reprod Fertil* 1994; **101**: 619–623.

77 Gosden RG, Baird DT, Wade JC, Webb R. Restoration of fertility to oophorectomized sheep by ovarian autografts stored at −196 degrees C. *Hum Reprod* 1994; **9**: 597–603.

78 Radford JA, Lieberman BA, Brison DR. Orthotopic reimplantation of cryopreserved ovarian cortical strips after high-dose chemotherapy for Hodgkin's lymphoma. *Lancet* 2001; **357**: 1172–1175.

79 Baird DT, Webb R, Campbell BK, Harkness LM, Gosden RG. Long-term ovarian function in sheep after ovariectomy and transplantation of autografts stored at −196 C. *Endocrinology* 1999; **140**: 462–471.

80 Oktay K, Buyuk E, Rosenwaks Z, Rucinski J. A technique for transplantation of ovarian cortical strips to the forearm. *Fertil Steril* 2003; **80**: 193–198.

81 Oktay K, Buyuk E, Veeck L *et al.* Embryo development after heterotopic transplantation of cryopreserved ovarian tissue. *Lancet* 2004; **363**: 837–40.

82 Donnez J, Dolmans MM, Demylle D *et al.* Live birth after orthotopic transplantation of cryopreserved ovarian tissue. *Lancet* 2004; **364**: 1405–1410.

83 Shaw JM, Bowles J, Koopman P, Wood EC, Trounson AO. Fresh and cryopreserved ovarian tissue samples from donors with lymphoma transmit the cancer to graft recipients. *Hum Reprod* 1996; **11**: 1668–1673.

84 Spears N, Boland NI, Murray AA, Gosden RG. Mouse oocytes derived from in vitro grown primary ovarian follicles are fertile. *Hum Reprod* 1994; **9**: 527–532.

85 Eppig JJ, O'Brien MJ. Development in vitro of mouse oocytes from primordial follicles. *Biol Reprod* 1996; **54**: 197–207.

86 Picton HM, Danfour MA, Harris SE, Chambers EL, Huntriss J. Growth and maturation of oocytes in vitro. *Reprod Suppl* 2003; **61**: 445–462.

87 Royal College of Obstetricians and Gynaecologists. Storage of ovarian and prepubertal testicular tissue. Report of a working party. London: Royal College of Obstetricians and Gynaecologists, 2000.

88 Ataya K, Rao LV, Lawrence E, Kimmel R. Luteinizing hormone-releasing hormone agonist inhibits cyclophosphamide-induced ovarian follicular depletion in rhesus monkeys. *Biol Reprod* 1995; **52**: 365–372.

89 Blumenfeld Z, Avivi I, Linn S *et al*. Prevention of irreversible chemotherapy-induced ovarian damage in young women with lymphoma by a gonadotrophin-releasing hormone agonist in parallel to chemotherapy. *Hum Reprod* 1996; **11**: 1620–1626.

90 Gosden RG, Wade JC, Fraser HM, Sandow J, Faddy MJ. Impact of congenital or experimental hypogonadotrophism on the radiation sensitivity of the mouse ovary. *Hum Reprod* 1997; **12**: 2483–2488.

91 Morita Y, Perez GI, Paris F. Oocyte apoptosis is suppressed by disruption of the acid sphingomyelinase gene or by sphingosine-1-phosphate therapy. *Nat Med* 2000; **6**: 1109–1114.

92 Hawkins MM, Draper GJ, Smith RA. Cancer among 1,348 offspring of survivors of childhood cancer. *Int J Cancer* 1989; **43**: 975–978.

93 Bonduelle M, Van Assche E, Joris H. Prenatal testing in ICSI pregnancies: incidence of chromosomal anomalies in 1586 karyotypes and relation to sperm parameters. *Hum Reprod* 2002; **17**: 2600–2614.

94 Hansen M, Kurinczuk JJ, Bower C, Webb S. The risk of major birth defects after intracytoplasmic sperm injection and in vitro fertilization. *N Engl J Med* 2002; **346**: 725–730.

95 Schieve LA, Meikle SF, Ferre C *et al*. Low and very low birth weight in infants conceived with use of assisted reproductive technology. *N Engl J Med* 2002; **346**: 731–737.

96 Gillick v West Norfolk and Wisbech Area Authority. All England Law Reports, 1985; 402.

97 Human Fertilisation and Embryology Act 1990. Chapter 37. London: HMSO.

98 Grundy R, Larcher V, Gosden RG. Fertility preservation for children treated for cancer (2): ethics of consent for gamete storage and experimentation. *Arch Dis Child* 2001; **84**: 360–362.

99 Wallace WH, Walker DA. Conference consensus statement: ethical and research dilemmas for fertility preservation in children treated for cancer. *Hum Fertil (Camb)* 2001; **4**: 69–76.

100 A strategy for fertility services for survivors of childhood cancer. Consultation document. British Fertility Society.

101 Wallace WH, Anderson RA, Baird DT. Preservation of fertility in young women treated for cancer. *Lancet Oncol* 2004; **5**: 269–270.

CHAPTER 14

Body image

M. Woods and L. Shearer

The style of this presentation will be informal, with Marc Woods introducing the presentation and then interviewing Lindsay Shearer.

Introduction

Marc: Who in this room is normal? It is a strange question isn't it? Society tends to measure people against what they consider to be normal or average.

From here I can see people who are bald. I can see people who some would say are a little overweight. It probably makes them feel a little uncomfortable when I say those things, when I make them think about their body image.

I have been fortunate enough to represent Great Britain at the Paralympics, but when I tell people, they say 'Why, what is WRONG with you? You look normal'. I tell them that nothing is wrong with me. I just have one leg.

Today Lindsay and I are going to talk about body image and we are going to do that by referring to our own personal experiences.

During this presentation we are going to look at body image from three different perspectives:

- the physical
- the social and mental
- and then finally in terms of relationships and sexual attraction.

Physical

Marc: Both Lindsay and I had cancer as teenagers and we both had a leg amputated. Lindsay, perhaps you would like to explain how you felt during this time.

Lindsay: Just like me you have all probably had a moment in your lives when you are not happy with the way you look. Often we all have

one part of our body (if not more) that we don't like. When
you are ill this feeling can be intensified – you start to scrutinize
yourself and place a greater emphasis on how you look and how
others perceive you.

When I was ill, friends would visit me and say things like 'Oh,
you look much brighter today' or 'You look good'. Look good, look
better, how? I have no hair; a nosebleed that won't stop as my
platelets are low; my eyes are all bloodshot; I'm tired and anaemic.
I have lines coming out of every possible vein. I can't walk and
I have lost so much weight I look like a boy! Just don't give me a
mirror, then I will really know what I look like – and whatever it is,
it isn't good!

There is more to body image than what you look like, more than
just accepting it. It is understanding yourself, loving yourself, being
yourself and adapting yourself to the environment and others. Yes,
it is all about me! But it is more than the physical image that meets
the eye: it goes much deeper.

As an adolescent, body image is a part of growing up, part of
human development. Fitting in and looking normal are sometimes
all that matters; it is the point in your life when you start to think
about make-up, fashion, height and weight and, of course, sexual
attractiveness. You want to fit in and not be teased or bullied, you
want to be liked. All this takes place when you are well; it is no
different when you are ill – you still want to fit in and be normal.
Having cancer might mean you can't wear the latest fashion or
join in the latest fad like rollerblading, or have the latest haircut.
All this can make a difference to feeling normal, but what is normal?
It is what we perceive it should be like.

Body image plays a large part in building our personality and self-
confidence as well as our relationships with others. How others
perceive us is important and our perceived abilities and disabilities
are often taken from a glimpse or first meeting, when all there is to
go by is what people see in front of them – body image. My body
image dominates my life; therefore my illness is never far behind
it – it is difficult to put the past to rest but it is possible to build on it
and take strength from it. A change in your body image is a constant reminder of your illness, be it temporary, like no hair; hidden,
like a scar, or on show like the loss of a limb.

Marc: Would you say that the physical side of body image was the most
difficult part to come to terms with?

Lindsay: The physical side of body image is probably the simplest and clearest
– it is either black or it is white – yet often it can be the hardest. You
know you look different from others and perhaps different from

how you perceived you would. Catching a glimpse of yourself in the mirror can be an upsetting part of being different. I would often forget that I was ill and had no hair or was so skinny. It didn't help that I was often mistaken for a boy. I still forget now that my body image is different from others, other than the fact that I walk on crutches I don't feel any different to everyone else. But when I catch my reflection in a window and see for myself how I walk I sometimes want to cringe, as I realize how different I do look, which can be hard to accept.

Marc: How did the medical staff prepare you for the changes in appearance that you were going to have to deal with?

Lindsay: My physical changes were all mentioned to me at the start of my treatment. I was told I would lose my hair, that I might lose or gain weight; I was also warned that if treatment didn't help I might lose my leg. I took it all on board and I accepted it from the start as I was lucky enough to be treated by people who spoke to me about my illness, but not my father. Staff were approachable and friendships and trust developed; they helped me to realize that everyday life went on. So it was all quite matter-of-fact, which helped me to take it in my stride, but I know that this is different in every case and some might prefer not to know, but I felt more in control knowing all the facts and theories! (As treatment doesn't always go to plan!) Scars were never really an issue for me – I knew I would have some, but it didn't really mean that much to me. Losing my hair wasn't really a trauma but I think to me it was all part and parcel of the illness. It could be very hard to accept as it is a constant reminder to you and others that life isn't quite going so well.

Marc: I find that if I wear shorts most people will stare at me and if I wear trousers they will not take a second glance. How does it make you fell when people react to the fact that you have one leg?

Lindsay: One of the hardest things to get used to was people staring at me. You don't mind young children as they are just being inquisitive; however, adults and elders can often be quite rude. I would feel obliged to explain why I looked different. To children I would say that my leg was poorly and the doctors took it away as they couldn't fix it. Ninety-nine per cent of the time when I am meeting new people I am happy to explain what happened – after all, it is part of what makes me Lindsay. However, people often assume it was an accident or from birth, and sometimes I will agree for a quiet life, especially if I am never going to see them again – that, or if they're annoying me I tell them it was an argument with a crocodile!

Marc: Why don't you wear an artificial leg? Wouldn't it make for an easier life?

Lindsay: Why don't I wear an artificial limb? To be honest it's because they're . . . not that good for a hindquarter amputee. I can do everything you can do on two legs with one, I can walk – albeit differently, but it is classed as walking – I can swim (maybe not as well as Marc!), I can play badminton and I can dance. But I cannot walk down the street and do my coat up at the same time when it starts to rain . . . It is small things like this that frustrate me, not what I look like. I am currently trying again at using an artificial limb, not for the way I look but more to look after the rest of me in preparation for ageing gracefully! I also want my hands back, as I sometimes feel that I haven't lost a leg but two arms! However, the limb is very restrictive. I can't play badminton in it, as I can just about get it to swing forwards and lock for me to put my weight on it; it is large and uncomfortable, and to be honest I feel more disabled when I wear it as I am more agile without it and I feel free and somehow normal!

Marc: There we are back to wanting to feel normal again! I wonder if we can now move on to some of the more social and mental issues. Do you feel that your treatment and operations affected your social development?

Social and mental

Lindsay: Depending on the age of diagnosis, your entire social development and education can be affected and drastically altered. Again, this deviates from the path that is perceived as normal and makes you feel different. Sometimes, ensuring you keep up with school work is a way of continuing routine and keeping in touch with friends and peers, keeping in touch with everyday life, reality. When I was ill it was like my life was on hold but everyone else around me carried on; I kind of felt left behind and in some cases forgotten. I sat some A-level exams whilst in hospital, as a great number of adolescents do.

I was eighteen, friends were going away to university, moving in with partners or following careers. I found this very difficult – socially I was being left behind but on the other hand I had to grow up faster. This image of uselessness and position of limbo made it difficult to meet new friends and keep in touch with old friends. However, now I have caught up. I went to university, which if it wasn't for my illness I wouldn't have done. I have since been back again and finished a master's degree. But again this was hard, meeting new people, making new friends, and conquering new challenges and environments to become accepted. As is the case in each major step in life, so my illness is never far behind me and my body image supplies the constant reminder.

Marc: How do you think your friends perceived you?

Lindsay: How I was perceived by even my closest friends varied. Some lost
               contact completely and felt they couldn't visit, as they wouldn't
               know what to say or if they would recognize me. Others said that I
               was still Lindsay and I was still there – you just had to look a little
               harder and talk a little longer to find me. Friends are an important
               part of adolescence – they provide social support and true friends
               will accept you for who you are, not what you look like. This is a
               first step in rebuilding self-worth and self-esteem; as people start to
               accept you, social anxiety is reduced and getting on with everyday
               life and fitting in becomes more achievable.

Marc: You say that friends had to look a little harder to find you. Do you
               think that your situation affected your ability to socially interact?

Lindsay: Having negative body image perceptions can affect social inter-
               action quite dramatically. Confidence is shaken, depression can
               occur and this can lead to psychological or psychosocial difficulties.
               I have always found it hard to meet new people but I would just
               throw myself into a situation and introduce myself even if inside
               I was feeling shy and embarrassed. Now I find it just as hard, and
               for a while at the back of my mind there was the question 'What
               am I doing? As if I don't stand out enough for being different
               now I'm drawing more attention to myself!' I have come to terms
               with this and I accept myself and I am usually the first to see the
               humorous side to things. People often have to look twice at me on
               a badminton court, as they aren't sure if they really saw someone
               with one leg.

Marc: You obviously love playing badminton now but was it initially
               difficult to start that type of activity?

Lindsay: At first it was difficult to take up social activities and be accepted,
               as again it was the initial image that I don't really look the type to
               play badminton! However, it was important to me to continue with
               my social interaction as I am quite an outdoors and active kind of girl
               but my body image doesn't communicate that message. This social
               and mental side of body image was a difficult hurdle for me as I felt
               I had to prove myself as capable, to others as well as myself. Since
               losing my leg I have taking up canoeing, done a tandem skydive,
               walked up and down Mount Snowdon and done a tandem paraglide
               – see, there I go again trying to prove myself capable! . . . I have
               had to make adjustments and find different ways of coping, both
               socially and mentally. I usually start an activity by dragging a friend
               along for moral support; however, I did make a conscious effort when
               I decided to have a go at water-skiing. I went along to the local
               centre on my own and gave it a go, which was a huge boost to my

self-confidence, despite the fact that I haven't been back. It made such a difference that now I don't think twice about trying new activities. I still feel awkward at times, but then I'll think 'why should I feel awkward – I'm the one who is getting out and enjoying life'. Just because I don't fit the mould doesn't mean I can't try things.

Marc: Earlier you mentioned that you sometimes make up stories as to how you lost your leg or you are happy to let people assume it was an accident. Is that because talking about cancer is another hurdle for you to climb?

Lindsay: Socially it is difficult, as once people hear the dreaded 'C' word they become worried they might upset you and clam up. Yes, C for Cancer – to you as an audience this is why we are here, and it has probably been said thousands of times in the last few days. But socially it is still not as accepted as we think. Especially in the same sentence as 'adolescent' or 'teenager'. Despite the increased diagnosis and public awareness, it still shocks people that as an adolescent you can suffer from cancer and how it affects your whole life, not just those few years of illness and treatment.

Negative thoughts or feelings about body image can lead to social avoidance. Research shows that a sense of euphoria is experienced immediately after treatment for beating the disease; this could be attributed to the positive physical changes occurring, such as hair growing back. However, these changes begin to slow and research also claims that several years after treatment the chances of negative body image, low self-worth and social anxiety are greater.

Marc: Is that something that you have found?

Lindsay: I found this to be the case as I analysed everything that was different in my life and how I couldn't follow the career I wanted due to my illness. I wanted to join the Royal Air Force, but this was not an option after my illness, and especially as my ill health was prolonged because of my leg. I was clear of cancer and was doing well in remission but I still couldn't put on weight as my leg made me quite weak. I couldn't see the end – it seemed my illness had gone but I was still ill. Being ill was easy; not being well was the hard part, as mentally I was still me but my body let me down and it put my life on hold.

There were times when I felt useless and worthless after my illness; I suppose in a way it was an anticlimax. After having the focus of my illness and working towards getting my health back for so long, I felt I had no focus and nothing to talk about – what had I done with my life? Oh yeah, it was on hold so nothing really for four years. I also felt I had failed with my physiotherapy. I had worked for so long to use my leg – and for what? It didn't work, I had no quality of life. Perhaps I blamed myself for being ill in the first place and for my leg not recovering as it should have.

Once I had decided to get a second opinion and agreed with my consultants that I was happy to take the option of amputation, I felt in control again. I thought the seriousness of the decision to amputate would affect me at certain points throughout the process, but each time it just felt the right thing to do, even on the morning of the operation.

Marc: Do you think that you tried to convince yourself that your life would just return back to normal?

Lindsay: In a way I did, but it is a different type of normal. Yes, it is normal because I do everything others do, but often it requires a little more grit and determination to do the simple things and find ways to adapt. Like carrying the ironing upstairs without needing to iron it all over again! This would sometimes get me down and trigger low self-esteem, as I would have to fail initially in order to go on and find another way of doing things. Ways which would sometimes make me feel different and negative, kind of like a freak. So for a while I blamed my body image for my failure, leading to feelings of low self-worth and increased social anxiety due to my perceived awkwardness. This, of course, was my perception of how others saw me, not how people actually perceived me.

It took a long time for me to change my mind-set to being more positive and sometimes I still have to lift myself out of the difficult times, just as everyone does in life. It took my interest in the outdoors to see that I could achieve much more through the challenge of finding ways to adapt. I decided to have a go at an obstacle course – yep, you know the ones, crawling under barbed wire, climbing over a wall and the old favourite, the cargo net. Well, I managed it and the fact I completed it gave others the inspiration to give it a go, despite their fear of heights. It was this that made me realize I can achieve more in my life through the challenge of accepting my body image and pushing it to the limits, just as any athlete does. This gave me the strength to accept myself as I am now, not as I thought I would be; that includes me accepting my body image before others can accept it – if I am positive so are others.

Relationships and sexual attraction

Marc: If it is okay with you I would like to ask you about relationships with friends and family. Have they changed?

Lindsay: Relationships with family and friends have changed. I know what is important to me and it is living my life my way, but I know my family have been through a great deal and I still think they find it hard to come to terms with my illness and how it has changed my life. My amputation is a stark and constant reminder, but it is often the centre of most jokes too. I am much closer to my father, brother and sister-in law. It was hard when I was ill, as when I was in hospital others would have their family visit them quite often, if not stay with them. However, my mother died when I was sixteen and I found this hard. We all know that the one person you turn to when you're ill is your mum, but I couldn't. My dad was great – he would visit when he could. I was treated in London so it wasn't like friends could pop in each day; my dad worked in London so when he was at work he could visit me in the evenings. It was hard for my family, as we had been through a similar thing with my mum and her illness. We are not a close family that lives in each other's pockets but we are closer now, and that means a lot.

My body image as others perceive it and as I think others perceive it, as well as my own perceptions of myself, have affected my relationships with friends and family. I know my family accepts me as I am and are grateful that I am still here to annoy them. I have true friends who will always be there for me. However, I find it quite difficult to make new friends as I feel protective of the real Lindsay and how I was before my illness – that part of my life is very important to me but do I hold on too much! Who knows?

I am conscious that my initial image of a disability, perhaps reliant on others, weak and awkward, does not portray the real me and it takes time to know the strong-minded, intelligent, adventurous, caring outdoor girl inside, who just wants to be loved and accepted as an equal.

Marc: Do you think that because people perceive you as a very strong-willed individual you have to act a certain way?

Lindsay: I do feel that I put on a much colder exterior and I find it difficult to let people in. I have had to cope with a lot but I am still vulnerable and I don't want to be hurt, so I can come across as confident and independent to the point that people think I want to be alone. Loneliness is a feeling that I have battled with throughout my illness. I have many friends and family but I can be in a crowded room and still feel alone. I believe this is due to the way I am, even if I hadn't been ill, but again it is increased through my situation. I find it difficult to express my feelings and most of all trust people. My illness and loss of confidence have attributed to the changes in the way I deal with people; I have and still get on well with my male friends. All my male friends have been great and encourage me to do mad things like walk up Mount Snowdon and go canoeing and caving, but they are quite protective too.

When it comes to relationships with a partner, well . . . I don't really have a great deal to say, as I am single and have been for the majority of the time since my illness. I don't know if this is due to my lack of confidence with my body image or if I am just very fussy! I think it is probably a mixture of the two. However, I find it difficult to approach guys; I feel very self-conscious about my body image when it comes to the opposite sex. I don't feel attractive and I appreciate it is a bit of a barrier. I know I would feel awkward and find it difficult if the roles were reversed.

Sex is an issue for adolescents anyway but when you don't feel very attractive it isn't really high on your priorities – but it is still important to address any worries or fears patients may have. It is not just the physical side to sex but the mental too. Sex was not on the agenda during my illness as again I was single throughout it and I didn't feel it was important at the time. But for others this might not be the case and having someone to ask those silly little questions is important. I was older, so perhaps this made it easier. After my illness I didn't find the physical side an issue – it was more the mental frustration again, lack of confidence and wanting to feel normal, instead of feeling awkward and unattractive.

If I am really honest I am probably apprehensive of the whole relationship thing, using my body image as an excuse to go along with me being too fussy. I am strong enough to realize that I don't need someone to make my life complete, but I know I want someone to share my life and future adventures with. Sometimes when I'm out with friends who are all either married, engaged or have a long-term partner, it brings it home and it will get me down, but only because they are times I want to share with someone special. Whenever we go out for a meal as a group of friends it is usually an odd number because of me. One frustration of this is that people don't mention it or comment – it is an accepted and expected fact that Lindsay will be going alone, but still I get the wedding invite which says Lindsay and guest! I suppose it is the easiest way for friends to deal with it.

Marc: And how do you see the future?

Lindsay: I am going to be 30 this year. I'm looking forward to it, firstly because there were times when I didn't think I would make it, so it is an important milestone in my life. Secondly, I am hoping it might just make me and others realize I am not ill or eighteen anymore! (Even though I feel it!) Thirdly, because it is a great excuse for a party! I often feel because I have been playing catch-up in life since my illness that I don't feel an adult, but that I am trapped in adolescence.

I am happy with myself and I wouldn't change for anyone, but sometimes I still feel left behind and alone whilst others have found someone to share their life with. I know this could be the case even if I wasn't ill and had two legs. Which brings me right back to blaming my body image for the way I am and wanting to feel normal, to be accepted and loved.

That said, I do care how people perceive me, but I just hope that one day I will meet someone special who will accept me and love me for being me.

Marc: Well I would like to thank you for being so frank and honest with us here today.

Lindsay: I hope that this has helped you realize that there is more to cancer than the illness itself – it never really leaves you, especially if your body image is altered. You just learn to adapt both mentally and physically to the environment and others. Some people find this easy, others may not, and those that you meet along the way can make it easier whilst others make it more of a challenge.

CHAPTER 15

The impact of cancer on adolescents and their families

K. L. Neville

Introduction

The developmental time span of adolescence reflects a tumultuous, challenging and complex time in life, beginning with the development of secondary sex characteristics and ending when young adult responsibilities and roles are assumed, some 10–12 years later. Adolescence is characterized by a complex interplay of several factors: biological maturation processes, psychological, cognitive and psychosocial development, and social change involving family, peers, school and workplaces.[1] It is classified into three phases: early (ages 11–14), middle (15–17) and late (18–20), each with a multitude of specific growth and developmental tasks to be achieved. When cancer strikes, adolescents face even greater difficulties, as illness-related stressors are superimposed on the normal physical and psychological stressors associated with this developmental period.[2] At a time when social emancipation, independence, autonomy, identity, peer relations and career goals are to be established, the diagnosis and treatment of cancer poses a significant threat to the achievement of these developmental tasks.[3]

As modern medical advances continue to improve the long-term survivorship of adolescents with cancer, attention to the psychosocial sequelae of having had cancer is ever more important. With more adolescents living longer and surviving cancer, there is an increased need to gain a better understanding of what the experience means and how that experience impacts on their lives, and that of their families, not just during their treatment but for long periods of time thereafter. This paper will reflect the components of a research programme devoted to examining the psychosocial impact of cancer on the adolescent during the period of diagnosis, 5–10 years after treatment, and in long-term survivorship.

In the initial study, which examined the impact of cancer during the diagnostic stage, a descriptive, correlational study was conducted to examine the influence of uncertainty and social support on psychological distress. An outcome of this initial work was the need to conduct an in-depth, qualitative inquiry with adolescent survivors of cancer to gain a more gestalt perspective of their cancer experience, rather than a mechanistic view of albeit critical variables pertaining to the psychosocial adjustment of adolescents with cancer. An in-depth inquiry, using the grounded theory approach, was conducted to examine the impact of surviving cancer on adolescent development more fully. Young adults who had survived teenage cancer described their experiences poignantly and how those experiences shaped their lives. Survivors of adolescent cancer described how social support and uncertainty in illness changed over time and, in general, how their lives were transformed by their cancer experience. As discovered during the in-depth interviews with young adult survivors of adolescent cancer, numerous family members expressed their strong desire to tell their stories about their experiences of having a child survive malignant disease. Research was carried out to investigate the family's perspective of the impact of their child's cancer experience on the family unit. Desire to revisit the experience through verbalization was varied; some family members communicated the need to discuss and share, while others expressed their desire to avoid discussing their experience at all. Although more detailed findings are reported elsewhere,[4-6] specific concepts and findings identified in this research programme will be addressed here.

Psychological distress

Although estimates of the prevalence of psychological distress among individuals with cancer cover a broad range, psychological distress is a frequent sequel to the diagnosis of cancer.[7] Despite methodological concerns regarding the measurement of psychosocial function in this age group, the prevalence of psychological distress has been described as similar to that in adults with cancer.[8] In the early years of psychosocial research, it was assumed that all adolescents diagnosed with cancer would manifest some form of psychological disturbance,[9,10] and over time researchers addressed distress as a frequent non-pathological sequel to cancer.[11] Current investigations of psychological adjustment in adolescents surviving cancer indicate that overall functioning is within normal limits, only some adolescents experiencing psychosocial difficulties. In an investigation of 60 adolescents recently diagnosed with cancer, the Brief Symptom Inventory[12] was used to measure psychological distress.[4] Psychological distress refers to 'dysphoric thoughts and feelings associated with a person's disorder and occurs as a direct result of the illness and its sequelae' (p. 73).[13] This measure consists of 53 items designed to tap the psychological symptoms of medical patients, psychiatric patients and healthy individuals, and has been used extensively in patients with cancer. Although this instrument focuses on determining a caseness for the presence or absence of psychological distress, the strong psychometric properties, ease of administration and use in adolescents without any apparent distortion[14] was the impetus for using this tool.

The findings revealed that few adolescents with cancer manifested psychological distress; in fact adolescents with cancer did not score differently from healthy adolescents.[12] This finding is consistent with reports in the literature supporting the contention that, despite difficulties, adolescents do fairly well in adjusting to cancer.[15–17]

Several factors warrant consideration of the above findings. Koocher and O'Malley,[18] in their classic research on childhood cancer survivors, identified that there are three ways in which children respond to cancer: high anxiety and other psychological adjustment problems as a result of living with constant fear of recurrence; believing that they were immune to cancer; and not thinking about it.[19] Other researchers[20] have identified that adolescents tend to deal with cancer by attending to daily tasks, school events and peer activities. When adolescents attempt to normalize their lives and not worry about their cancer, they are using adaptive denial, a strategy that calls for a positive, optimistic outlook in which an individual fills his mind with daily thoughts and concerns, rather than worries about illness (p. 196).[21]

A common problem in examining the psychosocial aspects of paediatric cancer is that of measuring the specific impact of the cancer experience.[22] While existing studies document strong psychometric properties of the instruments used to measure overall functioning of adolescents, they differentiate primarily between psychopathological states and normality.[22] Most adolescents diagnosed with cancer do not present inevitably with psychopathology, but rather are normal individuals who are facing what will probably be their most significant life stressor.

Another consideration for the low psychological distress scores and overall adjustment of adolescents with cancer pertains to methodological issues, whereby adolescents do not inevitably manifest psychopathological symptoms as such but may manifest difficulties in one or more areas of functioning, such as school phobias, separation anxiety and features of non-compliance,[8] which may be excluded from standardized psychosocial adjustment measures.

In summary, the assessment of psychological functioning in adolescents with cancer is a complex issue as developmental, clinical and methodological issues present real challenges to understanding how adolescents deal with the significant stressor of illness. Findings from this author's initial research identified the two factors of uncertainty and social support as important concepts related to the outcome of psychological distress, and will be briefly described.

Uncertainty in illness

Uncertainty has been identified as the single greatest psychosocial stressor to individuals and families faced with cancer[23–25] and a significant concern to adolescents with cancer.[26,27] Uncertainty is defined as the inability to determine the meaning of events, assign definite values to objects or events, or predict outcomes accurately.[28] Families awaiting information surrounding a cancer diagnosis in their child have identified the waiting and not knowing as the worst part of the experiences they went through as their child was being diagnosed with cancer.[23] Koocher and O'Malley[18] describe uncertainty as the Damocles' syndrome, named after a Greek myth involving the courtier Damocles who attended a feast where he sat beneath a sword suspended by one thread. The fears, anxieties, preoccupation with bodily function, and obsessive concern about the progression of disease are symptomatic of what has been termed the Damocles syndrome.[18] While medical advances have improved the long-term survival of paediatric cancer substantially, the ultimate fate and outcome of a child or adolescent with cancer remains uncertain.

Mishel[29] developed a theory of uncertainty in illness which explores how individuals process and derive meaning of illness-related events. Uncertainty regarding what will happen, what events mean and what the consequences of events may be are important to any individual faced with cancer. Managing the uncertainty about illness may be an important task in adaptation to those events.[30] The theory of uncertainty in illness asserts that, when uncertainty is viewed as a danger or an aversive event, coping efforts are employed to reduce uncertainty and, if these efforts are effective, adaptation then occurs. Difficulty in adaptation is congruent with psychological distress, poor psychosocial adjustment and family adjustment problems.[18] Uncertainty can also be viewed as positive. This can occur in the case of a downward trajectory, in which a negative outcome of a significant health threat is probable or highly likely. Attempts to maintain the state of uncertainty through the process of illusion may be made. In such cases, not knowing may be a preferred state.

Most people when faced with a significant health threat perceive uncertainty as a negative stressor and aim to either reduce uncertainty or to learn methods of coping with it, either alone or with social resources, including health-care professionals. Uncertainty in illness may be more difficult for an adolescent who is experiencing rapid developmental changes than for an adult who has obtained a relatively stable lifestyle.[18] While numerous bodily changes occur during adolescence, the adolescent with cancer has many additional bodily concerns resulting from treatment and/or illness.

According to Mishel's theory of uncertainty in illness,[31] uncertainty has a direct effect on psychological distress. Being unfamiliar with a large medical centre, often in a location unknown to an adolescent and his or her family, as well as with new health professionals and specialists, new technologically advanced treatment modalities and unfamiliar hospital routines, and even medical terminology, can generate a tremendous sense of uncertainty. Combined with the existential uncertainty experienced during the diagnostic phase of a life-threatening illness, uncertainty can be overwhelming and can generate psychological distress.

Uncertainty was a significant predictor of psychological distress among adolescents recently diagnosed with cancer.[4,32] While only a few adolescents manifested psychological distress, as determined by Derogatis's and Spencer's rule of caseness,[12] those with high levels of uncertainty regarding their illness had higher scores for psychological distress than those reporting low uncertainty.

The role of social support as a predominant factor in adaptation to illness has been investigated extensively, and researchers have supported the association between social support and psychological distress during adverse life events.[33] Investigators have also identified the need to explore the intervening factors associated with social support and psychological distress.[34,35] Using the uncertainty in illness theory, in addition to supporting strong relationships between uncertainty and psychological distress,[5,32] researchers have also supported strong relationships between uncertainty and social support.[30,36] As a result of the uncertainty experienced in illness, many individuals have an increased need to share their fears and concerns, to be reassured by others, and to clarify what is happening to them.[37] While this increased support is needed, many individuals experience difficulty in obtaining adequate support.[38]

Uncertainty has been identified as an intervening variable between social support and psychological distress among adult cancer patients.[32] Among adolescents with cancer, similar findings were identified. While a weak relationship between social support and psychological distress was noted, the most significant finding related to the combined effect of social support and uncertainty. Those adolescents who reported high levels of uncertainty about their illness, as well as low levels of social support, had the greatest psychological distress. By itself, social support was not a significant predictor of psychological distress, but when combined with uncertainty, adolescents who were the most uncertain and had the least social support reported the highest level of psychological distress. The combined variable became the most significant predictor of psychological distress for these adolescents recently diagnosed with cancer.[5]

In this study, all adolescents reported that their parents, especially their mothers, were the strongest supports, followed by extended family and then friends and peers.[4] Most adolescents described their friends' reactions as initially shocked and not knowing how to respond to them, with only a few instances of reporting that friends avoided them. One female adolescent poignantly described being stigmatized as the teenager in town with cancer. However, the majority of adolescents reported highly supportive responses from their peers during this phase of illness. Additionally, through observation during data collection, it became obvious that friends provided a sense of normalization to these ill adolescents. Conversations focused on peer activities, school and sport events, and other non-illness-related activities, which appeared to distract adolescents from the reality of their illnesses.

Guarded communication patterns

Despite describing parents as most supportive and helpful during the diagnostic phase of cancer, displays of guarded communication patterns were evident in this study. This protective or inhibited communication pattern has been recorded throughout research in paediatric oncology. Binger and colleagues[39] reported that even children as young as 4 years who were not informed of their diagnoses displayed evidence of their awareness of their grave illness and eventual demise. While some parents attempted to protect their children from what they believe to be harmful knowledge, older children reciprocated in this mode of communication to protect their parents. As a result of this lack of communication, Binger and colleagues showed that these were the loneliest children of all. Bluebond-Langner[40] identified the formation of a mutual pretence between children and their parents, whereby children would hide their knowledge about their prognosis and therefore avoid any communication about dying to their parents. In another classic study of dying children, Martinson[41] described how parents did not address and even avoided talking about death to their children, and subsequently these children learned not to pursue any information.

Among adolescents recently diagnosed with cancer, participants frequently described protecting their parents by not communicating all their concerns, fears and anxieties. Participants described how they wanted to spare their parents as many stressful events as possible, as they were already overburdened with fear, and concern for them. In many cases, they described a substitute person to communicate with, such as a boy/girlfriend, or an extended relative. As became evident in the next phase of research, which examined the impact of cancer on families, this altered communication pattern still continued, in which full disclosure was not always present among all family members.

The impact of cancer on adolescent development

Only recently has the expectation of cure become a reality for many individuals faced with cancer. Cancer survivorship is now a top international research priority[42] and, specific to adolescence, research is needed to ascertain just how cancer impacts on adolescent development:[43] does it slow down, speed up or redirect development? In response to this need, an in-depth qualitative investigation was conducted to explore how the experiences of cancer affected the achievement of developmental tasks of adolescence, and to identify common themes regarding the impact of cancer on adolescent development.[6]

Young adult survivors of teenage cancer were recruited from a long-term follow-up group in a children's cancer centre in the northeast corner of the USA. An unstructured interview of 1–2 hours was conducted at a mutually agreed private location. After consent was obtained, the interview began by posing the broad question of how cancer impacted on life, followed by specific questions related to the acquisition of developmental tasks. Theoretical saturation was used to determine sample size, such that when redundancies and patterns emerged, a sufficient sample size was achieved. In this study, there were six females and one male, and ages ranged from 23 to 30 years.

Based on these intensive, face-to-face interviews, constant comparison analyses revealed that cancer had affected their lives profoundly, as well as those of their families. While described in more detail elsewhere,[6] the predominant themes were catching up, focused career direction, return to pre-illness interests, increased maternal affiliation, resilience, and self-transcendence.

All participants described catching-up as a top priority for them as soon as treatment ended. Maintaining their academic standing was of crucial importance and was reported not to be difficult, as they received substantial support from inpatient and outpatient educators, and they reported having long periods of available time during treatment. With the exception of one male and one female, all of the participants described catching up socially as a most difficult endeavour because they had missed a most valuable time in adolescence, namely the formation of peer groups and the development of intimacy in relationships. Adolescents who were younger reported greater difficulty than older adolescents, who had presumably succeeded in these developmental tasks. For example, one 18-year-old participant was already engaged when she was diagnosed and did not report catching up socially as a problem. Many of the participants described themselves as 'still catching up socially', and recognized how much they had missed out on 'normal social activities'. While participants all described having substantial social support from friends, neighbours and family at the time of diagnosis, many participants described isolation and loss of friends over time. In many cases, the inability to participate in school and sports activities led to their gradual isolation and exclusion from peer-related activities. Many participants described feeling stigmatized as the teenager in town with cancer, and related having a fresh start in college, where no one knew about their illness unless they chose to inform others.

All participants described having a focused career direction as a result of their cancer experience. While some participants were attracted to the health professions, two reported an aversion to anything health- or hospital-related. All described having lots of time during treatment to plan and think about their career paths and, once recuperated, began a rigorous effort to make up for lost time. This finding of focused career path is consistent with previous literature identifying that adolescent cancer patients had a greater tendency to foreclose on a career path than did healthy adolescents.[16]

Another identified pattern in this research was a return to pre-illness interests. Participants had described how cancer interfered in their activities of adolescence, but many of them said that, many years after treatment, they sought ways to engage in their previous interests, even if they were altered. For instance, one female, who was an avid gymnast prior to her illness, returned to her interest by becoming a dance therapist. While altered, she believed she had worked out many of the issues related to her illness, and she was finally able to pursue what she wanted.

As was shown in the initial research during diagnosis, participants described their mothers as most helpful and supportive throughout their illness. Participants expressed an intense appreciation and affiliation for their mothers for all of their sacrifices and intense caring. Many participants spoke of devotion and support of their mothers, and an intense bond between child and mother as a result of the experience. After recovery, overprotectiveness was not identified as a problem.

As a result of their cancer experiences, all participants talked about how different their lives were as survivors. As in the diagnostic stage, if survivors had social support, they described having stamina and an ability to tolerate adversity. Exposure to others' demise (as was not uncommon for children in the early 1980s), pain and existential concerns all fostered the development of self-transcendence. All participants described themselves as changed, and of viewing life quite differently prior to their illness. Some spoke of an incongruency between their chronological and maturational years, as they felt much older than their chronological years, as if they had experienced so much more than their peers. It was common to hear of changed values, and an appreciation of the fragility and impermanence of life, so typically uncommon in this age group. Also, as a result of their cancer, there was residual fear and uncertainty – fear of recurrence and uncertainty regarding their health status.

It was during these rich, emotional interviews that families expressed their desire to be heard and to tell their stories. As a result, the third phase of this research programme was devoted to the psychosocial issues of adolescent cancer. In this study, entire family units were invited to participate in an investigation examining the impact of adolescent cancer on the family. A snowball sampling technique yielded intense in-depth interviews with six families, all of whom had a child or adolescent who had survived cancer. While concepts similar to those presented above were identified, the possibility of post-traumatic stress, as well as discrepant parental responses, were the key themes identified in this study.

Post-traumatic stress disorder

Historically, the term 'post-traumatic stress disorder' (PTSD) has its origin in wartime experiences, beginning with the Civil War in the USA and continuing through every war thereafter. PTSD has been well documented, but has been referred to differently with each American war. After the Civil War, due to autonomic cardiac symptoms experienced by soldiers, the term 'soldier's heart' or 'irritable heart' was applied to symptoms commensurate with what is now referred to as PTSD. In World War I, 'shell shock' was used to characterize the symptoms of PTSD, and the disorder was believed to have occurred after brain trauma from exploding artillery. Among World War II veterans, survivors of Nazi concentration camps and survivors of the atomic bombings in Japan, as well as survivors of the famous Coconut Grove nightclub fire in Boston, Massachusetts, similar symptoms (characteristic of PTSD) were referred to as 'combat neurosis', 'operational fatigue' or 'combat stress reactions'.[44] The term 'post-traumatic stress disorder' was first used during the Vietnam War and was recognized as a significant mental health disorder, affecting approximately 30% of Vietnam veterans.[44] These veterans' PTSD symptoms included recurrent nightmares, dreams, flashbacks, persistent re-experiencing of the events and general emotional numbness with constricted behaviours and affect.[45]

The fourth edition of the *Diagnostic and Statistical Manual of Mental Disorders* (DSM-IV) (1994)[46] describes PTSD as a set of typical symptoms that develop after a person witnesses, is involved in or hears of an extreme traumatic and overwhelming stressor.

Responses to the traumatic experience are fear, persistent re-experiencing or reliving of the event, feelings of psychological numbness and attempts to avoid being reminded of it. Symptoms of PTSD include re-experiencing the traumatic event through recurrent, intrusive recollections, repetitive play or distressing dreams; avoidance of associations with the event through restricted affect and feelings of detachment, and hyperarousal symptoms such as poor concentration, irritability, aggression; and physiological reactions to the trauma-related events.[47] PTSD has been shown to affect adults, as well as children from 2 to 19 years of age, and can result from many different types of traumatic exposure, such as death, injury or physiological threat to the self, family members or significant others.[47] Diagnostic criteria include exposure to a traumatic event, the symptoms of re-experiencing avoidance and hyperarousal which last more than 1 month. However, PTSD may not present for months or even years after the stressful event.[44]

In recent years, PTSD has been investigated in individuals and families of survivors of childhood and adolescent cancer, and evidence exists that such survivors, and their parents, manifest symptoms of PTSD.[48,49] The diagnosis and treatment of cancer, with its abounding uncertainty and fear, separation from family and friends, prolonged hospitalization and often intrusive and painful treatment, provide sufficient criteria for exposure to a traumatic event. In studies of families surviving childhood cancer, a small number of survivors of paediatric and adolescent cancer manifested moderate levels of PTSD, while increased incidences of PTSD were identified in mothers, fathers and siblings.[50] Clearly, the diagnosis of cancer in a child represents one of the most severe stressors faced by parents.

Although interest in the psychological sequelae of the cancer survivor experience and its association with PTSD is relatively recent, predictive variables have been identified.

Children and adolescents with higher levels of anxiety during treatment were more likely to manifest PTSD than those who were not anxious.[48] In addition, survivors' perception of their treatment intensity and life threat have been identified as predictors of PTSD.[51] Increased levels of perceived social support have been associated with lower levels of reported PTSD.[50] While age has not been investigated extensively, young adults are believed to be the most vulnerable to PTSD.[44] This vulnerability may be understood by the multiple developmental demands of this period and the effect of illness on delayed or altered acquisition of young adulthood tasks, or perhaps by the variable and often delayed symptomatic presentation of PTSD. Additionally, while some survivors manifest full criteria for the diagnosis of PTSD, many more survivors present with subclinical findings, such as the avoidance of painful reminders of the cancer experience.

While the initial aim of this in-depth investigation of families of survivors of paediatric cancer was not to identify PTSD, it is possible that subclinical aspects of PTSD might have existed. Many cancer survivors described how they avoided reminders of their illness, such as not liking to travel into the city where they were treated, or how even certain olfactory stimuli, such as alcohol, reminded them of their painful treatment. Other instances of avoidance were evidenced by the unwillingness, or lack of desire, to participate in the research describing their families' responses to illness. One parent described how he 'closed the door and does not look back' as his way of dealing with his daughter's cancer. Another mother of a survivor of 15 years described not wanting to 'go down that route and rehash all that negative stuff again – I just can't go there anymore'. While speculative, it is possible that these statements characterize the avoidance component of PTSD.

Parents are often relied upon to help the family adjust to the major stressors associated with a potentially life-threatening illness. How the family responds to this crisis can impact significantly on the overall functioning of the family. Research has focused often on and provided substantial information about a mother's responses and experiences when her child is faced with cancer, because she is often the primary caretaker.[52] Less research has been conducted on fathers, but consistent findings have been reported.[53] Fathers are less involved in the medical aspects of care,[54] they use increased denial and avoidance, engage in more instrumental tasks,[55] express less emotion than mothers,[56] and utilize less social support.

In a recent study of gender differences in parenting a child with cancer,[53] the authors report a different parenting experience among 124 parents. While mothers report handling the medical aspects of the illness as their most important parenting task, fathers, presumably because of their sex-role orientation, reported financial management as their most time-consuming activity. Spending time with family and communication with the extended family and friends were more important to mothers than fathers, and may support a gender difference in social support needs. Among parents who were interviewed regarding the impact of cancer on their families,[57] mothers frequently described their need to communicate with others, particularly other mothers of children with cancer. In this research, some fathers did not wish to participate, but sat in a nearby room when the interview was being held. This finding is consistent with the literature asserting that fathers are less likely to share their feelings or to seek help from others.

Two focus groups of fathers of children with cancer revealed the private nature of fathers' responses to the threat of their children's cancer, such that not even their responses could be shared with their wives.[58] Fathers reported the need to be strong and protect their wives, despite feelings of intense vulnerability. While not able to express themselves fully with their families, they were able to share their experiences with other fathers and benefit from it.

Fathers of seriously ill children have been referred to as 'forgotten parents',[58,59] and recommendations have been made for greater inclusion of fathers by health professionals. Although the traditional role of provider is of paramount importance and necessity, attention to the gender-specific needs of fathers warrants further inquiry. While fathers may not seek social support actively, is it logical to believe that, at the time of crisis when their child is facing a potentially life-threatening illness, and long after, additional paternal support is needed. Finding methods to provide this in an acceptable manner when it will be accepted graciously remains the health professionals' challenge.

Flexibility in appointment scheduling and communicating to both parents, rather than one, can be used to encourage more active participation, when feasible.

In summary, cancer survivorship is, most fortunately, becoming an increasing reality for many more children and adolescents than in previous years. Additional studies to more fully understand the unique and often difficult and long-lasting impact of cancer on individuals and their families need to be conducted so that appropriate interventions can be delivered. Common psychosocial responses to the diagnosis and treatment of cancer in adolescence have been identified, yet many young adult survivors believe their responses to cancer are abnormal. Using a model of recovery, survivors can be educated to understand the full impact of their cancer experience, to view their responses as normal, and to integrate this experience in their changed world.

In clinical practice, and certainly in paediatrics, a family is viewed as the centre of care. Thus, understanding a family's perspective is important for the provision of comprehensive and sensitive care. Although the methodological issues of conducting family research pose difficulties in understanding the gestalt perspective of the family, additional methods to facilitate inclusion of more family members are needed.

Lastly, since much of this research is qualitative there is an inability to generalize findings beyond these samples. Further research is necessary to generate theory, test theory through hypothesis formation, and ultimately to improve clinical practice.

References

1 Sieving, R, Bearinger, L. Health promotion of the adolescent and family. In Wong D, Ed. *Whaley & Wong's Nursing Care of Infants and Children*, 5th edn. New York: C.V. Mosby, 1995, pp. 825–861.

2 Baum B, Baum E. Psychosocial challenges of childhood cancer. *J Psychosoc Oncol* 1990; **7**: 119–129.

3 Novakovic B, Fears T, Wexler L *et al.* Experiences of cancer in children and adolescents *Cancer Nurs* 1996; **19**: 54–59.

4 Neville K. Psychological distress in adolescents recently diagnosed with cancer. *J Pediatr Nurs* 1996; **11**: 243–251.

5 Neville K. The relationship among uncertainty, social support and psychologist distress among adolescents recently diagnosed with cancer. *J Assoc Pediatr Oncol Nurs* 1998; **15**: 37–46.

6 Neville K. *Mature Beyond Their Years: The Impact of Cancer on Adolescent Development.* Pittsburgh: Oncology Nursing Press, 2000.

7 Ganz P. Patient education as a moderator of psychological distress. *J Psychosoc Oncol* 1988; **6**: 181–197.

8 Rait PS, Holland JCB. Pediatric cancer: psychosocial issues and approaches. *Mediguide Oncol* 1986; **6**: 1–6.

9 Lowenberg J. The coping behaviors of fatally ill adolescents and their parents. *Nurs Forum* 1970; **9**: 269–287.

10 Moore DC, Holten CP, Martin, GW. Psychologic problems in the management of adolescents with malignancy. *Clin Pediatr* 1969; **8**: 464–473.

11 Blotchy AD, Cohen D. Psychological assessment of the adolescent with cancer. *J Assoc Pediatr Oncol Nurs* 1985; **2**: 8–14.

12 Derogatis LR, Spencer P. *Administration and Procedures: BSI Manual I.* Baltimore (MD): Clinical Psychometric Research, 1982.

13 Derogotis LR. The psychosocial adjustment to illness scale. *J Psychosom Res* 1986; **30**: 77–91.

14 Derogatis L, Melisaratos N. The Brief Symptom Inventory: an introductory report. *Psychol Med* 1983; **13**: 595–605.

15 Baider L, Kaplan De-Nour A. Group therapy with adolescent cancer patients. *J Adolesc Health Care* 1989; **10**: 35–38.

16 Stern M, Norman SL, Zevon M. Adolescents with cancer: self image and perceived social support as indexes as adaptation. *Adolesc Health* 1993; **8**: 124–142.

17 Zevon MA, Tebbi CK, Stern M. Psychological and familiar factors in adolescent oncology. In: Tebbi DK, ed. *Psychological and Familiar Factors in Adolescent Oncology.* Mt Kisco (NY): Futura, 1987: 325–348.

18 Koocher GP, O'Malley JS. *The Damocles Syndrome: Psychological Consequences of Surviving Childhood Cancer.* New York: McGraw Hill, 1981.

19 Koocher, GP. Psychosocial care of the child cured of cancer. *Pediatr Nurs* 1985; **11**: 91–93.

20 Zeltzer L, LeBaron S, Zeltzer P. The adolescent with cancer. In: Blum RW, ed. *Chronic Illness and Disabilities in Childhood and Adolescence.* New York: Grune & Stratton, 1984: 375–395.

21 Weekes DP. *Adolescents with cancer. Correlates of intraindividual changes in types of coping strategy.* Doctoral dissertation, University of California at San Francisco, 1989.

22 VanDongen-Melman JE, Pruyn JF, DeGrout A *et al.* Late consequences for parents of children who have survived cancer. *J Ped Psychol* 1995; **20**: 567–586.

23 Clark-Steffen L. Waiting not knowing: the diagnosis of cancer in a child. *J Pediatr Oncol Nurs* 1993; **10**: 146–53.

24 Cohen M, Martinson I. Chronic uncertainty: its effects on parental appraisal of child's health. *J Pediatr Nurs* 1988; **3**: 89–96.

25 Halldorsdottir S, Hamrin E. Experiencing existential changes: the lived experience of having cancer. *Cancer Nurs* 1996; **19**: 29–36.

26 Bearison, DJ, Pacifici C. Psychological studies of children who have cancer. *J Psychosoc Oncol* 1984; **5**: 263–280.

27 Brunnquell D, Hall MD. Issues in the psychological case of pediatric oncology patients. *Am J Orthopsychiatry* 1982; **50**: 32–44.

28 Mishel MH, Braden CJ. Finding meaning: antecedents of uncertainty in illness. *Nurs Res* 1988; **37**: 98–103, 127.

29 Mishel MH. The measurement of uncertainty in illness. *Nurs Res* 1981; **30**: 258–263.

30 Mishel MH. Uncertainty in illness. Image. *J Nurs Scholarsh* 1988; **20**: 225–232.

31 Mishel MH, Hostetter T, King B, Graham V. Predictors of psychosocial adjustment in patients newly diagnosed with gynecological cancer. *Cancer Nurs* 1984; **1**: 291–299.

32 Mishel MH, Braden CJ. Uncertainty: a mediator between support and adjustment. *West J Nurs Res* 1987; **9**: 43–57.

33 Aro H, Hanninon V, Paronen O. Social support, life events and psychosomatic symptoms among 14–16 year old adolescents. *Soc Sci Med* 1989; **29**: 1051–1056.

34 Bloom JR. Social support accommodation to stress and adaptation to breast cancer. *Soc Sci Med* 1982; **16**: 635–637.

35 Holahan CJ, Moos RH. Social support and psychological distress. *J Abnorm Psychol* 1981; **90**: 365–370.

36 Scoloveno MA, Yarcheski A, Mahon N. Scoliosis treatment on selected variables among adolescents. *West J Nurs Res* 1990; **12**: 601–615.

37 Wortman CB, Dunkel-Schetter C. Interpersonal relationships and cancer: a theoretical analysis. *J Soc Issues* 1979; **35**: 120–155.

38 Wortman CB. Social support and the cancer patient. Conceptual and methodological issues. *Cancer* 1984; **15**: 2339–2359.

39 Binger CM, Ablin AR, Feuerstein MD *et al.* Childhood leukemia: emotional impact on patient and family. *N Engl J Med* 1969; **280**: 414–418.

40 Bluebond-Langner M. *The Private Worlds of Dying Children*. Princeton (NJ): Princeton University Press, 1978.

41 Martinson IM. *Home Care of the Dying Child: Professional and Family Perspectives*. Norwalk (CT): Appleton-Century-Crofts, 1976.

42 Fitch M. Creating a research agenda with relevance to cancer nursing practice. *Cancer Nurs* 1996; **19**: 335–342.

43 Hinds P. Revision theories on adolescent development through observations by nurses. *J Pediatr Oncol Nurs* 1997; **12**: 1–2.

44 Kaplan H, Sadock B. *Kaplan and Sadock's Synopsis of Psychiatry. Behavioral Sciences/ Clinical Psychiatry*, 8th edn. Baltimore (MD): Williams & Wilkins, 1998.

45 Horowitz M, Solomon G. A prediction of delayed stress syndrome in Vietnam veterans. *J Soc Issues* 1975; **31**: 67–80.

46 American Psychological Association. *Diagnostic and Statistical Manual of Mental Disorders, Fourth Edition*. Washington (DC). American Psychological Association, 1994.

47 Zink KA, McCain GC. Post-traumatic stress disorder in children and adolescents with motor vehicle related injuries. *J Soc Pediatr Nurs* 2003; **8**: 99–106.

48 Barakat I, Kazak A, Meadows A *et al.* Families surviving childhood cancer: a comparison of posttraumatic stress symptoms with families of healthy children. *J Pediatr Psychol* 1997; **22**: 843–859.

49 Stuber ML, Kazak AE, Meeske K *et al.* Predictors of posttraumatic stress symptoms in childhood cancer survivors. *Pediatrics* 1997; **100**: 95–64.

50 Kazak A, Meeske K, Penati B *et al.* Post-traumatic stress, family functioning and social support in survivors of childhood leukemia and their mothers and fathers. *J Consult Clin Psychol* 1997; **65**: 120–129.

51 Hobbie W, Stuber M, Meeske K *et al.* Symptoms of posttraumatic stress in young adult survivors of childhood cancer. *J Clin Oncol* 2000; **18**: 4060–4066.

52 Hovey JK. The needs of fathers parenting children with chronic conditions. *J Pediatr Oncol Nurs* 2003; **20**: 245–251.

53 Elliot Brown KA, Barbarin OA. Gender difference in parenting a child with cancer. *Soc Work Health Care* 1996; **22**: 53–71.

54 Alexander D, White M, Powell G. Anxiety of nonrooming in parents of hospitalized children. *Child Health Care* 1986; **15**: 14–20.

55 Keller C, Nicolls R. Coping strategies of chronically ill adolescents and their parents. *Issues Compr Pediatr Nurs* 1990; **13**: 73–80.

56 Koller PA. Family needs and coping strategies during illness crisis. *AACN Clin Issues* 1991; **2**: 338–345.

57 Neville K. Discrepant parental responses in pediatric cancer survivorship. In progress.

58 Sterken DJ. The adventures of superman: fathers of children with cancer: considerations for clinical practice: a focus group. *J Pediatr Oncol Nurs* 1996; **13**: 175.

59 May J. Family matters. Fathers: the forgotten parent. *Pediatr Nurs* 1996; **22**: 243–246.

CHAPTER 16

Resilience in survivors of teenage cancer: a life-adaptive approach

J. J. Spinetta

Introduction

Can having had cancer in one's teenage years actually be helpful rather than harmful for growth into adulthood? Is it possible that our long-term survivors might be better adapted and adjusted than their peers, and even be better prepared to face adult challenges? What might our role be as paediatric health-care professionals and parents in helping the survivors move towards that positive vision and growth? Is there a point in our dealings with the survivors of teenage cancer when we can help them shift from their view of cancer as a disease for which they have been successfully treated to viewing the cancer as an opportunity for life-sustaining growth and learning? These questions will be addressed in the context of the psychological study of adjustment and adaptation.

Paediatric oncologists have taken seriously their responsibility to continue following cancer survivors long after successful treatment. There is increased emphasis on the study of potential long-term effects many years later. The various researchers have made many recommendations: among these are improving the awareness of late effects and their implications for long-term medical and psychological health among childhood cancer survivors and their families; developing interventions to prevent or reduce late effects after treatment; furthering improvements in the quality of care to ameliorate the consequences of late effects on individuals and families; and increasing the efficiency of methods of follow-up, so that long-term sequelae can be documented more effectively.[1]

There is no dispute about the importance of a focus on the potential long-term medical and psychological sequelae of cancer treatment. This, after all, is the role of 'good' doctors. Whatever can be done should be done to reduce the risk of long-term complications. The effort is deemed successful when medical professionals can predict and help prevent potential medical and psychological sequelae.

As effective and important as these long-term studies of late effects are, there is a problem. The problem is that excessive emphasis for an increasingly longer period of time on the presence or absence of potential long-term damage can sometimes encourage the survivors to continue focusing on their past and distract them from making full use of their remaining, even if physically restricted, potential. Constant and repeated follow-up contact with medical professionals can keep the survivors focusing on the potential damage their cancer and its treatment may have inflicted instead of reflecting on their past experience and learning from it how to survive and endure future hardships. They ideally need to further develop their positive life-adaptive qualities.

After all, even after one discovers a specific long-term effect and prevents it or treats it medically, the survivor must still deal with having had the cancer and having gone through the cancer experience. Even those young adults who do have serious physical sequelae are capable of learning and growing from the experience and committing themselves to the pursuit of a full and effective adulthood, despite possible restrictions and limitations imposed on them by the disease and its treatment. Besides, while the therapies have put some survivors at risk of long-term medical and psychological difficulties, the majority of survivors of childhood cancer enjoy overall general good health.

The issue is not whether paediatric cancer health-care professionals are interested in the fact that survivors can learn positive coping strategies from their cancer experience and apply these learned strategies in their adult lives, but whether we, as parents and as health-care professionals working with long-term survivors, are actively helping them move on with their lives despite possible sequelae from their treatment or, by continuing to focus for years on potential sequelae, we are hindering their full commitment and movement toward their future.

A brief review of the psychological study of adjustment and adaptation may help to put these issues into context.

The psychology of adjustment

One of the world's leading authorities on the psychology of adjustment and adaptation, Richard Lazarus, after over 50 years of research in the field came to the understanding that there are two types of denial: problem-focused and emotion-focused.[2] One is bad; one is good. One is maladaptive; one is adaptive.

When one has a problem that can be fixed, be it physical or psychological, and one denies that there is a problem, that form of denial is maladaptive. If, for example, a person suffers pain in the chest while jogging and keeps on running just to prove to himself that it wasn't a heart attack, that person is engaging in problem-focused denial. Not a healthy thing to do. If, however, that same person goes to a physician and discovers that he has a heart condition and that he needs to follow a reduced physical regimen, take certain medications to control the heart condition, and comply with the physician's recommendations, the person has accepted the problem and done something about it. To deny the problem would be foolish, and this form of problem-focused denial is maladaptive.

However, once the person begins to treat the problem he is faced with an attitudinal choice. The person can choose to view himself as physically weakened, can become depressed and bitter over the life change involved and can effectively stop living as full a life as is still physically possible. While he may view his attitudinal choice as realistic, that particular choice can lead to a much less fulfilling life. His other choice is to say that, even with the necessity to adhere to a more controlled exercise regimen and to comply with the need to take medications, his life is still worth living and living with all the enthusiasm he can muster, despite the new limitations. This latter state of mind is what Lazarus calls emotion-focused denial, a very healthy, optimistic and hopeful view of life's difficulties that can make life not only bearable but fulfilling.

While this concept is not new – one can find references to a healthy and optimistic attitude toward life's problems dating back to the earliest human writings – there is within the field of psychology a current refocusing on attitudinal modification and on the possibilities and opportunities for growth rather than on viewing people as needing to be 'fixed'. The message of this approach to psychology is that a positive attitude is critical to a full and healthy life, that true happiness and fulfilment can come only when one can accept with non-bitter enthusiasm even life's setbacks, no matter how large they might be, and can move on in life with hope and optimism.[3]

It should be clear how this concept can apply to young adults who have survived cancer.

Adjustment and adaptation in the long-term survivor

What should the health-care professional do regarding young adult survivors? On the one hand, there is a serious responsibility to determine long-term sequelae so that they can be treated and/or prevented. On the other hand, survivors should be encouraged to move on with their lives. What is needed is a healthy balance between the two. Given the intense effort in recent years to pursue the long-term effects of cancer treatment for increasingly long periods, the pendulum seems to have swung too far in the first direction. Whether or not some of the current long-term effects can be modified or prevented altogether, the fact remains that both the survivors who are at risk for long-term complications and the majority of survivors who report overall good health have a golden opportunity to learn from their cancer. By helping the survivors to pay more attention to this aspect of survival – the enhancement of life-sustaining coping skills – we, either as parents or as health-care professionals, can help the survivors develop towards a mature and successful adulthood.

Not everything can be fixed. The fact that the survivors once had cancer as teenagers is an integral part of who they are. However, the past cancer should not be allowed to be used as an excuse to aim less high with one's life. We must ask ourselves, as parents and as health-care professionals, if in our own continued focus on potential long-term repercussions of the cancer we are expecting the survivors to do less and to strive for less. Are we passing that message on to the survivors?

With our help and focus on the issue, a teenager with cancer can learn early on one of the most valuable lessons in life: making the most out of restricted possibilities. The challenge both to parents and to health-care professionals is to help the young adult who has been treated for cancer and survived not to continue to dwell on the fact that they once had disease, but to learn from the cancer experience and develop and enhance their innate coping skills as they grow into as full, effective and committed an adulthood as is their right.

References

1 Hewitt M, Weiner SL, Simone JV, eds. *Childhood Cancer Survivorship: Improving Care and Quality of Life*. Washington (DC): National Academies Press, 2003.
2 Lazarus RS. *Emotion and Adaptation*. New York: Oxford University Press, 1991.
3 Seligman MEP, Csikszentmihalyi M. Positive psychology: an introduction. *Am Psychol* 2000; **55**: 5–14.

CHAPTER 17

Surviving with scars: the long-term psychosocial consequences of teenage cancer

M. C. Self

Introduction

Perhaps the most powerful testimony to the improved prognosis for the adolescent cancer patient is the fact that I can write this chapter from two perspectives. First, as a teenage survivor, having been diagnosed in 1983 with osteosarcoma of the femur, at age 17. Treatment consisted of amputation of my left leg and chemotherapy. In 1999 I developed a lung metastasis that was surgically removed. I have since remained well.

Secondly, I write as a doctor. I commenced my studies at Liverpool University 10 months after the diagnosis of cancer. I qualified in 1988, the year I celebrated my 5-year survival. The threat of cancer has been ever-present for more than half my life, uniquely shaping my physical, social and psychological world.[1]

The long-term psychosocial consequences of childhood and adolescent cancer – referred to as the Damocles' syndrome[2] – have become increasingly apparent as survivors live to recount their tales.[3] It is estimated that currently 1 in 1000 young adults aged 20–29 are survivors of childhood cancer.[4] In the 1960s a diagnosis of acute lymphoblastic leukaemia (ALL) represented imminent death; now 70% achieve a 'cure'.[5] The 5-year survival rate for all childhood cancers combined now exceeds 70% and several individual types of tumour have 5-year survival rates that exceed 90%.[6] Concurrent with improved outlook has come a shift in psychosocial emphasis away from preparing a youngster for death and towards achieving cure with a high quality of life. The uncertain nature of the diagnosis, the unpleasant nature of aggressive treatments and the multiple complications that may follow surgery, chemotherapy and radiotherapy, sometimes decades after completion, are all significant factors in future psychological functioning.

In order fully to understand the psychological and psychiatric morbidity that may follow a diagnosis of cancer in the adolescent, we must first appreciate the developmental challenges all teenagers face.

On being a teenager

Adolescence is the transition from childhood to adulthood and contains overlapping elements of both. There are major challenges for any teenager (see Box 17.1), let alone one facing the dual challenge of adolescence and cancer.[7]

Box 17.1 Key challenges of adolescence

Survivor speaks

There I was – seventeen and, as far as I knew, dying. My left leg had been amputated along with my healthy care-free future. Instead of exams, boyfriends and clothes, I was worrying about disability, sickness and death. Then came the poisons. The treatment seemed worse than dying when my hair started to fall out in handfuls. I felt like an ugly, mutilated freak – some bizarre alien life-form. How could anybody ever love me again? The question went round and round in my mind all day and all night. Then my periods stopped, my breasts shrank and my pubic hair fell out, stripping me of my newly discovered womanhood. Suddenly I was in this little girl's pink body again. A body I didn't want or recognize. I hated my violated body and yearned achingly for the future I had planned and the woman I wanted to be.   MCS

Control

Adolescence is a time when control is threatened as multiple physical, social and emotional changes occur. Maintaining control is seen as vital and loss of control is experienced as inherently stressful. Having negotiated normal physical changes, such as menarche and the appearance of secondary sexual characteristics, cancer treatment can then lead to further bewildering changes. These may include radical surgery, hair loss and sexual changes, such as delayed, reversed or even precocious puberty,[8] representing a frightening loss of control.

Self-esteem

Adolescence is marked by an all-consuming preoccupation with appearance, athleticity and physical prowess. Socializing and forming significant relationships becomes crucial. Body image and high self-esteem underpin success.[9] Psychological havoc ensues when hair loss, weight changes and surgical procedures threaten them. Negative changes in body image and a threat to body integrity can precipitate a profound lowering of self-esteem which may persist for decades.

Identity

Teenagers ask big questions, such as 'Who am I?' and 'Why am I here?' Cognitive processes become abstract and existential as new values, attitudes, morals and philosophies are adopted.[10] Parental influences are discarded in favour of those of the peer group. Losing childhood and embracing adulthood is a poignant transition for the average young person.[11] For the teenager diagnosed with cancer, the potential loss of new-found identity is an appalling possibility. To lose both remembered past and hoped-for future before discovering who one really is presents an intolerable confusion.

Independence

The teenager must separate from the family unit and become an individual with personal responsibility in order that future relationships may be secure and content.[11] Regression is a normal response to major illness, forcing an adolescent back into childlike dependency upon parents and caregivers. Hospitalization, invasive treatments and the inability to perform intimate tasks of daily living can be a source of resentment and anger.[12]

Communication

Adolescence involves mastering communication with parents and adults. Ordinarily, this may be turbulent. When a teenager is presented with complex and upsetting information of a life-threatening nature, difficulties in communication are accentuated.[12] The adolescent may be reluctant to disclose sensitive information or admit to unhappiness. A balance of space and support is required.

Relationships

Peer group approval and contact is of paramount importance to the teenager.[9] Hospital visits, prolonged treatment and repeated absences from school, along with ongoing threats to self-esteem, can threaten relationships, leading to isolation, withdrawal and anxiety. A proportion of peers will not be able to cope as their own views on mortality are challenged, and they may desert the teenager. A return to the peer group may provoke teasing or even bullying as a result of changed appearance. All these factors can contribute to future psychological difficulties.

Future direction

Teenagers imagine they can be anything, go anywhere and do anything, and nothing will stop them. The future seems full of possibilities, hope and the certainty of being indestructible . . . until cancer, when the future – if it exists at all – becomes a horrific prospect of painful and devastating treatments.[7] Most teenagers will equate a diagnosis of cancer with death. In them, life is suddenly no longer guaranteed.

Some will lapse into denial and become non-compliant with therapy. These patients often create inordinate challenges for their family and health-care team, let alone compromise their own survival.

> **Box 17.2 Seasons of survival**
>
> **Survivor speaks**
>
> I call them my 'ten-ton truck' days. Days when something quite small, and seemingly inconsequential, triggers the grief and it feels like I'm back there. I see that speeding truck racing towards me again. Pain and shock hit me like a juggernaut and leave me pulverized, bleeding, dying. I feel numb, broken and can hardly draw breath. But I'm learning to deal with the truck. Each time it knocks me down, it does less damage. I bruise less. I hurt less. My wounds are fewer. I recover more quickly. I get up and fight again. And I find new strength, new courage, fresh ability to survive. One day that truck is going to speed towards me and I shall simply side-step, put out my hand and stop it in its tracks. We shall be equal then. For I shall have lost my fear of the ten-ton truck.   MCS

The cancer journey

A diagnosis of cancer is not simply a single distressing life-event. It is a life-changing journey of survival involving uncertainty and change. It is also a journey of growth and discovery. There is no defined end-point to coping, for an adolescent is a dynamic being who will assimilate the evolving experience of cancer into adulthood. A teenager's experiences of cancer, together with personality make-up and individual circumstances, will affect reactions in the long term. The cancer journey has been likened to 'seasons of survival',[13] which encompasses the transitional nature of survivorship (see Box 17.2).

Acute survival (diagnosis and treatment)

The acute survival phase is the time of initial diagnosis and treatment. This will dramatically influence how a person reacts in the long term. If emotional well-being is neglected then it will impact deleteriously on future psychological health.[14]

All patients diagnosed with a life-threatening illness will undergo a period of adjustment in the acute survival phase. The reaction to diagnosis will depend on many factors – personality, level of social support, severity of illness, type of treatment and the perceived meaning of the illness. It may be difficult, if not impossible, in the early stages to differentiate between what is a normal healthy response to illness and a pathological one.[15] A variety of psychological responses can occur following diagnosis, including acute stress reactions and adjustment disorders. These are marked by a mixture of anxiety and depression. The responses are ordinarily transient, within the range of common experience and reversible. These disorders merge between a healthy response and an affective disorder; however, at the time they can be experienced as overwhelming. A proportion of at-risk individuals will go on to develop psychopathology.

The time surrounding diagnosis is marked by denial. Denial is a necessary defence mechanism, temporarily protecting an individual from distressing information and allowing time for gradual digestion of bad news. Denial is the commonest defence mechanism in this phase – so common that it has been found to occur in 99.1% of children, as described below.[14] It represents the first stage of a more gradual adjustment process that has been likened to a grief reaction,[16] continuing over weeks and months. Diagnosis of a life-threatening illness leads to an unacceptable loss of self-identity that results in utter confusion, and refuge is sought in this primitive defence mechanism. There may be times during treatment and in the cancer journey when the child or teenager will return to denial, particularly if bad news is received. Extremely prolonged denial is considered maladaptive, threatening treatment compliance and acceptance of diagnosis.[17]

In his study of defence mechanisms in childhood cancer, O'Malley and colleagues[14] looked at 111 children aged between 5 and 18 years diagnosed with various cancers, and found that 110/111 exhibited denial and 103/111 showed avoidance at the time of diagnosis. Coping mechanisms evolved with time from diagnosis and progressed to rationalization (95.5%), repression (70.3%) and reaction formation (42.3%). However, the defence mechanisms of a 5-year-old are very different from those of a 17-year-old, which the study did not take into account.

Guilt and self-blame can also be experienced.[18] Minor misdemeanours and past foibles can become the focus of inappropriate guilt, leading to silent misery. Attribution of blame in the acute phase of survival can contribute to depression later.

Extended survival (re-entry)

The extended season of survival is a time of re-entry. Treatment is completed and life begins again. Normalization takes place as the teenager returns to school, college or work. The cessation of treatment can be stressful as the safety net of therapy is withdrawn and the adolescent is faced with fighting cancer alone.

Independence needs to be regained and autonomy restored. The resumption of education and friendships with peers will enhance self-esteem, allowing the teenager to feel back in control. It also maximizes the chances of achieving cherished life-goals in the future, further increasing self-worth.[19]

It must be remembered that the adolescent with cancer wishes to be seen as a teenager first and a cancer patient second. Support and education are essential to help the adolescent cope with this season of survival and return to a normal environment. Ultimately, time and effort invested here will prove beneficial to future psychosocial adjustment.

Permanent survival (living life)

Permanent survival is about living life. There is no magic moment of cure in this phase, although many survivors will set a special marker in their minds, such as a 5-year cancer-free anniversary. Permanent survival is evolution into a phase where cancer is seen as permanently arrested.[20]

Multiple delayed challenges will occur within this phase.[12] Crisis points occur when cancer-related losses are felt afresh, such as cancer anniversaries. A recurrence of suspicious symptoms, similar to the cancer presentation, will induce extreme concern that is heightened by visits to clinics or by further investigations. Marker events such as graduation, marriage or childbirth cause a survivor to envisage the future. This can evoke bittersweet emotions as uncertainty is contemplated. Event-specific crises, such as job rejection or the confirmation of infertility, may cause fresh anxiety. Secondary adversities, such as growth retardation, neurocognitive deficits and limb amputations, will provide regular reminders of cancer's lifelong legacy.

All these life-events must be negotiated and integrated into the life-course of the permanent survivor. Whilst representing risk factors for future psychological distress, they also provide an opportunity for personal growth. Each uncertainty may be a catalyst for change, producing the potential for post-traumatic growth in the teenage cancer survivor.[21]

Psychological models of cancer survival

Increased interest in and justified concern surrounding the psychosocial well-being of adolescent cancer survivors has led to an increase in research and publications on the topic. One approach to the prevention of psychopathology has been to identify survivors who are at increased risk by measuring various psychosocial outcomes that are assumed to be markers of healthy psychological adjustment. Alternatively, one can look for the presence of psychiatric illness in survivors, such as rates of depression or anxiety. Another approach is to understand the psychological and social processes involved in accommodating the lifetime implications of cancer.[22]

Adjustment involves a lifetime process of adapting to multiple psychosocial challenges. 'Adjustment' suggests a point of completion but survivorship may be more accurately viewed as a continuous transition. Appreciating the adaptive psychological processes is the key to understanding where things may go awry.

Coping theory and stressors

Coping is the process of managing demands appraised as taxing and exceeding available resources.

Five styles of coping have been identified in adult cancer patients.[23] These are avoidance, fighting spirit, fatalism, helplessness–hopelessness and anxious preoccupation. Research has shown that the first two are associated with less psychological distress and the other three are more likely to predispose to depression.[24] However, these studies were conducted on adults and we must be cautious in extending this conclusion to teenagers. What it does show, though, is that different coping styles can influence the psychological outcome.

Coping styles vary with personality, maturity and progress within the cancer journey. Some forms of coping, such as denial, are temporary defences occurring in the early stages. Persistent denial can lead to an inability to accept bad news.[25]

Predominant coping mechanisms in adolescents with cancer are denial (99.1%) and avoidance (92.8%).[12] Celebrating survivorship and employing adaptive denial have been seen as effective forms of coping in the past.[26] Studies have shown that employing repressive styles of adaptation may be protective against psychological distress in the short term. In 1992, Canning and colleagues showed in a cross-sectional controlled study that only 5% of repressors developed depressive symptoms compared with 29% of non-repressors, which was statistically significant.[17] However, as adolescents become young adults they gain deeper insight into the implications of diagnosis. As the teenager matures, so do defence mechanisms, and flexible adaptation styles may prove beneficial. More complex mechanisms may be called for, such as 'searching for meaning' – attempting to find some higher purpose to surviving cancer. In the long term a rigid repressive style may make adjustment more problematic.

Coping theory states that successful adjustment is promoted by self-efficacy through problem-solving approaches, allowing survivors to regain mastery and control over their lives. Active coping mechanisms enhance self-esteem and restore life direction.[27] Whilst coping theory allows the use of practical measures to help survivors, it does not offer deeper insight into the subtle complexities of growing up with cancer.

Multiple losses and mourning

Elements of cancer can be understood by applying the model of grief and mourning. Any major life-event threatens individual core assumptions about one's personal world and brings about psychosocial transition – the changes necessarily occurring after a bereavement or major loss.[28] The greater the loss, the more protracted the mourning.

Cancer in adults can be viewed as a series of losses,[29] described as those of:
- security
- physical abilities
- body image
- strength
- independence
- self-esteem
- respect
- future.

Losses may differ and be more subtle in the adolescent, such as loss of peer friendships, education, life-goals or newly acquired secondary sexual characteristics. Secondary adversities represent significant areas of loss and may occur at a later date: loss of a limb, fertility, or further loss of health caused by therapy.

As with bereavement, cancer losses are gradually assimilated. Changes and modifications give rise to an accommodated state in which the new self is redefined as a cancer survivor.

In addition to the normal grief response, loss events contribute to the development of depression, anxiety, substance abuse and psychosomatic disorders in the adult in later years.[30]

The evidence for depression and anxiety occurring in survivors of teenage cancer is conflicting. In many studies of adolescent survivors no increased rates of depression/anxiety were reported.[9,31,32] The study of Teta and colleagues[32] used siblings of survivors as a control group, which may not be the most suitable control as siblings are also psychologically affected by a diagnosis of cancer in a family member. It included only those meeting criteria for a major depressive disorder and may have missed more minor depressive episodes. Additionally, many of these studies used self-report measures of depression. In adolescents who employ repressive styles of coping, under-reporting may occur.[17] Other studies show the opposite; for example, Zeltzer and colleagues[33] reported significantly more depression among ALL survivors than in their siblings. The highest rates were encountered in female and unemployed survivors. Lansky and colleagues also showed significantly higher rates of depression in a small population of survivors than in a general population control using a standardized structured interview technique.[34]

Other studies have shown that adolescent cancer survivors are less likely to exhibit illegal substance abuse and antisocial behaviour than their healthy peer group.[35] Rates of alcohol and tobacco use were observed to be no different between teenage cancer survivors and controls.[35]

Multiple trauma model

A diagnosis of cancer and events that follow may be seen as a series of multiple traumas, beginning with the life-changing diagnosis itself and continuing throughout the cancer journey.

Psychological distress occurs in response to trauma involving threat to oneself or a loved one. Post-traumatic stress disorder (PTSD) was initially described as a delayed psychological response to trauma experienced by combat veterans. In 1980, the American Psychiatric Association recognized PTSD as a response to traumatic events outside usual human experience.[36] In 1994, the fourth revision of the *Diagnostic and Statistical Manual of Mental Disorders* (DSM-IV) included a diagnosis of 'life-threatening illness' as a qualifying traumatic event for PTSD.[37]

The core features of PTSD include:
- experiencing or witnessing life-threatening events
- re-experiencing events (unwelcome intrusive memories, flashbacks or nightmares)
- avoidance of triggers reminding one of the event
- persistent symptoms of increased arousal (difficulty sleeping, irritability, hypervigilance, difficulty concentrating).

Symptoms can appear at any time following the trauma and can last from weeks to years.

Aggressive treatment and late side-effects can amount to a series of chronic traumas.[36] Follow-up and adversities like amputations, scars and infertility act as lifelong triggers.

As the adolescent matures, the significance and understanding of cancer-related traumas change. Meanings will be assimilated at a deeper level and full implications realized for the first time. Infertility may not be considered traumatic by a 14-year-old girl. Ten years later the perspective may well be different. As new stresses are faced that are due to the original cancer and its therapies, there is ample opportunity for retraumatization and the return of PTSD symptoms.

This model allows us to understand that the traumatic nature of diagnosis will inherently produce 'normal' responses in the majority of individuals – such as increased anxiety, emotional blunting, avoidance of cancer-related triggers and flashbacks. Again, there is a degree of overlap between the normal, healthy response to trauma and a pathological one. The distinguishing features of PTSD are in the duration and intensity of the symptoms experienced. It allows us to detect PTSD in the survivor and to intervene appropriately but does not fully explain why some adolescents find aspects of treatment and illness stressful for many decades.[38]

Multiple models and social cognitive transition theory

The social cognitive transition (SCT) theory of adjustment builds on all models previously described. It attempts to account for both negative and positive aspects of cancer, emphasizing the social context of an individual's experience.[22]

According to this theory, cancer survivors do not merely respond to a stimulus in order to protect themselves, but learn and develop from experiences. Emotions and plans change in their light. Meanings of events are constantly reorganized as new situations are encountered.

SCT theory encompasses four distinct stages:
- stress arousal
- denial/avoidance
- worry and cognitive adaptation
- core reformation.

When initially exposed to trauma, capacity to adapt may be temporarily overwhelmed with a high level of stress arousal. The struggle to accept leads to denial and avoidance. Worry and cognitive adaptation occur as the new threat is appraised. Core assumptions are reformed as a consequence, based on life trajectory, self-worth, attachments to others and existential concepts.

The advantages of this model are that it allows for both psychological distress and positive personal growth. The main difficulty is that no psychometric tool exists to measure changes in core assumptions.

Adolescence is precisely the age when core assumptions about the world and oneself are formed. Existential and spiritual questions of life are being

> **Box 17.3 Psychological models of cancer**
>
> **Survivor speaks**
> I am not sure if my experience of cancer can be made to fit into a single theory. I have lived with cancer now for more than half my life and grown up with it. All my formative life decisions have been taken with cancer somewhere in the background; whether I sat my A-levels; which university I went to; which type of career to choose; if and when to marry; whether we risked trying for children; how many children to have and when; what do we tell the children . . . the list goes on. There have been elements of grief, trauma and stress throughout the journey. But I have always come out the other side and managed to find a way forward and some meaning to the whole story. Now I can honestly say I'm a better doctor, wife, mother, friend and daughter and have a deeper faith because of cancer. I have no regrets. What theory can explain that?   MCS

deliberated, discarded and reformed. Transition occurs in every area of the teenager's world, quite apart from those caused by cancer. It is not difficult to understand why the teenager with cancer faces such a confusing emotional maelstrom.

The above models (see Box 17.3) enable us to understand the multiple intrapsychic and interpersonal psychological challenges posed by a diagnosis of cancer. Now we must look at the evidence base for existence of psychosocial morbidity in the adolescent cancer survivor.

Long-term psychosocial morbidity in adolescent cancer survivors

In the last 20 years, much research has been produced surrounding psychosocial sequelae of childhood and adolescent cancers. The evidence is complex and at times contradictory. The first major study, by Koocher and O'Malley[2] in 1981, resulted in the naming of 'Damocles' syndrome' to describe the long-term psychosocial effects of childhood cancer. This landmark study showed there was a significant level of maladjustment and psychosocial difficulty amongst survivors; 59% showed some degree of maladjustment, with 34% of those judged moderate to severe. Outcomes included self-esteem, social adjustment and standardized measures of anxiety and depression.[14]

Several studies in the 1980s[31,32,39] showed that survivors functioned at relatively good levels, although some psychosocial difficulties arose with time. Teta and colleagues[32] showed an increase in rejection from the US armed forces (80%) and a significantly higher level of rejection for life insurance (24 versus 19%). He showed no increase in lifetime prevalence of depression and a picture of normal adjustment, confirmed by later studies.[40,41] However, other studies showed that there was a small but significant increase in depression and anxiety.[33,34] It is difficult to compare these conflicting studies directly because they use different control groups and varying outcome measures and the inclusion criteria differ.

Workers showed a high level of employment problems in survivors[42] and significantly lower marriage rates; 50% of survivors married compared with 76% of Americans of the same age.[43] Other research showed that teenagers rated the side-effects of treatment worse than the disease itself.[44]

In summary, Lansky and colleagues[34] concluded in 1989 that, although severe psychopathology was rare, studies consistently found a subset of survivors who reported significant psychological distress.

In the following decade a trauma model was suggested to explain this subset of poorly adjusted survivors.[45-47] Studies showed increased rates of PTSD amongst childhood cancer survivors. Further research demonstrated that 35% of adolescent cancer survivors met lifetime criteria for PTSD, compared with 7% amongst adolescent survivors of abuse.[48] Workers pointed out that the more general screening tools used previously would not have detected the symptoms of PTSD.

This research provided a model which explained some of the conflicting results in previous studies. It also showed that the perception of threat to life and treatment intensity increased the risk of developing PTSD, as did female gender, other sources of stress, and poor family support. Older age at diagnosis posed increased risk of developing PTSD. Avoidance of triggers was thought to contribute to under-reporting of symptoms.[49]

It generated further questions for research, such as the significance of the repeated traumas inherent in a diagnosis of childhood cancer. What will be the life-course of survivors who develop PTSD, given that psychiatric co-morbidity occurs in 50–90% of sufferers with high rates of depression, anxiety and substance abuse? How does cognitive maturation and personal growth affect the course of PTSD?

These questions are the subject of ongoing research but there is substantial evidence for the development of PTSD in childhood cancer survivors. A study in 2000 showed that 10% of childhood cancer survivors met full PTSD criteria, 78% meeting partial criteria.[50] High levels of PTSD symptoms correlated positively with somatic symptoms, and somatic symptoms increased with severe or recurrent cancer-related traumas. In addition, the workers showed that psychological distress increased with higher levels of somatic symptoms. A repressive style of coping with high levels of avoidance was seen in those with somatic symptoms.

A recent study has also looked at the relationship between somatic concerns and the intensity of chemotherapy, and have revealed a positive association.[51] The same study showed a link between somatic symptoms and increased risk of depression. Another study has concentrated on the incidence of somatic symptoms, such as fatigue, aches and pains, and how this impacts on quality of life. A high level of somatic symptoms appears to reduce life quality.[52]

Studies in recent years have looked again at various markers of psychosocial adjustment, using a host of different scales and outcome measures. Results show that a subset of childhood cancer survivors have reduced academic functioning[53] and poorer friendships and love relationships,[54] and worry more about fertility and the health of their offspring.[55] We must consider how good these outcome measures are as markers of healthy psychosocial adjustment.

Recent reviews[55,56] have commented on factors that may contribute to the conflicting results and have suggested that further high-quality research is needed. These systematic reviews have drawn together some general conclusions from the wealth of literature, and these are summarized below.

- Most childhood cancer survivors function well psychologically.
- Older age at diagnosis, increased functional impairment and a higher number of relapses are adverse psychological risk factors.
- Educational difficulties are more likely in survivors of brain tumours and ALL.
- A significant number of survivors encounter problems with life and health insurance.
- The rate of marriage amongst survivors is decreased.
- The rate of parenthood is lower.
- Survivors worry more about fertility and the health of their offspring.

Implications for the future

Research

Recent reviews[54,55] have highlighted the need for further methodologically precise research, using multicentre prospective longitudinal studies with comparative control groups and clearly defined outcome measures. Various studies have used siblings, peers or other illness groups as controls. Siblings of survivors and youngsters with non-oncological chronic illness have their own psychological issues and may not be the best control groups. Myriad different research tools and outcome measures have been used and they may not be directly comparable. Studies are diverse in population inclusions, differing in age at diagnosis, type of cancer, intensity of treatment and time since completion of treatment. Studies with larger numbers of adolescents would increase the power of results.

Adolescent survivors exhibit more psychological distress than younger children and research methodology should take this into account. When considering the inclusion of cancer type, the relatively poorer psychological prognosis for ALL and brain tumour survivors should be borne in mind. The life course of the adolescent will change with maturity and the progress of disease; multiple assessments are needed to reflect the true lifetime prevalence of psychopathology. Childhood cancer survivors employ adaptive denial to reflect themselves in a good light and therefore self-report scales may not be accurate measures. This and the shift response – an altered perception of distress – may lead to under-reporting.

Time and resources need to be allocated to high-quality research: psychiatrists and oncologists would benefit from combining their expertise

Screening for psychological distress

The needs of the adolescent cancer patient must be considered holistically from the outset; physical, social and psychological issues should be addressed from the onset of care. If this is the case, teenagers will feel less threatened about psychological intervention in the long term. Additionally, support provided in the acute phase of survival can reduce distress and protect against psychiatric morbidity in the future. Those who are perhaps more vulnerable can be identified at an early stage of treatment and links with counsellors and psychologists established at an early stage.

As the needs of adolescents are unique, there is a growing body of opinion suggesting that teenagers should be managed in dedicated adolescent units.[57] This allows the centralization of skill and expertise in relevant specialties.[11] Adolescent units facilitate the maintenance of peer-group relationships, providing an informal level of support. They may also allow the teenager to have improved access to educational facilities; for example, through the provision of computers and of environments conducive to study. Specialist nurses and health-care workers with expertise in dealing with adolescents will aid communication and allow teenagers to vent distressing emotions. Autonomy and independence can also be respected, which will enhance self-esteem. Amongst the disadvantages are the fact that geographical access may be more difficult, further restricting access to peers, family and education.

It is possible to screen for psychological distress amongst adolescent survivors. However, this is not always practical in a busy oncology outpatient clinic; neither is the relevant expertise always available. Currently, follow-up clinics in the UK focus on the detection of relapse and the development of second malignancies. This, of course, is essential, but the needs of the cancer survivor in the acute phase are manifestly different from those in the long term.

Various workers have suggested the need for transition clinics[58] to address ongoing psychosocial problems. If the psychosocial barriers and symptoms of psychological distress are acknowledged and explained from a point early on in diagnosis, this can be a first step in helping to deal with survivors' reactions. Honest discussion of late effects of treatment is imperative, with referral to other specialties if necessary. Advice can be given on modifiable risk factors, such as smoking and diet, emphasizing controllable aspects of lifestyle.

Transition clinics could perform more complex screening for psychiatric morbidity such as PTSD.[58] This requires knowledge of the right questions to ask and which psychological tools to use. Adolescents with symptoms could then benefit from prompt referral to a psychologist or psychiatrist. A multidisciplinary approach would encourage closer links between specialties, facilitating research and education and improving patient care, allowing the survivor to anticipate and plan for many potential psychosocial life stressors – thus avoiding unnecessary future trauma.

Education

Health workers and survivors alike need to be aware of the long-term psychosocial effects of childhood cancer. Issues of survivorship are not always attractive to oncologists and they may not receive adequate training to deal with difficulties when they arise.[59] Health workers need to understand the emotional devastation that can occur in the wake of a cancer diagnosis. The best way to learn is by listening to survivors themselves. More formal education processes need to emphasize the growing importance and relevance of this area. Better liaison between oncologists and mental health-care workers would assist.

Educating adolescent survivors is another way of increasing awareness. If psychological health is discussed openly and routinely when treatment begins, it will not appear threatening; self-efficacy and effective coping measures can be promoted.

Interventions

There is an ongoing need for support and additional help as the adolescent survivor grows up. Various workers have suggested a re-entry programme.[59,60] Adolescents need peer group involvement, support to vent their emotions and empowerment by being equipped with knowledge.[61] Group therapy best serves teenagers' psychosocial needs.[40] Groups help maintain peer relationships, reduce isolation and improve self-esteem and confidence. As a group progresses, knowledge and expertise is shared and group wisdom grows. Role modelling can take place. Taboo topics can be discussed. Two-thirds of adolescent survivors worry about sexual attractiveness and reproductive ability but have never discussed this with their oncologist.[8]

Box 17.4

Survivor speaks

I found a lot of things out the hard way or by accident. I attended follow-up for 10 years. In that time nobody asked me how I was feeling. My chest got X-rayed and then I went home. Don't get me wrong – it was great to know I was 'clear'. But no-one ever discussed fertility with me and the first time I realized I was not infertile was when the dot turned blue on the pregnancy test! That was when I stopped going to follow-up. I realized I had PTSD 7 years ago when I started training in psychiatry. Until then I had assumed my terrible nightmares, tendency to depression and intrusive memories were to be expected. Another patient advised me to apply for life insurance as soon as I hit 10 years cancer-free. When I relapsed 7 years later I was grateful I had heeded her advice.   MCS

Teenagers feel comfortable with group facilitators as time progresses. It may be that oncologists can draw on skills of psychiatric nurses and social workers accustomed to running such groups. A therapeutic group allows staff to identify adolescents with more severe problems who need referral. Programmes evolve with time and maturity and may progress to include workshops, information leaflets, group activities and newsletters.[60]

The teenage survivor who exhibits symptoms of psychiatric illness will benefit from referral to mental health services for assessment and follow-up. Specific therapy, such as cognitive behavioural therapy, may prove an effective intervention.

Postscript and conclusion: living with Damocles

Cicero's anecdote poignantly speaks of life's fragility. The tyrannical emperor Dionysius trades places with his envious courtier, Damocles, to demonstrate the constant threat he lives under. Damocles' initial delight in being invited to take the place of honour at a royal banquet turns to fear as he notices a sword suspended over him by a single horse-hair. Realising the threat of an untimely death, Damocles gratefully returns to his former position of obscurity and safety – an option not open to the teenage cancer survivor, who will always live with Damocles' sword.

In conclusion, it should be emphasized that, whilst a subset of survivors encounter psychiatric problems, the majority of childhood and adolescent cancer survivors are remarkably resilient, despite huge setbacks, and achieve excellent psychosocial function. Additionally, most research to date has not sufficiently addressed the growing evidence that many childhood and adolescent cancer survivors report positive growth from their experiences.[21] Many go on not just to survive cancer but to strive for and attain an enhanced purpose in life. Whether it is possible to measure this by current research methods remains to be seen.

Box 17.5

Survivor speaks

I sometimes wonder – if I could go back and trade places, would I? Would I go back to my safe seat and be a mere onlooker? Or would I choose the sword with its legacy of pain and scars? Can the scars that make us different be made to make a difference? I have grasped the gleaming metal and found a keen blade that has shaped my life uniquely and carved out the pleasure of living the banquet of life. I have loved more intensely through knowing grief; laughed with deeper joy for sorrow overcome; lived with a zest enhanced by the drive for survival. My spirit – birthed in adversity – has glimpsed beyond the banquet's finale.   MCS

Acknowledgements

This chapter is dedicated to my husband, Dr Richard Self, who has always believed in my ability to survive and who unconditionally loves my scars.

I would like to thank Dr J. Bisson, Consultant Liaison Psychiatrist, University Hospital Wales, for his comments and advice on this chapter. I also thank Mr Rod Chaytor, author and journalist, for proofreading the final manuscript.

References

1 Self M. Personal view: the sharp edge of Damocles. *Br Med J* 1999; **318**: 339.
2 Koocher GP, O'Malley GE. *The Damocles Syndrome – Psychosocial Consequences of Childhood Cancer.* New York: McGraw Hill, 1981.
3 Self M, Chaytor R. *From Medicine to Miracle.* London: Harper Collins, 2001.
4 Kissen G. Late effects of treatment on the paediatric oncology patient. In: Selby P, Bailey C, eds. *Cancer and the Adolescent.* London: BMJ Publishing House, 1996.
5 Birch JM, Marsden HB. Improvements in survival from childhood cancer: results of a population based survey over 30 years. *Br Med J* 1988; **296**: 1372–1376.
6 Pediatric Oncology Group. Progress against childhood cancer: the Pediatric Oncology Group experience. *Pediatrics* 1992; **89**: 597–600.
7 Kellerman J, Zeltzer L, Ellenberg L *et al.* Psychological effects of illness in adolescence. I Anxiety, self-esteem and perception of control. *J Pediatr* 1980; **97**: 126–131.
8 Woolverton K, Ostroff J. Psychosexual adjustment in adolescent cancer survivors. *Cancer Invest* 2000; **18**: 51–58.
9 Eiser C. Long-term social adjustment after treatment for childhood cancer. *Arch Dis Child* 1994: **70**: 66–70.
10 Piaget J. *The Moral Judgment of the Child.* New York: Free Press, 1965.
11 Lewis I. Defining adolescence. *Br Med Bull* 1996; **52**: 887–889.
12 Koocher GP. Psychosocial care of the child cured of cancer. *Pediatr Nurs* 1985; **11**: 91–93.
13 Mullan F. Seasons of survival: reflections of a physician with cancer. *N Engl J Med* 1985; **313**: 270–273.
14 O'Malley JE, Koocher GP, Foster D *et al.* Psychiatric sequelae of surviving childhood cancer. *Am J Orthopsychiatry* 1979; **49**: 608–616.
15 Lloyd GG. Psychiatry in general medicine. In: Kendell RE, Zealley AK, eds. *Companion to Psychiatric Studies,* 5th edn. Edinburgh: Churchill Livingstone, 1996.
16 Ross EK. *On Death and Dying.* London: Tavistock, 1970.
17 Canning EH, Ganning RD, Boyce WT. Depressive symptoms and adaptive style in children with cancer. *J Am Acad Child Adolesc Psychiatry* 1992; **31**: 1120–1125.
18 Koocher GP, O'Malley JE, Gogan JL *et al.* Psychological adjustment amongst pediatric cancer survivors. *J Child Psychol Psychiatry* 1980; **21**: 163–173.
19 Roberts CS, Turney M, Knowles AM. Psychosocial issues of adolescents with cancer. *Soc Work Health Care* 1998; **27**: 3–17.
20 Gotay C. Quality of life among survivors of childhood cancer: a critical review and implications for intervention. *J Psychosoc Oncol* 1987; **5**: 5–23.
21 Parry C. Embracing uncertainty: an exploration of the experiences of childhood cancer survivors. *Qual Health Res* 2003; **13**: 227–246.

22 Brennan J. Adjustment to cancer – coping or personal transition? *Psychooncology* 2003; **10**: 1–18.

23 Watson M, Greer S, Young J *et al*. Development of a questionnaire measure of adjustment to cancer: the MAC scale. *Psychol Med* 1988; **18**: 203–209.

24 Watson M, Greer S, Rowden L *et al*. Relationships between emotional control, adjustment to cancer and depression and anxiety in breast cancer patients. *Psychol Med* 1991; **21**: 51–57.

25 Parkes CM. Bereavement as a psychosocial transition: process of adaptation to change. *J Soc Issues* 1988; **44**: 53–65.

26 Muzzin LJ, Andersen NJ, Figueredo AT *et al*. The experience of cancer. *Soc Sci Med* 1994; **38**: 1202–1208.

27 Brennan J, Sheard T. Psychosocial support and therapy in cancer care. *Eur J Palliat Care* 1994; **1**: 136–139.

28 Parkes CM. Psychosocial transitions: a field for study. *Soc Sci Med* 1971; **5**: 101–115.

29 Parkes CM. The dying adult. In: Parkes CM, Markus A, eds. *Coping With Loss*. London: BMJ Books, 1998.

30 Parkes CM. Introduction. In: Parkes CM, Markus A, eds. *Coping With Loss*. London: BMJ Books, 1998.

31 Mackie E, Hill J, Kondryn H *et al*. Adult psychosocial outcomes in long-term survivors of adult lymphoblastic leukemia and Wilms' tumour: a controlled study. *Lancet* 2000; **355**: 1310–1314.

32 Teta MJ, Del Po MC, Kasl SV *et al*. Psychosocial consequences of childhood and adolescent cancer survival. *J Chronic Dis* 1986; **39**: 751–759.

33 Zeltzer LK, Chen E, Weiss R *et al*. Comparison of psychological outcome in adult survivors of childhood acute lymphoblastic leukemia versus sibling controls: a cooperative Children's Cancer Groups and National Institute of Health study. *J Clin Oncol* 1997; **15**: 547–556.

34 Lansky SB, List MS, Ritter-Sterr C *et al*. Psychosocial consequences of cure. *Cancer* 1986; **58**: 529–533.

35 Verrill JR, Schafer J, Vannatta K *et al*. Aggression, anti-social behaviour and substance abuse in survivors of pediatric cancer: possible protective effects of cancer and its treatment. *J Pediatr Psychol* 2000; **7**: 493–502.

36 Rourke MT, Stuber ML, Hobbie WL *et al*. PTSD: understanding the psychosocial impact of surviving childhood cancer into young adulthood. *J Pediatr Oncol Nurs* 1999; **16**: 126–135.

37 American Psychiatric Association. *Diagnostic and Statistical Manual of Mental Disorders, Fourth Edition*. Washington (DC): APA, 1994.

38 Kazak AE, Stuber ML, Barakat LP *et al*. Assessing post traumatic stress related to medical illness and treatment: the impact of traumatic stressors interview schedule (ITSIS). *Fam Syst Med* 1996; **14**: 365–380.

39 Meadows AT, McKee L, Kazak AE. Psychosocial status of young adult survivors of childhood cancer: a survey. *Med Pediatr Oncol* 1989; **17**: 466–470.

40 Fritz GK, Williams JR, Amylon M *et al*. After treatment ends: psychosocial sequelae in pediatric cancer survivors. *Am J Orthopsychiatry* 1988; **58**: 552–561.

41 Kazak AE, Meadows AT. Families of young adolescents who have survived cancer: social–emotional adjustment, adaptability and social support. *J Pediatr Psychol* 1997; **22**: 249–258.

42 Mellete SJ, Franco PC. Psychosocial barriers to employment of the cancer survivor. *J Psychosoc Oncol* 1987; **5**: 97–115.

43 Gogan JL, Koocher GP, Fine WE *et al*. Pediatric cancer survival and marriage: issues affecting adult adjustment. *Am J Orthopsychiatry* 1979; **49**: 423–430.

44 Zeltzer l, Kellerman J. Psychological effects of illness in adolescence: II. Impact of illness in adolescents – crucial issues and coping styles. *J Pediatr* 1980; **97**: 132–138.

45 Barakat LP, Kazak AE, Meadows AT *et al*. Families surviving childhood cancer: a comparison of post traumatic stress symptoms with families of healthy children. *J Pediatr Psychol* 1997; **22**: 843–859.

46 Kazak AE. Post traumatic distress in childhood cancer survivors and their parents. *Med Pediatr Oncol (Suppl)* 1998; **1**: 60–68.

47 Stuber ML, Meeske K, Gonzalez S *et al*. Post traumatic stress after childhood cancer: I. The role of appraisal. *Psychoncology* 1994; **3**: 305–312.

48 Pelcovitz D, Goldenberg L, Mandel F *et al*. Post traumatic stress disorder and family functioning in adolescent cancer. *J Trauma Stress* 1998; **11**: 205–221.

49 Stuber ML, Kazak AE. Is post traumatic stress a viable model for understanding responses to childhood cancer? *Child Adolesc Psychiatr Clin N Am* 1998; **1**: 169–182.

50 Erickson SJ, Steiner H. Somatic symptoms in long-term pediatric cancer survivors. *Psychosomatics* 2000; **41**: 339–346.

51 Zebrack BJ, Zeltzer LK, Whitton J *et al*. Psychological outcomes in long-term survivors of Childhood Leukemia, Hodgkin's Lymphoma and Non Hodgkin's Lymphoma: a report from the Childhood Cancer Survivors' Study. *Pediatrics* 2002; **110**: 42–51.

52 Zebrack BJ, Chesler MA. Quality of life in childhood cancer survivors. *Psychoncology* 2002; **11**: 132–141.

53 Langeveld NE, Stam H, Grootenius MA *et al*. Quality of life in young adult survivors of childhood cancer. *Support Care Cancer* 2002; **10**: 579–600.

54 Newby WL, Brown RT, Pawletko TM *et al*. Social skills and psychological adjustment of child and adolescent cancer survivors. *Psychoncology* 2000; **9**: 113–126.

55 Stam H, Grootenhuis MA, Last BF. Social and emotional adjustment in young survivors of childhood cancer. *Support Care Cancer* 2001; **9**: 489–513.

56 Langeveld NE, Ubbink MC, Last BF *et al*. Educational achievement, employment and living situation in long-term adult survivors of childhood cancer in the Netherlands. *Psychoncology* 2003; **12**: 213–225.

57 Barrett A. Where should patients be treated? In: Selby P, Bailey C, eds. *Cancer and the Adolescent.* London: BMJ Publishing House, 1996.

58 Meeske KA, Ruccione K, Globe DR *et al*. Post traumatic stress, quality of life and psychological distress in young adult survivors of childhood cancer. *Oncol Nurs Forum* 2001; **28**: 481–489.

59 Links PS, Stockwell ML. Obstacles in the prevention of psychological sequelae in survivors of childhood cancer. *Am J Pediatr Hematol Oncol* 1985; **7**: 132–140.

60 Stalker M. Supportive activities requested by survivors of cancer. *J Psychosoc Oncol* 1989; **7**: 21–31.

61 Jamison RN, Lewis S, Burish TG. Psychological impact of cancer on adolescents: self-image, locus of control, perceptions of illness and knowledge of cancer. *J Chronic Dis* 1986; **39**: 609–617.

Part four
Palliation

CHAPTER 18

Whose dying is it anyway? Palliative care in adolescence

R. Hain

Palliative care: its philosophy and nature

Give me a doctor, partridge plump,
Short in the leg and broad in the rump
An endomorph with gentle hands
Who'll never make absurd demands
That I abandon all my vices
Nor pull a long face in a crisis,
But with a twinkle in his eye
Will tell me that I have to die.

W. H. Auden[1]

Only a small proportion of patients are poets, but most poets will at some time or another find themselves as patients. Whilst he may be able to articulate it more clearly than most, Auden probably speaks for many patients in this poem. He gently chastises the medical profession for its emphasis on trying to change his lifestyle in a futile attempt to extend his life. At the same time, he welcomes the presence of a physician who, with kindness and even with humour, can accompany him through his difficult last days.

Coleridge seems to have less patience with us. His comment[2] was that doctors '. . . are *shallow* animals, having always employed their minds about Body and Gut, they imagine that in the whole system of things there is nothing but Gut and Body'.

Both are, in their own ways, trying to make a similar point. If we are to meet the needs of our patients adequately, we need to lift our eyes from the somewhat narrow horizons of simple physical illness and symptomatology and embrace the broader dimensions of human experience. Just as all objects in a physical universe can be described in the three spatial dimensions of depth, breadth and height, so all human experiences can be said to exist in the three dimensions of physical, psychosocial and spiritual (or perhaps better, existential).

This philosophical perspective becomes a particularly important one during the phase of an illness when there is no prospect of a cure. It is a time when physicians, used as we are to dealing with physical problems by providing physical solutions, can feel we have little to offer. Yet, as Auden points out, by considering the other dimensions of what our patients are enduring it is often possible for us to recognize new ways of supporting them and improving the quality of their life. It is important to remember that symptoms, like all experiences, exist simultaneously in all three dimensions. There are not, for example, symptoms that have only physical aspects any more than there are objects that possess only length. All symptoms need to be considered as far as possible in all dimensions. This multidimensional or holistic approach is a fundamental principle on which palliative medicine in children and young people is based.

The nature of palliative care

Physical

The physical aspects of a symptom are often considered by the young person in terms of the question 'What is happening?' followed closely by 'What can be done to stop it?' These are the questions with which, perhaps, physicians feel most comfortable. We are used to a model that identifies a problem, analyses it and provides a solution. In attempting to encompass a broader understanding of symptoms, it is important not to lose sight of the centrality of physical issues for many. For example, adequate management of the pain of metastasis from osteosarcoma necessarily includes adequate diagnosis and appropriate management. Unrelieved pain with a major physical component will make attention to wider issues extremely difficult.

Psychosocial

The psychosocial dimension links two aspects of a symptom. The first can be considered by asking 'How will this affect my life?' It therefore invokes issues about functioning and the role of an individual in family, school, university, or society generally. The second aspect is that addressed by the question 'How do I feel about it?' This invokes an individual young person's *response* to a change in function. The move from a role as elder sibling, for example, to dependent child involves a process of adjustment and loss which young people may find very difficult. Thus, it is not enough simply to consider factually the impact of symptoms on a young person's functioning: one should also consider how he or she feels about and responds to that impact.

Spiritual or existential

In some ways this is the aspect of an experience that can be most difficult to define and is certainly the most personal. Spirituality is often confused with religion, and indeed the two are often closely related. At the same time, the concepts that lie behind spirituality are quite distinct from those of any specific formalized religion. Spirituality refers to the way an individual attempts to develop a construct of reality that explains his or her experience. It is therefore characterized by the questions 'Why is this happening to me?' and 'What does it mean?'. A specific religious framework may provide an answer. Some of these may be unhelpful; for example, if illness or pain is blamed on lack of faith or on punishment by a vengeful god. Others may be extremely valuable, providing explanations in terms of benefit to others or personal spiritual growth.

It is important not to make assumptions about spirituality based on an individual's religious conviction. Atheism, based on a firmly held but unprovable belief that there is no god, is as much a faith as any other and just as liable to be questioned in the last days and weeks of life. Young people with no belief in God may put their trust instead in healthy eating and exercise and feel betrayed and aggrieved if they nevertheless become ill. These are spiritual issues.

In short, spiritual aspects of symptoms should not begin, still less end, with formal religious belief. Spirituality is a characteristic of human beings which, however it is manifested, needs to be acknowledged in working with young people during the palliative phase of their illness.

The nature of palliative care in children and young people

So the philosophical premise of palliative medicine is a holistic understanding of human experience, including symptoms. This ambitious and all-encompassing approach was applied to children and young people by the Royal College of Paediatrics and Child Health in 1997.[3] The RCPCH/ACT document defined palliative care as '. . . an active and total approach to the care of children, embracing physical, emotional, social and spiritual elements'. Based on this definition, the Royal College defined four groups of life-limiting conditions in which children and young people might need palliative care. The four groups are shown in Table 18.1.

Table 18.1 Conditions that may need palliative medicine in adolescents and young people

Group 1: Life-threatening conditions for which curative treatment may be feasible but can fail. Palliative care may be necessary during periods of prognostic uncertainty and when treatment fails (eg cancer, cardiac anomalies).	***Group 2***: Conditions in which there may be long periods of intensive treatment aimed at prolonging life and allowing participation in normal childhood activities, but premature death is still possible (eg cystic fibrosis, muscular dystrophy).
Group 3: Progressive conditions without curative treatment options, in which treatment is exclusively palliative and may commonly extend over many years (Batten's disease, mucopolysaccharidosis).	***Group 4***: Conditions with severe neurological disability which may cause weakness and susceptibility to health complications, and may deteriorate unpredictably, but are not considered progressive (eg severe cerebral palsy).

The significance of this publication was two-fold: firstly, until publication, it had often been considered that once cure was no longer possible, physicians had nothing further to offer in the management of young people with life-limiting conditions. While affirming the role of other professionals in their care, the Royal College document underlined the important role that the physician can and should play in the care of young people with life-limiting conditions.

Secondly, the Royal College extended the definition of palliative care well beyond what had previously been considered. It now includes, for example, non-malignant conditions that are nevertheless terminal. Previously, the adult model of palliative medicine, based almost entirely on the understanding of symptoms in cancer, had often been extrapolated to children and young people. Suddenly, in the wake of the RCPCH publication it was clear that here was a different and much larger constituency whose needs needed to be considered by those expert in their care. Ramifications of the 1997 RCPCH publication are still being felt. Service development in palliative care services to children and young people is assuming greater priority nationally and internationally.

Adolescents and palliative care

Adolescents and young people are over-represented among those with life-limiting conditions, both malignant and non-malignant. Among those with cancer, this is because the nature of solid tumours in childhood is such that those occurring in adolescence, such as osteosarcoma and rhabdomyosarcoma, often carry a poor prognosis. In leukaemia, adolescents are more likely to die than younger children because their leukaemia is of a more drug-resistant phenotype.

Adolescents and young people are also over-represented among those with non-malignant life-limiting conditions. This is largely a result of the natural history of these conditions. One of the commonest is Duchenne muscular dystrophy. The trajectory of this disease means that its palliative phase typically falls in late adolescence or early adulthood.

The specific needs of adolescents should therefore have some priority in considering how to develop and expand palliative medicine services.

Emotional needs

Although a great many different definitions of the term 'adolescence' have been used, perhaps the most useful are those that consider it a period in life characterized by the need to achieve a series of goals.[4] The essential task of adolescence is to become an autonomous adult by severing ties with parents and the exploration and discovery of self. For the adolescent with normal intellectual function the palliative phase occurring during this task is characterized by a number of paradoxes. As the condition progresses, the young person becomes increasingly dependent, rather than increasingly autonomous, in direct opposition to the natural progress of development into an adult. At the same time, there are aspects of the process of dying that can actually facilitate the achievement of autonomy. Many young people have identified that the process of dying has helped them to 'grow up' and to begin to see things from the perspective of an independent adult at an earlier age.[5] As an adolescent seeking to exert influence over family, many find that, by virtue of their condition, they are given much more control. Adolescents dying from cancer find themselves curtailed in physical activity but at the same time more able to influence the actions of others around them.

Lastly, there is of course a sense in which dying represents ultimate independence: the adolescent who is dying is preparing to leave the family for ever.

Physical

Adolescents and young people are distinct from younger children and from older adults in a number of important physical ways. They are substantially larger than children and indeed physically often resemble adults. At the same time, their renal function is rather better than that of most adults and resembles much more closely that of children. This may be important, for example, when considering the dose of opioid analgesics, which are largely excreted renally. It is not clear whether dosing regimens should be extrapolated from data in children or in adults. In practice, it usually depends on the background and experience of the physician writing the prescription.

Adolescents are much more likely than younger children to be able to articulate symptoms accurately and with abstract understanding. This is partly because adolescents simply have better abstract capabilities than younger children. It is also because adolescents needing palliative care include a high proportion of those suffering from conditions that do not affect intelligence, such as cancer and Duchenne muscular dystrophy. By contrast, younger children with cerebral palsy or neurodegenerative conditions are often unable to articulate symptoms clearly.

Once again, therefore, it is clear that adolescents and young people are distinct both from adults and from younger children. Whatever their chronological age and however they may physically resemble adults, they are in reality quite distinct and need to be considered as such.

Spiritual

Figure 18.1 is a drawing by a 14-year-old girl dying from acute myeloid leukaemia. It shows the figure of an adolescent girl inside a bubble. In places she has broken through the bubble and there are fragments of cracked and shattered glass.

This picture illustrates the central contradiction of adolescence generally, not just adolescence with a life-limiting condition. On the one hand, the artist is trapped. The impression is that she is struggling to break free, and indeed she has begun to succeed; her limbs and head are beginning to break out.

At the same time, there is a clear sense that the figure is ambivalent about her hard-won freedom. She draws herself naked and vulnerable. There is the impression that the bubble does not simply trap her, it also protects her. There

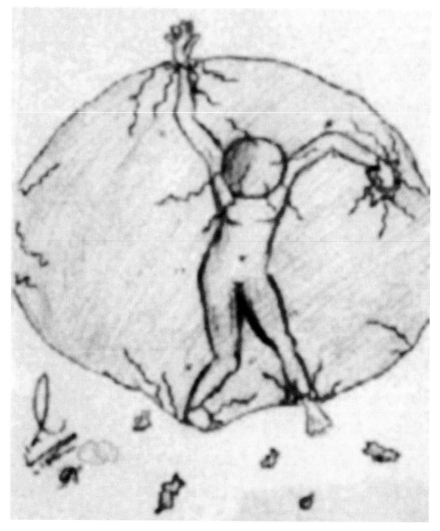

Fig. 18.1 Self-portrait by Sharon, a 14-year-old girl dying from acute myeloid leukaemia. (Reproduced with permission from her family and from Myriam Weyl Ben Arush, Associate Professor in Pediatrics, Pediatric Hematology Oncology Department, Meyer Children's Hospital, Rambam Medical Centre, Haifa, Israel.)

is a violence about the way she has broken free, and the jagged fragments that have resulted, that suggests she finds the process of breaking free traumatic and painful.

It is perhaps true for all human beings that autonomy is exciting, but also frightening. The challenge in caring for adolescents and young people is that they simultaneously require and repel the support of family and professional carers. Sometimes this may require the careful and sensitive balancing of benefits. For example, many young people would prefer not to take regular morphine when they are told to do so, even if the result of not taking it is an increase in their physical pain. Perfect physical pain control might be possible, but if it is at the expense of overriding his or her autonomy, then to the adolescent it may not be worth the cost.

Social

There is, of course, infinitely wide variability in the issues that affect an adolescent socially. Social dimensions of human experience are concerned with issues of an individual's role within relationships, family and perhaps society. Three aspects perhaps have particular importance for adolescents and young people.

Self-image

Self-image goes well beyond issues of sexuality. Adolescence is a time of immense sensitivity to personal appearance. During the palliative phase, dramatic changes can occur with frightening rapidity, leaving little time to adjust. Adolescent boys with Duchenne muscular dystrophy find they are becoming painfully thin while their normal peers are becoming more muscular. Girls may lose their hair as a result of chemotherapy, or their figure as a result of steroids. Many find the insertion of gastrostomy tubes or central lines difficult to adjust to.

Oddly, however, other adolescents report positive benefits of terminal illness in self-image.[5] These often focus on weight loss and perhaps reflect rather sadly on the priorities of modern image-makers. Individuals who have been concerned by minor physical flaws may feel quite differently when confronted with the possibility of the need for amputation. It is important to remember that adolescents and young people needing palliative care are adolescents first and dying patients very much second. Their image of themselves owes much more to their affinity with their peers and icons than to the stereotypes of their condition.

Sexuality

Inherent in the achievement of autonomy during adolescence is the discovery of one's own sexual identity. Sexual activity is not necessary in order to establish one's identity, but in practice the two usually go together. For adolescents and young people with life-limiting conditions, opportunities for sexual activity are usually limited. It is often tempting to address this in superficial ways; for example, simply by facilitating sexual experience. Whilst this may be very helpful for some individuals, of itself it is not enough. Sexual identity is not simply the capacity to perform sexual acts; it is the way in which we as individuals relate to others as individuals, based on our gender. We attempt to elicit responses that inform and reassure us of our own identity as sexual beings. This process, largely independent of sexual practice, continues for most adolescents during the palliative phase. Again, young people with life-limiting conditions have much more in common here with other adolescents than with other people with life-limiting conditions. Like other individuals of their age, they need the opportunity to develop and express sexuality, but also need to have appropriate boundaries.

'Function'

In achieving autonomy during adolescence, a young person has to review his or her role in life. Young adulthood will shift the emphasis from being primarily a son, daughter, brother or sister to being principally someone's partner or friend. The emphasis may move from being the recipient of care in the home to being the provider, from being pupil to being employee. Superimposed on this shifting sense of personal responsibility the adolescent with cancer will have to face a change from being strong and healthy, perhaps caring for siblings or even elderly parents, to needing the care of others.

Ethical issues

Because it is a period of transition that largely defies precise definition, adolescence is characterized by a number of ethical issues that need to be considered during palliative management. Two important ones are consent and confidentiality.

Consent

The question of whether an individual young person has the right to consent to treatment has by tradition been left largely to doctors. Because it is based on case law and therefore can be changed by subsequent rulings, the legal position is not always clear. The assumption of many doctors, on the other hand, is that the law is a machine into which a problem can be fed at one end and a solution retrieved at the other. This is far from the case.

Children who are 16 years and over are treated in essentially the same way as adults. The Family Law Reform Act of 1968[6] says that the '. . . consent of a minor who has attained the age of sixteen years to any . . . treatment which in the absence of consent would constitute trespass to his person, shall be as effective as if he were of full age . . .'. However, it is also recognized that children who are less than 16 years may nevertheless be perfectly competent to give consent. The often ill-understood concept of 'Gillick competence' was summarized in 1992[7] in the following way: '. . . Gillick competent child can consent, but if he or she declines to do so . . . consent can be given by someone else who has parental rights or responsibilities'. In other words, a child who is under 16 but competent can give consent but may not necessarily be able to withhold it. At the same time, the judgment went on to say '. . . refusal of a Gillick competent child is a very important factor in the doctor's decision whether or not to treat . . .'. In other words, as physicians we cannot override the stated wishes of a child who is 16 or over any more than we could if they were adult. We can override the wishes of a Gillick-competent child if we have parental permission, but if we do so we would have to be prepared to show the courts that we have taken the child's wishes very seriously into account.

Those working in palliative medicine may therefore find themselves having to advocate for adolescents and young people in their determination to refuse interventions. Sometimes this advocacy may also be against professional colleagues. Despite its efficacy, some boys with Duchenne muscular dystrophy will choose not to have non-invasive nocturnal ventilation. It may be our job to ensure that young people are not coerced into a procedure with which they are not comfortable.

Confidentiality and collusion

Physicians have a tendency to assume that parents have an automatic right to access information about their children. This is not the case. This was clarified recently by the British Medical Association[8] in the following way: 'All patients, regardless of their age . . . are entitled to expect that information about themselves . . . discovered in the course of their health care will not be revealed to others without their consent'. In other words, a child is entitled to the same right of confidentiality as an adult. In practice, of course, it is generally taken as read that a child is happy for his or her parents to have access to medical information about him or her. This is clearly the only practical approach. It would be perverse to imagine that parents could exercise their responsibilities in any realistic way without being granted such access.

The right to confidentiality becomes much more challenging in practice when an adolescent or young person is in the palliative phase. Professional carers often find themselves discussing management with parents. As the disease progresses and the news becomes grimmer, it is more and more tempting for parent and professional alike to hold discussions in the young person's absence, and selectively to feed back filtered information. This is a transgression of the right to confidentiality and should be avoided. It is also practically undesirable and makes good palliative medicine extremely difficult.

Parents may want to withhold information from their adolescent offspring for many reasons:
- to protect him or her from painful news
- fear that he or she will give up on hearing the news
- to avoid the personal pain of discussing a difficult topic
- to avoid facing the truth themselves.

Many of these reasons have the young person's best interests at heart, and most parents feel they are benefiting their child by not passing on bad news. However, it is essential that we as professionals acknowledge that it is not their information to withhold in the first place. Parents have access to their child's information because the child, implicitly or explicitly, gives them permission to do so. The information belongs to the young person, who may then choose to share it with their family, not vice versa.

How do we avoid this? Generally, at diagnosis the care team communicates with the family and adolescent as though they were a single unit, assuming that communications between young person and family are good. As the care team gets to know the young person better, they may communicate with family and young person independently. Provided there is good communication between adolescent and family, this does not matter. However, as the news becomes more difficult for the care team to discuss with the adolescent they may unconsciously begin to communicate with the family alone. At the same time, the family will typically find it increasingly difficult to discuss issues with the young person. As time passes, communication becomes largely or exclusively between the care team and the family and the adolescent becomes increasingly isolated. This process in which information about the young person is freely discussed by the care team and family, with or without reference to the adolescent, is known as 'collusion'.

To avoid this, the care team should ideally concentrate its communications energies on the adolescent. Provided communication between the young person and family is good, there will be free flow of information. If communication between family and adolescent becomes less open, the care team should, with the adolescent's permission, open up channels of discussion with the family. The effect of this is to put the young person in charge, and affirm their rights over their information. An adolescent has to be given the chance to choose how to share his or her information. This supports the young person in attaining the goal of autonomy.

In practice, this can best be done by involving the young person from the start, when the news is not so bad and is less difficult to share. All new information should be given to the patient and family simultaneously, and families should be encouraged to discuss issues openly. It can be helpful to allow parents to explain their perception of a situation in the presence of the young person him or herself, so that any misunderstandings can be corrected. The effect of this is to emphasize the care team's role as information source without compromising the unspoken contract of care with the family or young person.

Although it is usually unhelpful for families to withhold information from young people, it is important that professional carers should recognize and respect genuine coping strategies. For some families, not discussing it with the young person is the right thing to do after all. Insisting on a communication strategy that is more open than the family (including the young person) can deal with is intrusive and counterproductive.

How do we meet these needs?

There has been a growing awareness over recent years of the distinct needs of young people for palliative care. A superb summary has been provided by the Association for Children with Life-limiting or Terminal Conditions and their Families (ACT) working with the National Council for Hospice and Specialist Palliative Care Services and the Scottish Partnership Agency for Palliative Cancer Care. Their 2002 publication *Palliative Care for Young People Aged 13–24 years*[9] summarizes much of the research done in this area and sets out a number of important steps that need to be taken. These are:

- recognition of young people needing palliative care as a distinct group
- involvement of young people themselves in decision-making
- multidisciplinary and multi-agency services
- provision of link and key workers
- joint health and social service planning
- development of psychological and spiritual services
- transition planning from children's services
- specific training in palliative care and in management of young people among those working in this field.

Summary

Adolescents have unique needs and this is equally true in the palliative phase of a life-limiting condition. Service development in palliative care for young people should reflect this uniqueness. Adolescents should be treated with the same respect as adults, even if they sometimes use their autonomy to choose to act as children.

References

1 Auden W. *Collected Poems*. Washington (DC): Vintage USA, 1991.
2 Coleridge S. On doctors. 1776. Letter to Charles Lloyd, Sen. 15 October 1796. Quoted by R. Porter in *The Greatest Benefit to Mankind: A Medical History of Humanity*. Harper Collins, 1997.
3 Baum D, Curtis H, Elston S *et al. A Guide to the Development of Children's Palliative Care Services*, 1st edn. Bristol: ACT/RCPCH, 1997.
4 Erikson EH. *Childhood and Society*. London: Penguin, 1965.
5 Hodgson AE. *'Everything has changed' – experiences of young people with recurrent metastatic cancer*. MSc thesis, University of Wales College of Medicine, Cardiff, 2003.
6 Family Law Reform Act (6) 1968 Section 8(i).
7 Re: R (A minor) Wardship: consent to treatment. In: Fam 11 at 12; 1992.
8 British Medical Association. *Consent, Rights and Choices in Health Care for Children and Young People*, 1st edn. London: BMJ Books, 2001.
9 Joint Working Party on Palliative Care for Adolescents and Young Adults. *Palliative Care for Young People Aged 13–24 Years*. Bristol: ACT, 2001.

CHAPTER 19

The parent's perspective of teenage cancer

R. Kanarek and V. Riley

The following presentation, which is in narrative format, explores some universal themes amongst parents whose teenagers battle cancer. Two nurses discuss it from different perspectives. One nurse, Mrs Robin Kanarek from the USA, lost her 15-year-old son after a 5-year battle with acute lymphocytic leukaemia and describes her family's tribulations. The other nurse, Ms Vikky Riley, shares what she has learnt from parents whilst working as a nurse on the Teenage Cancer Trust Unit at the Middlesex Hospital, London.

Robin Kanarek: *Why did the chicken cross the road? Seventeen!*

> This may seem ridiculous to you, but that was the way my 4-year-old son, David, told his first joke. While he had mastered the form of telling the joke, the substance had still eluded him. He knew that following the answer to the question came an avalanche of laughter. He had not yet made a connection that the answer needed to be appropriate to the question.
>
> During the years our family battled David's cancer, we witnessed numerous situations where the substance of the treatment was perfect but its delivery form did not always take the family into consideration. So while David, as a toddler, missed the substance of the story, the medical team sometimes misses the nuances of the form.
>
> My name is Robin Kanarek and I lost my 15-year-old son David to acute lymphocytic leukaemia in 2000, after a 5-year battle with the disease, including chemotherapy and a stem cell transplant. I have also been a registered nurse in the United States for the past 25 years. I have been asked to speak today by the Teenage Cancer Trust (TCT) organizers to present a different point of view of teenage cancer treatment. I worked on a TCT committee with Mrs Myrna Whiteson and Mr Simon Davies, 1 year after our losing David, to develop an educational brochure for parents whose teenagers were recently diagnosed with cancer. It is there that I

met Vikky Riley, my co-presenter today. When we served on this committee together, she told us about many of her experiences with her patients. I was astounded by her insight into the psyche of teens undergoing treatment. She understood what I went through with David and knew about all the intimate issues of care we as a family had experienced. She had a keen and very deep sense of what it was all about. I wish David had had a 'Vikky' throughout his experience to help provide him the guidance and support he needed.

My husband, Joe, and our daughter, Sarah, are here today and have provided me with the strength and support to share our story. By sharing some of our personal ordeals, we hope to shed some light on the impact cancer has on the entire family.

As David's mother, I look back on what he experienced throughout his short life and I am in awe at how well he adapted to the effects of the disease and the treatment.

Sarah, my daughter, who is now 13, also had to endure a great deal throughout David's illness. She was 5 when David was diagnosed and spent much of her early years in the shadow of his illness. Sarah was 10 years old when David relapsed and was the only suitable candidate for a stem cell donation. Initially, she was terrified of all the procedures she was to undergo to facilitate the transplant. David patiently explained what would happen to her and reassured her throughout the entire process. They were very close. Through David's experience, Sarah now has an insight and maturity well beyond her years.

Vikky Riley: I am a nurse who has specialized in adolescent oncology for over 12 years and during this time completed an MSc in Counselling and Psychotherapy. I am also a mother of a 4-year-old son. Robin has explained how we first met, but at our first meeting I felt like a fraud. I had been asked to provide an expert's view on a parent leaflet we were working on, but was acutely aware that two of the women at the meeting had lost their beloved sons to cancer. They had lived the experience I only choose to work within. I am not only in awe of the young people I meet, but also their parents. By listening to the parents and hearing their experiences, I have learned so much and I hope to represent their perspective today.

We have deliberately chosen not to concentrate on the specific issues for parents when their teenage child dies. Firstly, we think that this would have been almost impossible for Robin to do. Secondly, the actual death of one's child is not the part of their life that you want to remember, in fact, the majority of parents describe trying desperately to restore happy memories to the front of their minds rather than the painful ones associated with death. It is our hope, therefore, to present the significance of a process that begins at diagnosis. If the process is instituted as we advocate from time of diagnosis, the parents, though devastated, will not be left with unnecessary hurt and regrets after death of their teenage child.

We do not profess to speak on behalf of all parents. However, after many hours of discussion, we have identified four recurring themes. You may already be aware of what we will discuss, but what we want to convey is its impact and how it carries into the family's life. The four themes are as follows:

- Cancer is more than an illness.
- The impact a cancer diagnosis and treatment has on parents.
- The complex issues faced by parents.
- Strategies for health-care professionals.

Cancer is more than an illness

- A cancer diagnosis has cultural, religious, social and psychological implications and parental adaptation is challenged by feelings of failure, punishment and fear of death.

Even in the 21st century, for many a diagnosis of cancer holds fear and dread. When a young person is diagnosed with cancer, it can be a truly terrifying experience for everyone involved. The parents who need support have developed their own attitudes and beliefs about cancer through past experiences and the influence of the media and literature. Unless health-care professionals recognize the complexity of a cancer diagnosis, they will be ineffective when seeking to provide support to their patients and parents.

From a cultural and religious perspective, cancer as an illness holds different meanings. *A Turkish mother described her terror and explained that cancer was so feared in her community that many people would not even say the word 'cancer'.*

A Nigerian mother who was expressing guilt over her daughter's cancer explained to me *'It is difficult for you to understand, but my child having cancer is my punishment for having been bad.'*

A Catholic mother expressed what I have heard many times, *'When I got pregnant I considered an abortion. Now I wonder if I am being punished.'*

Despite medical advances it is also essential from the parent's perspective to recognize that cancer continues to carry the spectre of death. *'Death is like a shadow or ghost that hovers all around. It haunts you all the time'* – a father's view.

Robin Kanarek: The oncologist entered the room and told me that David had leukaemia. In that moment, my whole world was torn apart. Joe was at work and I asked the doctor to call Joe to give him the news. She was very calm when speaking to him and told him that she was most confident that David's leukaemia was treatable and curable. That was all Joe had to hear. The doctor had told him that David would be OK and that was enough for him to hear to mentally prepare for what lay ahead.

The doctor and I then had to tell David the news. Amazingly, David was relieved when he was told that there was a name to his problem. He had no idea what cancer was. His response to the diagnosis was *'Well as least we know what the problem is and now we can treat it'*. I was stunned. It wasn't until several months later when we had to put our 10-year-old dog to sleep because she had cancer that David finally understood the severity of his condition.

Throughout that first week of treatment, the oncologist constantly reassured us that David's prognosis was a good one. I was numb for several days following the diagnosis. I was unable to retain whatever the nurses and doctors told us. Books, videos and pamphlets were constantly being given to us and all I did was put them aside. All I wanted to do was shout *'Stop, this cannot be happening!'*

After being in the hospital for 3 days I went home to see Sarah. I listened to the answering machine and received numerous messages from friends and family who had heard the news and told how devastated they were for us. At that moment, the reality of what was happening finally set in.

Vikky Riley: At the time of greatest distress we might seek to provide unrealistic reassurance. This is dangerous because of the unpredictable nature of cancer. The process of truthful communication, however difficult, between the teenager, parent and health professional needs to be handled with compassion and sensitivity.

The impact of a cancer diagnosis and treatment upon the teenager and their family

- Family life: Robin will describe the impact that David's leukaemia made upon David and her family.

Robin Kanarek: The first few weeks following the initial diagnosis until David reached remission was an unbearably difficult time for us as a family. Our first priority was, of course, David – learning about all his medications, side-effects, signs of adverse reactions and daily care. For me as a nurse, this was not a difficult transition. But I can't imagine how stressful this would be for parents with no medical training. I met many parents in the waiting room of the oncologist's office and many told me of their difficulties with insurance companies, lost wages and the juggling of care for their other children. Luckily, I had family and friends nearby. Many families do not have this available to them. We quickly learned to re-establish our family's priorities and only focused on what was most important – which of course was David and ourselves.

Over the course of those first 2 years of David's protocol, we were constantly reminded that we could not look too far ahead. The future was a scary place. We took each day as it came. Our time as a family was precious and by knowing that there was a possibility of losing him, everything became more meaningful and special.

David relapsed three and a half years after his initial diagnosis. He was absolutely devastated and felt betrayed. We had no idea how we could bear watching David suffer through the treatment again. But we had no choice. We needed to be strong and to go forward with him. This is when one learns the strength of the human spirit. Our family depended on each other for support and encouragement. My husband and I found solace in one another. We worked together as a team and it brought us closer than I could ever imagine. Those special memories provide a tremendous source of comfort to us now.

Vikky Riley

- Social isolation

Cancer alters relationships and can lead to social isolation for the young person and their family. This can lead to a sense of abandonment and can compromise the teenager's and parents' ability to cope. Throughout our lives we establish support networks and if these fail at the time of greatest stress it can be extremely destabilizing. For most young people, their main social network is school or college. When these networks fail, parents experience further guilt, anger or frustration, as they want to protect their child from further hurt.

Robin Kanarek: Many friends could not handle the cancer diagnosis and never made contact with us after David became ill. Then, there were those special few, who through their own personal experience knew what we were going through and, without asking, took it upon themselves to help us. Of those who avoided us, some have reconnected, but many have not. I understand and don't hold it against them.

Luckily, David's closest friends supported him through his first bout with leukaemia; only when he relapsed and underwent a stem cell transplant did his friendships wane. He was in strict isolation for weeks and even when he returned home those who visited him had to wear a mask. This must have been terrifying to 15-year-olds. David's best friend was there every bit of the way and I still keep in touch with his family. I am sure that the loss of David will forever have an impact on how he views life.

Vikky Riley

- Sense of loss

The vast majority of us have hopes and dreams and we spend our lives planning for the future. Having a child intensifies these hopes and dreams but a cancer fills the future with fear. The sense of loss, and the need to grieve for what has been lost, following a child's cancer diagnosis cannot be emphasized enough. *'Everyone expects me to be strong. I find I am the one saying "it will be okay". But, it's* my *heart that is torn apart'* – Parent.

Parents are faced with a colossal challenge. Whilst separated from family and friends they have to juggle finances, travel arrangements and care of other children. They have to find the strength to witness the loss of their child's health and dreams as their child undergoes countless procedures. They witness their child's body being invaded and made ill by the very medicines that are meant to be making them well. They watch as their child's hair falls out and then have to find the energy to support their child as they return for another session of debilitating treatment.

It is not a surprise that after 12 years in the specialty, I remain in complete awe of parents who do the best they can in the most difficult of circumstances.

The complex issues faced by parents whose teenager is diagnosed with cancer

- Child versus adolescent

'I wish he was little again, four or five. Then I could make the decisions, cuddle him and keep him safe' – Mother.

Robin Kanarek: David was 11 years old when he was diagnosed. When he relapsed in 1999, he was just shy of his 15th birthday. His reaction to his diagnosis at 11 was very different from the one at 15. At 11, he had no experience with cancer and he had no expectation of what he was to endure. My husband and I cared for him around the clock and made every decision for him. By the time he relapsed, he knew the medications, side-effects, prognosis, treatment plan and what was entailed to get him into remission. He wanted some control over what was happening to him and became an active participant in his care. He still wanted my husband and I to make the really difficult decisions. Although he was more capable and interested in understanding what was going on, he wasn't as mature as an adult. He was an adolescent going through puberty and fluctuated between child and adult.

The following is an account that will illustrate this point. After relapse, David had to take numerous pills throughout the day. I would prepare and leave them for him to take. One day, I happened to be emptying the waste bin when I noticed several pills lying at the bottom. How could *my* responsible, intelligent son do such an illogical thing? When confronted, he sulked like a child caught in the act, and responded, *'I don't know – I just didn't want to take them.'* I am sure he wanted to get caught, or else he would have disposed of them in a less conspicuous place. I realized he was not an adult – he was a teenager and entitled to have moments of irrational behaviour. From that moment on, we took turns watching him take his medication.

In contrast, David had moments of being wise beyond his years and had a deep understanding of life. We learned a great deal during that time, especially about priorities and the importance of family. There were times when my husband and I were overwhelmed with responsibility. We tried to hide this from David, but of course he picked up on it. It was during these times we would find David consoling *us* and telling us that he was going to be just fine.

Vikky Riley: Robin has eloquently described the differences between a child with cancer and a teenager. Adolescence is a complex time and because a cancer diagnosis can interrupt the transition from child to adult it is vital that the process must be negotiated with sensitivity and understanding. One minute a teenager may feel and behave like a child and yet in the next moment demonstrate maturity and wisdom.

- Privacy, legal rights, social and ethical implications

The teenager's privacy, dignity and social independence are all jeopardized, and as health professionals it is of importance that we understand the significance of this.

We have to help parents see the importance of their role in helping their child, however unwell or regressed, to adapt to the diagnosis and to enable the teenager to reclaim their identity, independence and control. Parents need to be supported through this process as it can be extremely challenging and vary from moment to moment. One mother bravely admitted '*I feel guilty but it is like having my baby back. I can do things for her again and actually spend time with her. I feel needed again.*'

We also have to consider the ethical issues we confront every day in order to be able to deal with the philosophical challenges we face. Who does the information belong to? What if the young person really does not want his parents to know about his illness? What if he wants to stop his treatment? None of these dilemmas have clear-cut answers, but as health professionals we must be aware of the difficult area in which we choose to specialize and be able to cope with these complexities.

Strategies for the health-care team to help parents cope

- Why professional and personal self-awareness/boundaries are essential to be an effective practitioner in adolescent cancer care

Traditionally, many health-care professionals have adopted the distant professional image to resist becoming emotionally involved. This way of practising is unhelpful to everyone involved. It does not allow the professional to consider what cancer means to parents and how their work impacts upon them and those they seek to help. As health professionals, we may not be aware of how our choice of words and actions, or lack of, can haunt parents forever.

I will never forget when an oncologist told a 14-year-old girl in front of her mother that they were too close and needed a '*motherectomy*'. Symbolically, the word is hard enough to hear, how much harder for the mother whose child was undergoing a transplant.

Robin Kanarek: When David relapsed, we had to choose a paediatric cancer centre to have his stem cell transplant performed. Our oncologist favoured a particular institution, so we went to the centre with David to discuss the probable treatment plan. David was in a wheelchair and too weak to walk. We met with the head of the transplant team. The doctor immediately began going into detail about the complexities of the case. Graphs and statistics were provided to demonstrate the outcomes of their programme, with an emphasis on the complications and mortality rates. My husband and I looked at David; his eyes were facing downwards, his hands were covering his ears. We were mortified that this highly regarded physician could be so insensitive as to how David would respond to what she was saying. The insensitivity of the doctor to David's presence in the room enraged us. I am sure she did not display this behaviour intentionally and had no idea how it would affect us, but if the head of the department was this unaware of the results of the words she chose, what would the rest of the team's tone have been like?

Vikky Riley: Adolescent oncology is often traumatic and sad. We witness the beauty and the fragility of life every day. We see at first hand intimate family interactions and it is difficult to remain unmoved, but that is why self-awareness and maintenance of boundaries are so crucial. Alternatively, over-involvement is equally damaging to the health-care professional and those we seek to support. As health-care professionals we must be alert at all times to what we are feeling.

I remember a charismatic young man called Danny. He developed a close rapport with one particular nurse and they had great fun bantering and teasing one another. Their relationship became blurred and Danny viewed her as a friend not a professional. He soon relapsed and was admitted extremely unwell. As this nurse entered the room, he shouted, '*No, I want a nurse to look after me – not you!*'

We know it can difficult to balance professional boundaries in adolescent oncology. To be effective requires maturity and self-awareness, but to illustrate the importance I turn to the wise words of Debbie, a mum: '*It makes me feel special that you all care. But it is scary when I see some nurses cry. Who is going to be in control and support me?*'

• Parental support and involvement is crucial

The aim of most adolescent health-care models is the promotion of independence from parents and a sense of control over their medical condition for the teenager. But when a teenager is diagnosed with cancer, it is different. Cancer can interrupt adolescent transition, as it does normal life, with potentially devastating consequences. We must be alert to this, but at a time of crisis teenagers diagnosed with cancer turn to those closest to them, and that is usually their parents. Parental support and involvement is therefore crucial if the teenager is to adapt to the impact of their cancer diagnosis. It is imperative that support for the parents be readily available.

On the Teenage Cancer Trust Unit where I work, a multidisciplinary team strives to work as a united team whilst respecting each other's different roles when seeking to provide support for patients and their parents. One-to-one support is provided as well as a weekly parents' group. We recognize the importance of community and local hospital staff as they work closely with parents and often visit them at home. Liaison is crucial between all the health professionals involved with the teenager and their family, so that concerns can be discussed and appropriate interventions implemented. Many health professionals believe in arranging support by linking parents with parents who have been through a similar experience. Parents understand each other better than anyone, but that does not negate the need for effective professional support, as demonstrated by Robin's story.

Robin Kanarek: After David relapsed, we explored a stem cell transplant as a treatment option. Throughout this time, a local chapter of a cancer organization wanted to help us. The organization found a mom who was willing to talk to me. She called and told me how well her son was doing 2 years post transplant. Over the course of a few minutes, though, she slowly divulged that not all was actually well. Her son had developed graft versus host disease and it was having a profound effect on the quality of his life. He was not able to go to university, lived at home as a hermit and had few friends. Upon hearing this I panicked. I needed to hear hopeful, successful accounts, not the burdens and long-term effects. I quickly interrupted the conversation and told her I had to answer the front door bell. I could not continue listening to her. I never called her back. I cried for days afterwards.

Vikky Riley

- Acknowledge that parents usually know their child best

It is vital to acknowledge that though parents may not know their teenage child like they knew their toddler, they do know what makes their child who they are and how they cope with adversity.

Robin Kanarek: David was 2 weeks post stem cell transplant and was in strict isolation. It was a lonely time for David and he only had a handful of visitors. His sister and friends could not visit, and his activities were also limited because of the strict isolation he required. Understandably, David became depressed, edgy and began to verbally challenge not only the health-care team, but also my husband and I. The nurses and doctors felt this was normal; they had seen many of their patients respond similarly to being so isolated. After a few days of this behaviour, my husband and I realized something was very wrong. David had never displayed confrontational behaviour towards us; it wasn't his nature. We soon realized that David was frightened of possibly dying and did not want to burden us with his fears. We requested a child psychiatrist to start a dialogue with him about the topic. He ignored our request. Finally, one of the transplant doctors, whom David was very fond of, admitted that he too was concerned with David's emotional state. We voiced our concerns and pleaded with him to talk to David about his fears of dying and death. The doctor spent 3 hours at David's bedside. We are forever grateful that this gentle, compassionate and sensitive man took the time so that David could vent his deepest fears. What a difference it made in David after this discussion! His demeanour improved, he appeared more relaxed, was smiling and appeared as though the weight of the world was off his shoulders.

Vikky Riley

- Listen

The previous story demonstrates how essential the art of listening is.

Listening to the parent about concerns and changes in their child's behaviour should be taken seriously and never dismissed. Listen and you will learn not only about the young person but also discover how individual parents cope and how they all interact as a family.

Robin Kanarek: During a very difficult time for David, right after his transplant, the same child psychiatrist met with David several times. David asked to discontinue the sessions. David told us that instead of dealing with the current crisis, the psychiatrist kept probing about '*what mom did, and did not do, when I was a baby*'. Since that type of approach did not help and seemed to annoy him, we requested that the psychiatrist be replaced. Unfortunately, he was the only one available and having found out about our concerns, expressed his strong displeasure.

We decided to ask a friend of ours, who was an adult psychiatrist and who knew David well, for help. He spoke with the doctor in question. During their discussion, the child psychiatrist expressed his dismay about being dismissed and claimed that '*David's parents caused a major portion of his anxiety*'. To make the point, he told our friend that we were the only parents that he knew of that would leave their child for a short period during the night, under the sole care of the medical team mind you, to get a few hours of sleep. In addition to this comment, he remarked, '*The only other time that I have seen parents leave the child's bedside was when the parents were incarcerated.*' Assuming for a moment that this statement was true, how heartless it was of a man who takes care of our emotional needs to make such a statement. His comment haunts me to this day and still leaves me guilt-ridden.

Vikky Riley: Parents already feel helpless and guilty so be careful not to be judgemental. As health professionals we often assume the position of power and expertise, but that does not give us permission to shatter fragile coping mechanisms.

- Respect the individuality of each parent and their coping mechanisms

All parents are individuals and in the traditional family men and women often cope differently. We have a responsibility to help parents recognize their own coping mechanisms and use them effectively so that they adapt to face their greatest challenge.

Regardless of the relationship that exists between the parent and child, it has to be our responsibility to try our best to support the parent so they in turn can support their child. Children look to their parents, and if their parents are coping well they may handle the journey a bit easier. This is illustrated by the following story.

Kelly was 18 years of age. She had been in care for most of her life and was volatile and occasionally violent. She was also terrified and vulnerable. Her mother described herself as the worst mum in the world; her life had been practically destroyed by alcohol and violence. Following Kelly's diagnosis, through the support of the multidisciplinary team, they slowly re-established a relationship. Eventually Kelly died peacefully at home in her mother's arms.

'*Through the unit's support, I was given another chance at being her mother. From something so awful, we found each other*' – Kelly's mum.

The entire multidisciplinary team supported Kelly, which is a feature of the care and teamwork in the Teenage Cancer Units. Age-appropriate care, appreciation of the impact of a cancer diagnosis and environment are crucial. But so is a team approach. Each member brings different skills that complement one another and ensure that both patient and family are supported.

Humour is often used as a coping mechanism. Initially, parents are often shocked at the amount of laughter and fun evident on the Teenage Cancer Unit. Their world has been turned upside down and they think they will never laugh again, but they do. Humour is a wonderful mechanism to release tension and it is also the way some parents and children communicate and show affection to one another.

Robin has told me a great deal about Joe and David's shared sense of humour.

Robin Kanarek: There are no right or wrong ways to relieve the pressure of your child undergoing cancer treatment. One of the ways that was very helpful to us was humour. We had all learned (including, and even led, by David) to joke about the disease and the treatment. It was obvious that laughing at the situation relieved a great deal of pressure for all of us and we laughed a great deal. The following story will give you an idea of how David could find humour even during the darkest moments.

While in intensive care during the last week of his life, David's body was retaining fluids, causing various, severe difficulties. In order to reduce the level of liquids in his body a diuretic was introduced. The urgency to urinate was so great that David was often incontinent. The solution to the problem was obviously the insertion of a Foley catheter. Since David had so many tubes in him already, the medical team decided on a non-invasive 'Texas catheter'. As the luck would have it, all the Texas catheters available were, wouldn't you know it, Texas size – while David was Rhode Island size! David made a suggestion to the medical team on how they would fit him to the large condom-like device. Baffled, they turned to hear David as he calmly responded with a big grin, *'Just give me some Viagra . . . that will do the trick!'*

Vikky Riley: To conclude, we hope that through our joint presentation we have demonstrated how a parent and health professional can work together. In the quest to support the teenager with cancer we must take the greatest care not to overlook parents.

After many hours of talking with Robin, she showed me a wonderful video of David. It was a beautiful and yet humbling experience. I was moved to tears not only by David but also Sarah, Joe and Robin. What I had witnessed was the message I want to convey. Although I had spent a considerable amount of time with Robin and heard her family's story, it was only when I saw the video that I felt I met David. Up until that point, he was Robin and Joe's son, Sarah's brother and he had died tragically from leukaemia. David was more than his illness. He was more than his death. He was a vibrant, funny, young man who was loved and cherished. As I watched the video the depth of love shone out. It is like that in our practice. We have to remember that we only meet the young person and family when their lives have been ripped apart by cancer. Parents know their child in a way that we will never know them because they have watched their child grow. We need to be vigilant that we do not exacerbate their difficult situation with careless words or actions that may haunt parents forever.

We must be considerate, patient and sometimes challenging. We must seek to establish a relationship based on respect and openness. If we support the parents, they can focus on doing the best they can for their child.

In the depth of winter, I finally learned that within me there lay an invincible summer.

Albert Camus

Part five
Controversies

CHAPTER 20

Who should care for young people with cancer?

J. Arbuckle, R. Cotton, T. O. B. Eden, R. Jones and R. Leonard

During the Second International Teenage Cancer Trust Conference a debate addressing the question of who should care for young people with cancer allowed professionals from different disciplines to present their perspectives.

A paediatric oncologist's perspective

Most care for teenagers and young adults with cancer is not provided by doctors but by nurses, parents, social workers and, of course, the patients themselves and their friends. Consequently, conflicts between paediatric and adult oncologists concerning the management of these patients are simply unnecessary. We should apply a team approach, stop competing and recognize that both groups of physicians have something to offer.[1]

Over the last 40 years, survival for children with cancer has advanced from 20% to more than 80% in Europe, America and other resource-rich countries. In the UK the number of children treated at specialized centres rose from 77% in the years 1980–1984 to 89% in the era 1990–1994. This allowed more of them to be enrolled on clinical trials and thereby enjoy a survival benefit. For 1980–1984, 70% of patients in acute lymphoid leukaemia (ALL) trials survived compared with 64% off trial. A decade later the figures were 84% compared with 68%.[2] In 2004 over 90% of children aged 0–15 years are now treated at the 22 UK Children's Cancer Study Group (UKCCSG) centres, with a mean of 75% of patients treated on trials (over 90% for leukaemia). Centralization of care has been shown to improve survival for a range of tumours,[3] and to prevent overtreatment.[4] Centralization of care and trial enrolment has enabled more consistent and thorough audit of toxicity, the sharing of information on risk and improved compliance, and has facilitated international collaboration. In North America only 20–35% of 15- to 19-year-olds are treated in either adult or paediatric specialist centres.[5] No such reliable figures exist yet for the UK, but only approximately 100 new cases among those aged over 15 years are registered annually with the UKCCSG, clearly a small proportion of the totality of cases. Only 10% of 15- to 19-year-olds and 1% of 20- to 29-year-olds in the USA are entered in clinical trials compared with 60% for those under

Table 20.1 Percentage of all eligible patients entered into the Medical Research Council Acute Lymphoblastic Leukaemia Trials UKALL X and Xa(7)

Age group (years)	Percentage entered into trials
1–9	78%
10–14	77%
15–19	62%
20–39	46%

Trial X was for children and Trial Xa was for adolescents/adults aged 16 or older. Trial X ran from 1985 to 1990 and Xa continued until 1992.

Table 20.2 Outcome by age (MRC UKALL X/Xa trial)

Age group (years)	10-year disease-free survival	10-year overall survival
1–9	62%	81%
10–14	49%	72%
15–19	35%	60%
20–39	29%	43%

15 years of age.[6] Adult entry into UK trials has reached 10% as the result of a huge effort by the new National Cancer Research Institute.

Leukaemia trials, seen as the flagship of cancer trials, show a rapid decline in entry with age, as illustrated in Table 20.1. Outcome by age showed a similar decline in this trial (see Table 20.2).[7]

The reasons for the worse outcome in older patients have been examined. Disease-related factors are very important. Pui and Evans[8] reported a decrease in the favourable features of cytogenetic hyperdiploidy and TEL-AML1 rearrangements, and an increase in adverse features, including BCR/ABL fusion genes, hypodiploidy and T-cell lineage disease. Some evidence of reduced steroid and antimetabolite sensitivity has been reported. As a result, remission rates were slightly lower (96 versus 98%), early death rates higher and marrow relapses more frequent (35 versus 22%) in the five adult and four childhood trials analysed by Pui and Evans.[8]

Patient and doctor compliance also appears to alter with increasing patient age. In the MRC UKALL X adult trial, 22% of adult physicians were protocol-non-compliant, giving more intensification and bone marrow transplants (not as part of the protocol), whilst only 2% of paediatricians deviated from protocol.[7] It is far more difficult to confirm patient non-compliance, although estimates put a figure of about 10% on paediatric ALL trials during the maintenance phase of therapy. It is said to be higher with increasing age as the patients become more responsible for their own medication. Non-compliance is a frequent reason cited for adolescent patients not being entered into clinical trials, but we do not have good evidence to back up this assertion.

It is clear from leukaemia trials that less favourable biology, non-entry into trials for whatever reason, protocol deviation and non-compliance all go some way to explain poorer outcome for adolescents than children.

Nachman and colleagues[9] have reported that treating ALL and acute myeloid leukaemia patients in paediatric Children's Cancer Group trials in the age range 16–24 years improved outcome compared with treatment in adult trials. More investigation is required to explain why this is so and what components of therapy make the difference.

The bottom line is that to treat young people with leukaemia and solid tumours successfully, both paediatric and adult oncologists need to work together. If we fragment our activities we will never know the true incidence of disease, optimize treatment, improve survival and provide the ideal environment where young people can feel most comfortable to receive their therapy. Whenever asked, teenagers and young adults have requested not to be treated alongside younger or older patients – each group needs their own age-appropriate environment.

An adult oncologist's perspective

There is clearly a problem to face in terms of the significant number of teenagers and young adults with cancer and an apparent rise in incidence. What is less clear is the definition of who is a teenager. The biology of disease may change very significantly from, for example, a 13- to 14-year-old compared with a 22- to 23-year-old, even with the same ostensible tumour. Clearly, there are differences in the relative tumour incidences with progression of age through the teens and early twenties.

It is acknowledged there is a great deal of relevant medical expertise in both adult and paediatric units: the expertise is disease- rather than practice-orientated, which in itself is an issue. During the conference a major focus has been on psychosocial issues but there has been little discussion on genetics, and this clearly is a very important aspect that requires focus if we are to understand tumour biology and how patients respond to therapy.

The 14–24 age group is very suitable for defining common cancers, such as leukaemias, lymphomas and sarcomas, so allowing the development of disease-specific expertise. What is far less clear is whether tumours across this age spread are biologically homogeneous. Furthermore, in this age range much is happening in terms of individual physical and emotional development, so teenagers and young adults are not psychosocially homogeneous either. The paediatric model of 22 centres is one way to deal with these circumstances, but the population across the UK is not limited to 22 cities. Most adult cancer units deal with populations of 500,000 or more and the number of adolescents treated in each centre is low. It has been estimated and presented that the number of adolescents entering into trials in the UK is less than the number of children but greater than the number of adults. The reason for these differences needs to be looked at jointly by all those who treat such patients. It is quite clear that in order to understand the cancers that afflict this age range, we must recognize that biology matters; that understanding the characteristic diseases is important; and that expertise and experience is important as we cross the 'boundaries' from adult to paediatric care.

The effect of the Chernobyl nuclear accident – which induced an approximate hundred-fold increase in thyroid cancer in children resident in the highest contaminated area at the time of the accident with a longer latency than other tumours presenting at an older age – goes some way to explain the rise in young adult cancer.[10] Adult oncologists are clearly interested and frequently involved in the sequelae of childhood cancer treatment. Nowhere is this more clear than in Hodgkin's disease, given the earlier treatment involving extensive field radiotherapy, which has led to an excess of breast cancer in particular, but also thyroid cancer and, later in life, lung cancer. This is an area of study that has not been given sufficient attention. For example, the greatest risk of breast cancer appears to be for those treated around the time of puberty with a 12.4-fold relative risk compared with 1.6 for women treated over the age of 25. It would appear that there is a window of time during which particular tissues are more susceptible to the carcinogenic effect of cytotoxic drugs or radiotherapy. The greatest risk of subsequent thyroid cancer appears to be in early childhood, whilst for breast cancer it appears to be the early to mid-teenage years. Adult oncologists frequently see the late consequences of paediatric and teenage cancer therapy even if they have not been the physicians involved in the initial care.

Much emphasis has been placed on the right environment within the hospital for teenagers and young adults, and we must also consider the environment outside the hospital as well as the influence of the family caring for the young person. Teenage Cancer Trust units around the country do not care for everyone; for example, in Edinburgh and in Swansea, where patient numbers are too small to justify a specialist unit because of the relative revenue costs. A survey was undertaken in Edinburgh to assess patient satisfaction, comparing those treated in a specialist adolescent unit and those treated either in adult or paediatric units. There seemed to be little difference in terms of patient satisfaction according to where they were treated, but the most significant advantages for the specialist adolescent unit were reported to be the 'companion' effect of being treated with others in the same age group and having an age-appropriate social area in which to relax and study.

Clearly, specialist units are important for a proportion of the population, but other types of services need to be developed, such as regional support teams and outreach from hospitals into the community. Just building specialist units in big population centres is not the only answer. A mixture of paediatric and adult approaches is needed. More research is needed, not only in biology and optimal treatment, but also in health-care delivery. We need to collect better data on outcomes as well as performing true audits of the value of treatment in different settings in order to produce a variety of loco-regional solutions as to how to manage and support teenagers and young adults optimally.

An adolescent unit nurse's perspective

Hutton described the adolescent as 'One of the most difficult patients to care for within the hospital setting'.[11] One of the main objectives of the Teenage Cancer Trust is to provide any young person, with cancer, access to a hospital environment appropriate to their age and disease. But the age range of these patients raises the question of who is the best qualified to look after a young person with cancer. The care of an adolescent in hospital may be delivered by staff who particularly enjoy looking after this age group or by those who fear contact with an adolescent due to feelings of intimidation, inadequacy or just plain indifference. Indeed, Burr[12] found that the majority of nurses in an adult setting perceived adolescents as being no different from adults.

There has been much discussion between paediatric and adult oncologists as to who is best qualified to care for this age group, but the debate is just as relevant for nursing staff. After all, it is the nurses that administer the chemotherapy, the antibiotics and the anti-emetics. It is the nurses that usually get shouted at by patients around lunchtime for waking them up too early and more importantly, nurses are the people who have to answer questions at two o'clock in the morning such as 'Why did *I* get cancer?'

Paediatric nurses

The training of paediatric nurses provides appropriate guidance in communication skills and family-centred care as well as in the physiological and psychological changes during adolescence. The issue of family-centred care is relevant in caring for patients who, due to their age, require a parent or guardian to give consent for treatment, as well as those patients over the age of 15 who regress and allow their parents to take control over their care. Nurses with paediatric experience may feel more comfortable in caring not just for the patient but the parents and any siblings too. Viner stated 'The more individual approach of adult staff can be seen as threatening to young people and their families . . .'.[13] The paediatric nurse is likely also to have greater experience of helping parents who need support, in being open and honest with their child, particularly when painful decisions or outcomes arise. Furthermore, research does suggest that paediatric nurses are best equipped to provide the psychological support that adolescents need when faced with a cancer diagnosis.[14]

Adult nurses

Nurse training currently offers little in the way of adolescent theory to those undertaking an adult nursing course. However, nurses working in an adult environment are likely, albeit infrequently, to come into contact with adolescent patients, particularly in areas of the country not served by a specialist unit. Older adolescents may be considerably more independent than their younger peers; many will have left home for university or moved in with a spouse or partner. Indeed some may be parents themselves. Therefore, the need for family-centred care (i.e. care of patients, parents and siblings) may be considerably less for the older adolescent. But it is also important for nurses to be able to recognize the significance of friends to the adolescent, who in some cases may have a greater impact on their life than parents or siblings.[15] Adult trained nurses may find it more difficult to initiate effective communication with younger adolescents, particularly those who have been treated previously on a paediatric unit. Barrett[16] suggests that, in this setting, parents are often more demanding and anxious and can take the nurse's attention away from establishing good rapport with the patient.

It is clear that both paediatric and adult trained staff can bring qualities needed to care for adolescents, yet several studies have come to the conclusion that nurses undertaking mental health courses are actually in the best position to fully understand the needs of an adolescent in hospital, mainly due to the emphasis they place on psychological care.[17]

Other factors

The Action for Sick Children report *Youth Matters*[18] highlighted several factors that it felt were important for the effective nursing of an adolescent in hospital. The age of the staff is one such factor considered. For example, several adolescent units take patients up to the age of 25, which in many cases is likely to be similar to the age of the junior members of staff caring for them. Patients may identify instantly with younger members of staff and come to see the nurse as a peer; this can lead the inexperienced nurse to inappropriately befriend a particular patient and may lead to contact out-side of the ward environment, believing it to be a natural progression of this friendship. This problem can be exacerbated by the relaxed environment of an adolescent unit, where familiarity and liveliness are juxtaposed with sadness and bereavement.[19] It is also highlighted that older members of the nursing staff are as susceptible to infringement of boundaries as their younger colleagues, for they may see qualities or characteristics in the adolescents similar to those in their own children, or may indeed develop maternal or paternal feelings towards the patients.

Nursing remains a female-dominated profession and yet the need to main-tain a balanced team of nurses in any adolescent unit is important. Positive role models of both sexes are vital to all adolescents' development, but when the adolescents are undergoing treatment for cancer and their very identity and independence are compromised the need is all the greater.

Conclusion

It is clear that caring for adolescents with cancer requires certain attributes in nursing staff. Compassion, empathy and approachability are all essential if the nurse wants to be able to provide adequate psychological support to his or her patient. But all of these need to be controlled by a measure of emotional detachment to protect both nurse and patient. A good sense of humour is of great benefit, as is a good all-round knowledge of youth culture and pastimes, including football, music and soap operas!

Whilst the definition of when adolescence begins and ends differs markedly, as long as units such as those funded by the Teenage Cancer Trust continue to acknowledge that a 13–24 age range can constitute a 'young person', both paediatric- and adult-trained nurses are able to provide the necessary qualities. The overwhelming issue in caring for these patients is the desire to meet their needs. Essentially, what matters is not how the nurse was trained but how the nurse practises.

A social worker's perspective

Before we look at who or where is best to treat young people with cancer, we need to look at the specific needs of this age group, and the developmental tasks they face that can be disrupted and sometimes delayed by their treatment. This can have both immediate and long-term consequences.

Young people are at a stage which is between dependent childhood and independent adulthood. It is a time of change, both physical and psychological, and many young people find it difficult enough to manage this transition without the added complication of a cancer diagnosis and the effects of its treatment. One of the main challenges for this age group is in establishing an individual, social and sexual identity and the social and interpersonal skills necessary for their emerging independence and autonomy. A cancer diagnosis increases young people's dependence at the very time they are trying to become more independent.

All young people need to be treated as individuals, and with respect. Referring to someone as 'the osteosarcoma in Ward 5' defines the young person by their disease rather than by who he or she is. Young people require an honest and direct approach from medical professionals, and are capable of deciding how they want to be involved in the process of their treatment. Some professionals are wary of removing hope for young people by being too direct, but sensitive and honest communication allows feelings to be expressed and explored. A lack of control and choices leads to a feeling of helplessness, which is far more likely to lead to a loss of hope. Young people's individual information-processing and decision-making skills depend upon their level of independence, individual coping mechanisms and their role within their families. Simply asking how they want to receive information (for example, directly or filtered through parents, in detail or basic facts only, the big picture or stage by stage) involves them in the process and gives them choices. This provides an element of control, which is desperately needed when we expect them to hand over the control of their body to strangers. Addressing issues such as consent to treatment and rights to confidentiality also respects them as young adults.

Young people need privacy and space, but they also need to be able to interact with their peers. Long, complex, intensive treatment programmes in either a children's hospital or an adult hospital isolates them from other young people. Unless they are in specialist treatment units for young people, they are often the oldest or youngest on the ward by years or even decades. To be able to identify with and be accepted by their peers at this socially crucial age is vital for self-esteem.

Gaps in education and employment at this age can have a major impact on future career development. Coping with changes such as hair loss, weight loss and gain, and undergoing major surgery can affect a young person's body image adversely. This, as well as effects on fertility, can make it more difficult to form and maintain future relationships.

Young people need support from their family, friends and professionals, and support also needs to be in place for their families so that they do not have to shoulder this responsibility alone. Readjusting to life after treatment involves all of these issues, plus altered perceptions about body, health, mortality, 'survivor guilt', and learning how to live with the fear of relapse and to build a different picture of the future. These are issues that the average young person does not expect to have to deal with.

There are no types of cancer exclusive to young people, but the range of cancers common in this age group include both more typically childhood cancers and more typically adult cancers. As a result, it makes sense to combine the expertise of both areas of medicine to create a specialist area.

The young people I have worked with in my role as a Sargent Social Worker have not expressed a preference as to who treats them, although the majority do feel very strongly about where they are treated. They want to be treated in an age-appropriate environment with their peers, and by professionals who have experience of working with their age group.

It is equally likely that adult physicians and paediatricians who do not have experience of this age group will overlook some of their specific needs and sometimes label them as non-compliant. Many adults regress when they are ill but young people are experiencing the dependence of childhood and the accelerated maturity which a serious illness brings, and are far more likely to swing between these stages. It is easy but unhelpful to dismiss this as either stroppiness and demanding or clingy and childish behaviour. Adult physicians who are more used to dealing with the upper end of the age spectrum may be less aware of the psychosocial and educational needs of young people, and unaware that certain life tasks have not been completed and that support networks and coping mechanisms are not always in place. In contrast, paediatricians, who are more used to dealing with younger children, may be used to coping with some of the more childlike responses of young people's behaviour, but less comfortable with some of their more adult responses, including addressing issues such as body image, sexuality and fertility. Anyone working with young people needs to be aware that adopting a maternal or paternalistic approach can be perceived as patronizing.

In order to improve young people's experience of cancer treatment, the professionals who are treating them would benefit from sharing their expertise and from receiving joint training about psychosocial needs. Training needs to deliver an understanding of the developmental tasks and specific requirements of young people, and how a cancer diagnosis and treatment can impact on these. Young people often find communication difficult and need to be drawn out of themselves by skilled communicators. Training for this is important, especially for those staff who lack confidence in the area. Young people often minimize physical effects and symptoms out of a sense of embarrassment, invincibility or fear, so good communication helps with the treatment process. Training also needs to address issues such as body image, fertility, late effects, fear of relapse and life after treatment, as this is often a time when the full impact of what has happened to them hits young people.

Expressing empathy whilst maintaining boundaries and an ability to reflect and develop a flexible approach when working with young people are all very important issues for training.

Conclusions

In conclusion, shared disease expertise combined with an increased knowledge of the psychosocial needs of young people, delivered within an age-appropriate environment, is likely to produce the best outcomes for young people with cancer.

As we are now seeing all over the country, environments can be changed by the creation of specific treatment units for young people, and attitudes can also be changed by education and training.

It is useful to conclude with some quotes from young people obtained in a questionnaire study collating the views of young cancer patients in Edinburgh, which was completed in May 2002. Hospital staff in both the adult and children's hospitals were praised and appreciated for their high levels of care, but unfortunately, few of the respondents felt that they understood the needs of young people:

- 'It took a long time to get them to talk to me instead of my parents.'
- 'Some didn't seem to understand teen moods and how to cope or solve problems that arose with these.'
- 'They don't always tell you all the information they would tell you if you were an adult, and they don't seem to like you to express your own views.'
- 'To be treated as an individual, that's the most important thing.'

References

1 Jeha S. Who should be treating adolescents and young adults with acute lymphoblastic leukaemia. *Eur J Cancer* 2003; **39**: 2579–2583.
2 Stiller CA, Eatock EM. Patterns of care and survival for children with acute lymphoblastic leukaemia diagnosed between 1980 and 1994. *Arch Dis Child* 1999; **81**: 202–208.
3 Stiller CA. Centralised treatment, entry to trials and survival. *Br J Cancer* 1994; **70**: 352–362.
4 Pritchard J, Stiller CA, Lennox EL. Overtreatment of children with Wilms' tumour outside paediatric oncology centres. *Br Med J* 1989; **299**: 835–836.

5 Bleyer WA. The adolescent gap in cancer treatment. *J Registry Manage* 1996; **23**: 114–115.

6 Bleyer WA, Tejeda H, Murphy SM *et al.* National cancer clinical trials: children have equal access, adolescents do not. *J Adolesc Health* 1997; **21**: 366–373.

7 Chessells JM, Hall E, Prentice HG *et al.* The impact of age on outcome in lymphoblastic leukaemia, MRC UKALL X and Xa compared: a report from the Medical Research Council Paediatric and Adult Working Parties. *Leukaemia* 1998; **12**: 413–473.

8 Pui C-H, Evans WE. Acute lymphoblastic leukaemia. *N Engl J Med* 1998; **339**: 605–615.

9 Nachman J, Sather HN, Buckley JD *et al.* Young adults 16–21 years of age at diagnosis entered onto Children's Cancer Group acute lymphoblastic leukaemia and acute myeloblastic leukaemia protocols. Results of treatment. *Cancer* 1993; **71**: (10 Suppl.) 3377–3385.

10 Shibata Y, Yamashita S, Masyakin V *et al.* 15 years after Chernobyl – new evidence of thyroid cancer. *Lancet* 2001; **358**: 1965–1966.

11 Hutton A. The private adolescent: privacy needs of the adolescent in hospitals. *J Pediatr Nurs* 2002; **17**: 67–72.

12 Burr S. Adolescents and the ward environment. *Paediatr Nurs* 1993; **5**: 10–14.

13 Viner R. Bridging the gaps: transition for young people with cancer. *Eur J Cancer* 2003; **39**: 2684–2687.

14 Smith S. Adolescent units – an evidence-based approach to quality nursing in adolescent care. *Eur J Cancer* 2004; **8**: 20–29.

15 Albritton K, Bleyer WA. The management of cancer in the older adolescent. *Eur J Cancer* 2003; **39**: 2584–2599.

16 Barrett A. Where should patients be treated? In: Selby P, Bailey C, eds. *Cancer and the Adolescent.* London: BMJ Publications, 1996.

17 Blunden R. An artificial state. *J Pediatric Nurs* 1989; **1**: 12–13.

18 Viner R, Keane M. *Youth Matters – Evidence-based Best Practice for the Care of Young People in Hospital.* London: Action for Sick Children, 1998.

19 Whelan J. Where should teenagers with cancer be treated? *Eur J Cancer* 2003; **39**: 2573–2578.

CHAPTER 21

Patterns of care for teenagers and young adults with cancer: is there a single blueprint of care?

I. Lewis

Introduction

Cancer in adolescence is relatively rare and yet presents challenging management problems, both medical and psychosocial. In recent years, questions about how teenagers and young adults with cancer should be managed have become more prominent and have generated some controversy. A perception has grown that traditional models of care are not adequately meeting the needs of teenagers and young adults. In the UK, a national charity, the Teenage Cancer Trust (TCT), was originally set up with the explicit aim of championing the needs of teenagers with cancer, principally by promoting the concept of, and providing capital for, specific in-patient facilities. A number of such sponsored units have opened in major cancer centres during the past decade, but as yet there has been limited formal evaluation of them. The concept of such units is still the subject of professional controversy.[1] To some extent, this controversy exists because of the lack of evidence of benefit and because some clinicians doubt the need to consider teenagers and young adults as an identifiable and separate group. They think that cancers occurring in this group should be managed within the context of site-specific teams.

This chapter sets out to address some of these issues and in particular to consider whether there might be a uniform model of care that could be applied to most, or all, young people with cancer.

Aims of care

The aims of care for any patient, irrespective of age or type of cancer at diagnosis, should be identical; that is, to maximize the chance of survival whilst minimizing the physical, psychological and social cost of that survival.

This bald statement conceals much additional complexity. It is not yet, and may never be, possible to treat all cancers or patients with curative intent. Some patients wish, for a variety of reasons, to exert their autonomy in choosing treatment that may not maximize their chance of cure. Others may wish to choose intensive or experimental treatments that have significant additional risks whilst only offering very limited prospects of success. A key requirement of cancer care must be to provide appropriate information within a supportive environment so that patients with cancer and their carers can be heard in a climate of openness and consent.

What might this mean for a teenager or young adult with cancer? Maximizing the chances of survival implies that patients are best advised and treated by clinicians expert in their particular cancer. Minimizing physical, psychological and social costs for teenagers and young adults implies that care might be best provided in an environment where the behaviours and needs of this client group are understood and can be met. Hence, there might appear to be an apparent tension between achieving the twin aims of care. Is this important and can the tensions be reconciled?

Teenagers and young adults have special needs

Working with teenagers and young adults can be both stimulating and challenging. These young people are experiencing a period of life when they are initiating major life tasks, including establishing their personal identity, establishing independence, making occupational choices and developing philosophical and lifestyle choices.

Cancer challenges the young person's sense of self-esteem, leading to feelings of loss of control at a time when self-image is pivotal to normal development. Periods of hospitalization and illness may contribute to increased dependence on parents, who quite naturally feel protective and may want to take over care, with loss of the young person's independence. In contrast, peer contact will decrease at a time when peer group acceptance is crucial. Reliance on family for financial support and on health-care professionals for treatment further contributes to a feeling of lack of independence. Treatment effects of chemotherapy, surgery or radiotherapy will affect identity and self-esteem.[2] These effects, combined with treatment effects on fertility, may also affect the young person's sexual confidence, identity and expectations.

Illness and treatment clearly change the lifestyle of teenagers. Education can be disrupted and future occupational plans may be changed, either because of treatment or because of a real or perceived threat to life.

In the UK, the special needs of young people and the requirement for service provision addressing these needs have been recognized in a number of formal publications by government and professional organizations.[3–5] There have been similar formal recommendations for young people with cancer. In 1995 the Expert Advisory Group in Cancer to the Chief Medical Officer of

England and Wales[6] recognized these needs and recommended the formation of specialist units for adolescents with cancer.

Current practice

In considering models of care for teenagers and young adults with cancer, it is important to have an understanding of factors influencing current practice. These include basic epidemiology – that is, which cancers occur in this group – and patterns of how, where and by whom teenagers and young adults are currently treated. This chapter will largely focus on practice in the UK. It is apparent that teenagers are subject to a lottery of care in which decisions about referrals and patterns of care have developed in an apparently ad hoc manner.

Descriptive epidemiology

The classic descriptive epidemiology of cancer in adults described using the *International Classification of Diseases*[7] categorizes cancers according to the site of origin within 5-year age bands. It has long been recognized that this approach is inadequate for reflecting the diversity of cancer in children and an alternative scheme based on histology with morphology and site-specific subgrouping has been developed.[8] Many authors of studies of cancers in teenagers and young adults have commented that they too are poorly described using a site-specific classification and have recommended a similar classification to that used for children. Recent epidemiological studies of teenagers and young adults use such a system.[9]

The incidence of cancer increases through the three age bands 10–14, 15–19 and 20–24 years. There is also a change in the types of cancer that occur in different age groups. This data is summarized in Table 21.1. In early adolescence leukaemias and brain tumours predominate, whilst epithelial cancers are rare. However, in 15–19 and 20–24-year-olds lymphomas account for around a quarter of all cancers and epithelial malignancy becomes increasingly

Table 21.1 Cancer in teenagers and young adults: relative incidence in different age groups

Age (years)	10–14 (%)	15–19 (%)	20–24 (%)
Leukaemia	25	10	10
Lymphomas	18	25	25
Brain/spine	25	10	12
Bone	13	15	5
Soft tissue sarcoma	6	6	6
Gonadal/germ cell	3	10	10
Epithelial	5	18	23
Others	5	6	10

Excludes cancer of the cervix *in situ*.

common. Bone sarcomas are seen quite frequently in those aged 10–19 but become relatively less common in older patients. Germ cell tumours, by contrast, are uncommon below 15 years of age but commoner in those aged 15–24 years. In younger adolescents, the epithelial cancers that most commonly occur are carcinoma of the thyroid and nasopharyngeal carcinoma, whilst it is unusual for the commoner adult-type carcinomas, such as colorectal, ovarian, cervical or breast cancer, to occur in those under 20. However, they are seen with increasing frequency in those over 20.

Patterns of care

It is important to understand both the epidemiology and some recent history in order to understand current patterns of care. These have varied for different ages and pathological diagnoses. The variety in management is depicted pictorially for several diagnostic categories in Fig. 21.1.

Teenagers and young adults under 15 years of age

In the UK, nearly all children and young people below 15 years of age are now referred to one of the 22 major paediatric oncology centres for management. This has been an incremental change. Prior to the mid-1970s, when children's cancer began to be recognized as a separate specialty, most children received their treatment locally, under the care of general paediatricians or surgeons. Following the establishment of children's cancer centres there was a rapid change in referral patterns, such that by the early 1980s the majority of children aged 0–9 years were treated centrally.

Interestingly, it took up to a decade longer before the majority of young adolescents aged 10–14 years achieved similarly high referral rates to children's cancer centres. As an example, in the period 1992–1994 only 58% of 13- and 14-year-olds and 73% of 10- to 12-year-olds were registered with UKCCSG centres compared with 85% of those aged 0–9 years. Although never formally analysed, it is now accepted that during this time adult specialists were treating many young teenagers in adult settings. There was only gradual (and sometimes grudging) acceptance by these specialists that young people would gain benefit from being treated in an environment more generally designed for them and where staff were more likely to understand their developmental, psychological, educational and social needs. Perhaps more importantly, paediatric oncology centres and teams also became more expert in treating the cancers that occur most commonly in this age group and in providing patients with access to appropriate clinical trials.

Fifteen to nineteen years

Paediatric oncology teams
Throughout the past 20 years there has been a small but increasing cohort of young people over the age of 15 years managed by paediatric oncology teams. This cohort can largely be divided into three.

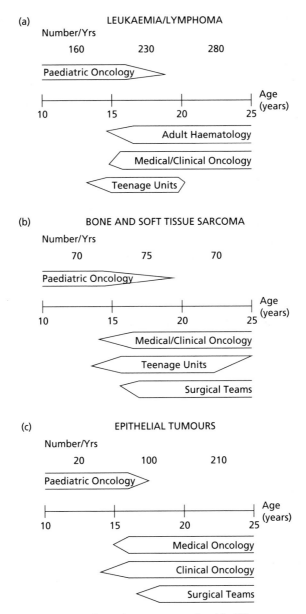

Fig. 21.1 Indicative patterns of care for young people with different types of malignancy, demonstrating the range of possible different medical teams that might be involved at different ages. 'Number/Yrs' refers to approximate numbers of expected cases in the UK by 5-year age band. (a) Leukamia/lymphoma. (b) Bone and soft tissue sarcoma. (c) Epithelial tumours.

First are patients initially diagnosed under the age of 15 years and treated in a children's cancer centre but who suffered disease relapse as an older teenager or young adult. These young people and their families often request treatment in a familiar environment by the team known to them and trusted by them.

The second group has been of patients over 15 years and newly diagnosed with cancers deemed to be paediatric in nature, most commonly bone sarcomas and acute lymphoblastic leukaemia, or the rare diagnosis in this age group of embryonic tumours.

The last group is of patients over 15 years but deemed to have paediatric needs. In some geographical areas formal service guidance has included the requirement for patients aged 16 years or more who are in full-time secondary education to be treated in a children's setting. Elsewhere the direction of referral has been determined by the referring clinician. The reasons given why older teenagers are referred can vary, but are often accompanied by a perception that the young person is relatively immature. This can often be determined by the size of the young person – a six-foot 15-year-old boy may be thought capable of treatment in an adult environment whilst a five-and-a-half foot 17-year-old might be deemed more appropriately treated within a children's service. The direction of referral often takes place without any structured assessment of educational capability or social support mechanisms.

The number referred to paediatric teams has been a minority. In 1995 fewer than 100 young people 15 years or older were registered as being treated at UKCCSG centres. Since then the number registered has increased, but as there has been a growth in units specifically designed for teenagers during this period it has not been possible to disentangle those referred to children's teams from those referred to teenage and young adult units that happen to be co-located with paediatric oncology units.

Adult oncology teams

The majority of young people over 15 continue to be managed by teams most of whose work is with older adults. To a large extent, this is determined by the pathological diagnosis, but even here a range of factors, some of which might be thought to be more rational than others, have determined the team taking the lead in treating young people.

As the first example, the most common malignancies in 15- to 19-year-olds are lymphomas. These are treated by a variety of teams. Most patients with lymphoma are managed by clinical haematology teams but a substantial number are managed by medical oncology or clinical oncology teams, depending on the setting or personal interest of the clinicians involved. The type of team can vary between hospitals or even within individual hospitals. Many young people are referred to cancer centres but a sizeable number continue to be managed in more local settings, where a teenager with cancer is a relative rarity.

A similar pattern is seen in young people with leukaemia, although most patients are managed by adult or paediatric haematology teams.

Adult teams treat most young people with sarcomas or germ cell tumours, although patterns of care vary. The adult oncology community has clearly demonstrated the value of centralized treatment for testicular tumours in young men. Nowadays structured multidisciplinary teams within cancer centres manage the majority. In contrast, many young women with ovarian tumours are managed by predominantly surgical gynaecological teams, often in district hospitals.

There is a similar pattern for sarcomas. In England and Wales, the majority of young people with bone sarcomas have their diagnostic and definitive surgery in one of two specialized surgical centres, and whilst chemotherapy may be delivered in paediatric, medical or clinical oncology settings, in the main this is given in cancer centres. In contrast, soft tissue sarcomas are often initially investigated and treated in district hospital settings by surgical teams. They may only be seen in cancer centres or by specialist teams if deemed to be more complex or if disease recurrence occurs.

Epithelial tumours appear to be mainly managed in local units. In a study by Selby and colleagues[10] of patterns of referral for young people aged 15–23 years in Yorkshire, only a small proportion were treated in a hospital that was not in their own district. This implied that only the minority of carcinomas were referred to specialist centres. Nasopharyngeal cancer and breast cancers were referred more frequently than other epithelial cancers, reflecting the importance of radiotherapy in accepted management. There is little evidence in the literature to suggest that patterns of care have changed significantly in more recent years.

Twenty years and over

In the main, treatment for most young people over 20 years is very similar to that observed in the 15–19-year age group, the majority being managed in adult units and very few being managed in children's services. There is a perception (but little hard data as yet) that a small but increasing number of young people under 30 are being managed in teenage and young adult units.

Teenage and young adult units and teams

The first unit specifically identified as being for adolescents with cancer was sited at the Middlesex Hospital in London. This 10-bed unit was first opened in 1990 and predominantly focused on the care of young people with bone sarcomas.[11] Since then about eight other units have opened, each reflecting local influences that have determined which cancers are managed within these adolescent units and which remain outside them.

Some of these teenage and young adult units opened as an adjunct to the local adult oncology unit; for example, those at the Middlesex Hospital in London and the units in Sheffield and Birmingham. Others have developed predominantly as an adjunct to paediatric oncology units; for example, those in Newcastle and Cardiff. It has been less common for units to be developed by joint collaboration between adult and paediatric oncology teams but examples of this are those in Leeds and Manchester.

Irrespective of their origins, it is commonly recognized by those staffing these units that care for this client group is challenging for staff and demands special skills. As yet, though, there is little in the way of formal guidance or training for staff undertaking this work.

The impetus for the formation of these units has come from a combination of professional awareness, patient pressure and lobbying by the voluntary sector, the last being mainly by the Teenage Cancer Trust. Despite notable successes to date, it is worth pointing out that it is still only the minority of cancer centres in the UK that have any specific facilities for young people. Even where they exist, there is often disagreement between different groups of professionals about the value of such units. Interestingly, clinical haematologists are the medical professional group that seems to have most difficulty with the concept of managing young people within age-specific facilities.

Most of these units started with a combination of professional goodwill and charitable support. Funding from formal National Health Service sources has been sporadic, dependent upon local champions harnessing evidence and sympathetic commissioners of health-care being prepared to listen. As a result, there has been no standard package of funding or pattern of development. Some units continue to exist on staff expanding their roles voluntarily from their original remit whilst others have had varying degrees of specific funding which may have included nursing staff, medical staff and other support staff. There is currently a national review of services to children and young people with cancer by the National Institute of Clinical Excellence which encompasses those up to their mid-20s (www.nice.org.uk: Child and adolescent cancer). It is to be hoped that this will give guidance to all commissioners of health services, thereby creating greater equality of access.

Interestingly, whilst the UK may have taken the lead in initially developing adolescent cancer units, units are now being developed in a number of other countries.

Paradigms of care

There are quite marked differences in how teams from differing disciplines interact with patients, and this can have a marked effect on how relationships and trust develop between young people, their families or partners and the professional teams. These differences are illustrated in Fig. 21.2.

Children's teams

Paediatric professionals work within the classic triad of professionals, parents and patient. Clearly, very young children are not usually able to express complicated ideas verbally, and whilst they can be enormously expressive in a number of ways, most of the complex discussion and decision-making tends to take place between professionals and parents or carers. Paediatricians and children's nurses are trained to observe and listen to children at the same time so that some assessment of their views can be made. As children get older, their individual contribution to decision-making becomes more apparent;

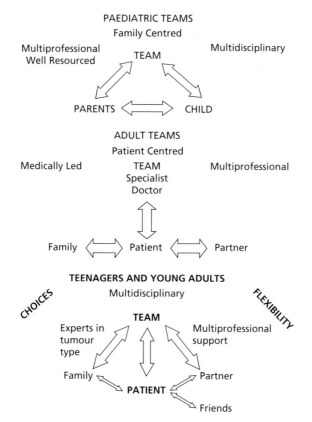

Fig. 21.2 Paradigms of care. Diagram indicating varying approaches normally used by different teams in oncology.

yet, by and large, decisions and discussions are an intricate process in which parents' views tend to predominate.

Paediatric oncology teams have been relatively well resourced, with quite a high staff/patient ratio. A culture of multidisciplinary and multiprofessional working has become embedded into practice, which should be family-centred in approach. It is axiomatic that this approach, combined with extensive multicentre, national and international collaboration in the development of clinical trials and studies, has been the reason why advances have been rapidly incorporated into practice and outcomes improved.

Adult teams

Professionals working with adults who have cancer tend to work much more within a classic medical model of a lead doctor interacting directly with the patient. This doctor–patient relationship is at the core of practice and is based on confidentiality and consent. The patient rather than the family is at the centre of this particular care paradigm and other family members or partners largely interact with the professional team through the consent of the patient.

Medical, clinical and haematological oncology practice tends to be strongly medically led, other professionals having a greater supporting role. Historically, much of the focus of adult teams has been on older patients. There is much logic in this as the number of older patients who develop cancer is large. The emphasis, therefore, has often been on treating largely with palliative intent whilst paying particular attention to unwanted side-effects.

In contrast to paediatric oncology, resources have been more stretched and staff/patient ratios smaller. This often implies less time for complex inter-action and less reliance on professional support. Historically, the proportion of patients entered into multicentre clinical trials is much lower, although increasing this proportion in adults is a key objective of the National Cancer Research Institute and Network in the UK.

Teenage and young adult teams

Patterns of care for teenagers and young adults with cancer are really only just emerging, but the evidence is starting to increase. It is clear that teenagers and young adults do not fit easily into either the classic paediatric or adult paradigms of interaction.

Teenagers and young adults are experiencing an evolution of personal independence whereby they gradually separate from their parents or carers and establish their own identities. New partners or friends tend to be more important but it is evident that these changes occur over time. Cancer nearly always interferes with these normal processes and often throws newly independent young people back on their families for support. It is paramount, therefore, that professionals dealing with teenagers and young adults develop knowledge of and sensitivity to these issues, whilst recognizing that enormous flexibility is required to meet the needs of each individual.

This largely requires an approach that uses elements of both classic paediatric and adult models. Professionals should predominantly interact with the patient himself or herself. They should, however, be sensitive to the needs and wishes of each individual and actively encourage patients to be accompanied and supported. For younger teenagers this is virtually always parents, legal carers or other family members, but for older teenagers or young adults it could be partners, friends or any combination of these. It is not uncommon to have a number of people accompanying teenagers or young adults with cancer. It should be appreciated that individual choices can change. The 14-year-old who comes accompanied by her parents and who largely defers to their wishes may well develop into the 18-year-old who brings her boyfriend and who may wish to override the advice of all around her. At 20, however, she may wish her parents to come as well and also to take and listen to advice from those around her. This therefore demands an approach that is both flexible and offers choices. It is almost impossible for this to be feasible without an extensive multiprofessional and multidisciplinary team.

Typically, patients in this age group have had a much lower percentage of entry into trials than children. The reason for this is likely to be multifactorial, but one important factor has been the perceived difficulty of engaging young people in complex discussion. In fact there is no reason for thinking that teenagers and young adults should be less likely to consent to clinical trials than any other group.

Is there, or should there be a single model of care?

Patient pathway

It is possible to develop a patient pathway that provides a fairly uniform structure of the potential key elements of diagnosis and treatment. Figure 21.3 demonstrates such a pathway, as seen from a professional viewpoint.

The first part of the pathway outlines the referral process, which in the UK is most commonly from general practitioner to general physician, surgeon or paediatrician and is usually followed by further referral to an oncology specialist.

The next element describes the formal medical evaluation of the patient for histological diagnosis, disease staging, and the assessment of underlying medical status and identification of any perceived physical problems.

The following step describes the need to inform the patient and family about these findings, to advise and decide on an initial treatment plan, and to discuss entry into a clinical trial if this is thought appropriate. This presumes an informed consent process.

At this point treatment commences. This will obviously vary considerably depending on the diagnosis and staging, but for many patients it might include one or more of chemotherapy, radiotherapy, surgery, or even high-dose therapy. This all demands close collaboration and multidisciplinary teamwork. For some patients treatment can continue for many months or even years. Patients require a range of supportive care, both medical to treat or prevent major treatment-related effects and psychosocial to help and sustain them and their families

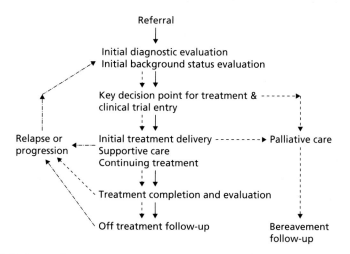

Fig. 21.3 Patient pathway.

through immensely stressful and challenging experiences. It is to be hoped that treatment will be successful and patients can then embark on follow-up having completed an end-of-treatment evaluation.

Many patients are then followed up and may require assessment and treatment of any long-term or late effects of therapy. Examples include cardiac toxicity following treatment with anthracyclines, neurological disability following treatment for a brain tumour, and infertility following exposure to, for example, alkylators.

Sadly but obviously, treatment might be either initially unsuccessful or disease may recur either on treatment or some time after completion. Usually, patients will require further evaluation of disease and then discussion about the treatment strategy. For many this will involve trying further therapy with curative intent, but for some further treatment will not be curative and they embark on a palliative course which may be brief or last many months, or even years. It can thus be seen that patients might continue to follow this pathway until they survive their disease or die as a result of it.

Is this pathway of relevance to teenagers and young adults? Maximizing survival, minimizing cost

It can be seen from the patient pathway discussed above that it is possible to describe various steps in the management of any patient with cancer. This particular path is rudimentary and gives little detail of the specific requirements of any single patient or tumour type, and needs to be expanded to indicate what services may need to be provided at each of these stages. Pathways for children with cancer, for example, need to recognize their particular supportive care and treatment requirements and the needs of the family. Even within paediatric oncology, a specific pathway for leukaemia will differ from that of a child with a brain tumour. The specifics of these children's pathways will look very different from those for adults with a range of tumours. However, the broad outline will remain the same.

Is it possible therefore to flesh out a single pathway for teenagers and young adults that is more than that described earlier?

It is clear that currently a young person with cancer might have many different experiences depending on disease, place of residence, pattern of referral, clinical team and the local availability of a teenager and young adult unit or staff proficient in managing this group.

In considering any pathway it is important to reflect, firstly, on what criteria should be used to measure success and, secondly, what elements to include to achieve the most successful outcome possible.

As described at the beginning of this chapter, the main aims of care should be to maximize the chance of survival whilst minimizing the physical, psychological and social cost of that survival. How, then, might survival be increased or maximized? How can the basic pathway be expanded to help achieve these aims?

Centralization and access to clinical trials

There appears to be fairly strong evidence from paediatric oncology that centralization of care improves outcome for rare tumours or those requiring complex treatment.[12–14] Further evidence has been published to support the benefits of specialized cancer care in adults.[15] There has also been evidence to support the contention that patients entered into clinical trials often have higher survival rates, especially in less common cancers. Trial entry has never been found to be associated with lower survival rates.[16] The evidence for teenagers and young adults is mixed. There is evidence that patients with testicular tumours have better outcome with centralized care.[17] Stiller and colleagues in 1999[18] looked specifically at teenagers and young adults with leukaemias in the UK between 1984 and 1994 and concluded that, although improvement had occurred over time, survival did not vary with the category of hospital. This study, of course, was prior to any significant development of specific teenager and young adult units. Wilkinson and colleagues, studying teenagers and young adults with cancer aged 15–24 years in Yorkshire between 1984 and 1994, demonstrated differences in outcome between geographical areas.[19] Whilst the exact reasons were unclear, it was possible to hypothesize that one factor may have been different patterns of care, in that fewer patients were referred to the specialist centre from the area with poorest outcome. There is also evidence to suggest that centralized care might reduce physical late effects. A study of Wilms' tumour demonstrated that children not treated in specialist centres might be overtreated.[20]

There is therefore some evidence supporting the contention that centralized treatment and access to clinical trials should be important elements of care for teenagers and young adults in order to maximize survival.

Cancer-specific and teenager and young adult-specific teams: is there a conflict?

Psychological, social and educational outcomes are other important factors that need to be taken into account. It is intuitive that these particular outcomes are likely to be improved if teenagers and young adults receive care in an environment designed for young people, where they can meet others of similar age and where staff are expert in and can focus on the needs of adolescents. However, there is little firm evidence of this and studies are needed to compare results of teenagers and young adults treated in different settings. Similarly, access for young people to an experienced professional team might also be expected to result in improved access to fertility advice and services.

Nevertheless, possible tension continues to exist between providing centralized care in a unit specializing in a particular malignancy or in a unit specializing in the care and needs of young people in general. To some extent it appears as though this tension is spurious, perpetuated by different clinical or medical factions. It might be thought that the best solution for young people is to create an environment that combines these elements, so that teenagers and young adults benefit from both. This requires individual clinicians and teams to commit to working in new ways, thereby providing teams expert in both the specific cancers and the needs of young people.

In the absence of clear evidence of improved outcome, it might also be reasonable to measure benefit by looking at process outcomes. These should include comparison of the rapidity of diagnosis, the clarity and quality of information received, choices about treatment, access to trials, access to psychological and peer support, access to education and access to facilities designed for young people.

Whelan uses similar arguments to promote the case that, where possible, the optimal model should be for specific units designed for young people and staffed by a skilled multiprofessional team expert in the care of both teenagers and young adults and their diseases.[21]

What do young people think?

In my talk on this subject at the Teenage Cancer Conference (London, March 2004), I used the analogy of Professor Tolkien's book and recent film trilogy *The Lord of the Rings* to describe some of the issues facing young people with cancer. The analogy is based on the principal character, Frodo, a young hobbit who looks remarkably like a teenager or young adult, being unexpectedly burdened with a magic ring. In order to rid himself of this burden he has to embark on a journey into the unknown. He has to face numerous dangers, unpleasant experiences and new places, all with the distinct possibility that he might not survive these events. Many others help him in these adventures, each bringing their individual skills and personality, but perhaps most support is given by his closest and long-standing friends. Although I would not want to overextend the analogy, one important reason why I think this is of relevance is that the story is told from Frodo's position. Thus, it gives a small insight into, and an appreciation of, a difficult personal journey.

The importance of this should be obvious. All too often services have evolved in an unplanned way with the result that they appear to serve the needs and predilections of professionals rather than service users who have to fit in. This is not unique to any particular group, so in many ways teenagers and young adults with cancer do not differ from large numbers of people using health-care systems. In designing and delivering services it should be essential to take the experiences and views of patients and their carers into account. In considering a pathway for teenagers and young adults, patients' and carers' views are indispensable.

There is an interesting, although not extensive, literature which reveals some insights into the concerns of young people with cancer and how management might be improved. Major elements of the direct cancer experience that concern young people include the possibility of disease recurrence, changes in body image, personal relationships with friends, family or partners, reintegration into education, and job prospects.[22–26] Whilst some issues are cancer-specific, others are shared by many young people who do not have cancer. Teenagers and young adults with cancer need to be seen firstly as young people and only then with cancer.

One key element identified in a number of publications is the requirement for clear, appropriate and comprehensive information at all stages. This allows participation and a level of control in decision-making, factors that relate positively to self-image and help with adjustment.[25,27,28] Patients need to be able to make choices for themselves.

Dunsmore and Quine[27] also reported on the qualities of health professionals that young people thought facilitated communication. These included the ability to listen, the ability to express concern, professional expertise and honesty. In contrast, an impersonal manner, excessive jargon, haste and a perceived generation gap impaired communication.

There are not many studies of young people's experience of health services in the UK. Wilkinson carried out a qualitative study as part of his thesis, some of which has subsequently been published.[29] In addition, evidence has been gathered at three Teenage Cancer Trust-sponsored events that have brought together several hundred young people with cancer who have experienced treatment in a range of settings. In ranking those factors deemed to be important by adolescents with cancer, by far the most important was to 'get better', a desire to be 'cured' and return to normal. This was followed by treatment in a specialist centre and the need to keep up with education. Whenever asked, young people want to be able to access family and friends and if possible to be at home or close to home. This desire is strongly outweighed by the willingness to travel to specialist centres if this means that outcome might be improved.

Lastly, one very important factor, which has often been identified but for which evidence is sparse, is the widely expressed perception of significant and avoidable delay in the initial diagnosis and referral. Many young people, particularly those with solid tumours, provide stories of numerous attendances and assessments before referral for investigations leading to a correct diagnosis. This causes them enormous concern, often expressed as 'I don't want other people to experience this.'

What might a single pathway for teenagers and young adults look like?

It is apparent that currently there is little predictable in the experiences of teenagers and young adults and there are many elements of chance in any one patient's journey. A pathway should be evidenced-based if possible and take into account the expressed wishes and experience of those undertaking the journey. Figure 21.4 is an attempt to unify these factors into a single pathway based on competencies and needs rather than particular places, people or professional interest groups.

The first element of the pathway reflects the need for as early a diagnosis as possible. This imposes responsibility on young people themselves to learn how to recognize symptoms or signs of concern and then seek appropriate professional help or advice. It also demands that professionals listen to young people and make early referrals for specialist assessment. An example of the

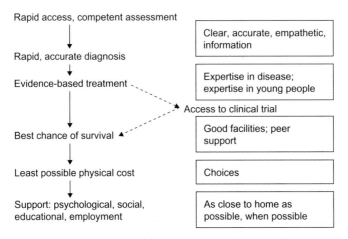

Fig. 21.4 Patient pathway based on views of young people. This is based on competencies and requirements.

former is creating public awareness amongst young men of the importance of testicular self-examination. An example of the latter would be evidence that patients are being referred rapidly from primary or secondary care to specialist cancer services and a reduction in time from initial symptoms to commencing treatment.

Much of the rest of the pathway might appear self-evident yet the evidence from the literature and the reports of many young people's personal experiences tell a very different story.

As outlined earlier in this chapter, young people find themselves managed by a wide range of medical teams, many of whom have little understanding of their needs. Both in the USA[30] and the UK, only a minority appear to be given the opportunity to participate in clinical trials.

For many patients it is not known if late physical effects of treatment are taken appropriately into account when treatment is planned. However, it is recognized that many young people report not having adequate information about fertility risks at the time of starting treatment and many 'adult' treatment protocols pay little regard to cardiac, renal and audiological toxicity monitoring.

Many young people report not being encouraged to continue with their education through treatment and are sometimes actively discouraged by well-meaning professionals. In addition there are often less than adequate resources available to adult teams to provide the psychological and social support needs of teenagers and young adults.

It is perhaps for these reasons that there has been such strong pressure and movement towards providing specialist facilities and teams. Young people need to be offered the opportunities so that they can choose, if they wish, to have their management coordinated by a professional team that is expert in young people and in the cancers from which they suffer. They should have access to a team that has adopted age- and developmentally-appropriate methods of communication and can provide the necessary support. They should be able to undergo treatment in facilities that meet their very particular needs, where they can meet other young people similarly affected and where the needs of parents, partners, family and friends can also be addressed. They should be given the opportunity to spend as much time as possible at home or close to home whilst still receiving the benefit of expert supervision and access to clinical trials.

I think that this means that it is feasible to outline a single generic pathway for teenagers and young adults with cancer. Obviously, the pathway will require tailoring for each individual and their personal disease and circumstances. I believe this will provide optimal care for young people and is worth striving for, but that will only happen when the grip of professional ownership is loosened and the needs of young people are addressed as the primary concern.

References

1 Lewis IJ. Cancer in adolescence. *Br Med Bull* 1996; **52**: 887–897.
2 Thompson J. Adolescents with cancer. In: Tiffany R, Webb H, eds. *Oncology for Nurses and Health Care Professionals*, Vol. 2. London: Harper and Row, 1988: 254–261.
3 Department of Health. *Welfare of Children and Young People in Hospital*. London: Department of Health, 1991.
4 Department of Health. *The National Service Framework for Children, Young People and Maternity Services. First Module – Standard for Hospital Services*. London: Department of Health, 2003.
5 Intercollegiate Working Party on Adolescent Health. *Bridging the Gap: Health Care for Adolescents*. London: Royal College of Paediatrics and Child Health, 2003.
6 Department of Health. *A Policy Framework for Commissioning Cancer Services. A report by the Expert Advisory Group on Cancer to the Chief Medical Officer of England & Wales*. London: Department of Health, 1995.
7 World Health Organization. *The International Classification of Diseases for Oncology (ICD-0-3)*. Geneva: WHO, 2000.
8 Birch JM, Marsden BB. A classification scheme for childhood cancer. *Int J Cancer* 1987; **40**: 620–624.
9 Birch JM, Alston RD, Quinn M, Kelsey AM. Incidence of malignant disease by morphological type, in young persons aged 12–24 years in England, 1979–1997. *Eur J Cancer* 2003; **39**: 2622–2631.
10 Selby P, Rider L, Joslin C, Bailey C. Epithelial cancer. In: Selby P, Bailey C, eds. *Cancer and the Adolescent*. London: BMJ Publishing, 1996: 39–53.
11 Souhami RL, Whelan J, McCarthy JF, Kilby A. Benefits and problems of an adolescent cancer unit. In: Selby P, Bailey C, eds. *Cancer and the Adolescent*. London: BMJ Publishing, 1996: 276–283.
12 Stiller CA. Centralisation of treatment and survival rates for cancer. *Arch Dis Child* 1988; **63**: 23–30.
13 Stiller CA. Centralised treatment, entry to trials and survival. *Br J Cancer* 1994; **70**: 352–362.

14 Peppercorn JM, Weeks JC, Cook EF, Joffe S. Comparison of outcomes in cancer patients treated within and outside clinical trials: conceptual framework and structured review. *Lancet* 2004; **363**: 263–270.

15 Selby P, Gillis C, Haward R. Benefits from specialised cancer care. *Lancet* 1996; **348**: 313–318.

16 Stiller C. Epidemiology of cancer in adolescents. *Med Pediatr Oncol* 2002; **39**: 149–155.

17 Harding PJ, Paul J, Gillis CR, Kaye SB. Management of malignant teratoma: does referral to specialist units matter? *Lancet* 1993; **341**: 999–1002.

18 Stiller CA, Benjamin S, Cartwright RA *et al.* Pattern of care and survival for adolescents and young adults with acute leukaemia – a population based study. *Br J Cancer* 1999; **79**: 658–665.

19 Wilkinson JR, Feltbower RG, Lewis IJ, Parslow RC, McKinney PA. Survival from adolescent cancer in Yorkshire, UK. *Eur J Cancer* 2001; **37**: 903–911.

20 Pritchard J, Stiller CA, Lennox EL. Overtreatment of children with Wilms tumour outside paediatric oncology centres. *Br Med J* 1989; **299**: 835–836.

21 Whelan J. Where should teenagers with cancer be treated? *Eur J Cancer* 2003; **39**: 2573–2578.

22 Roberts CS, Severinsen C, Carraway C *et al.* Life changes and problems experienced by young adults with cancer. *J Psych Oncol* 1997; **15**: 15–25.

23 Pendley JS, Dahlquist LM, Dreyer ZA. Body image and psychosocial adjustment in adolescent cancer survivors. *J Pediatr Psychol* 1997; **22**: 29–43.

24 Lynam MJ. Examining support in context: a redefinition from the cancer patient's perspective. *Sociol Health Illness* 1990; **12**: 169–194.

25 Evans M. Interacting with teenagers with cancer. In: Selby P, Bailey C, eds. *Cancer and the Adolescent*. London: BMJ Publishing, 1996: 251–263.

26 Eiser C. The impact of treatment: adolescents' views. In: Selby P, Bailey C, eds. *Cancer and the Adolescent*. London: BMJ Publishing, 1996: 264–275.

27 Dunsmore J, Quine S. Information, support and decision making needs and preferences of adolescents with cancer: implications for health professionals. *J Psychosoc Oncol* 1995; **13**: 39–56.

28 Jamison RN, Lewis S, Burish TG. Psychological impact of cancer on adolescents: self-image, locus of control, perception of illness and knowledge of cancer. *J Chron Dis* 1986; **39**: 609–617.

29 Wilkinson J. Young people with cancer – how should their care be organised? *Eur J Cancer Care* 2003; **12**: 5–70.

30 Bleyer WA. Cancer in older adolescents and young adults: epidemiology, diagnosis, treatment, survival and importance of clinical trials. *Med Pediatr Oncol* 2002; **38**: 1–10.

CHAPTER 22

Managing professional relationships across the services

S. Morgan

Introduction

Developing services for teenagers and young adults with cancer is challenging and may be fraught with difficulties. This is an area of medicine which, if we are to succeed, needs to be forged from the paediatric and adult disciplines within cancer centres. It is an evolving specialty which crosses many boundaries and will challenge many entrenched beliefs and ways of working.

The case for specialized care for teenagers with cancer has been well demonstrated.[1-3] Wherever possible, young people should be provided with their own space, so that they can mix with their own peer group in an age-appropriate environment and have experienced professionals who will care for them and are able to help them with their individual needs.[4]

In the UK the Calman-Hine Report[5] recommends that 'purchasers should look for opportunities for developing treatment of adolescents with cancer'. They present special medical and psychological problems and require specialized care in the cancer centre. But we only have to listen to the voices of these young people to know what they want. When asked why teenagers with cancer need a specialized unit, Ross, a boy aged 16 years with an osteosarcoma, said 'Because I don't want to be with screaming babies and I don't want to be with old fogies!'

Teenage Cancer Trust Units have been created in ten separate centres around the UK, and these, along with the pioneering work of the national charity after whom the units are named, have created the impetus to develop services. It is very clear that, alongside the development of specific units, we must develop the ethos of building upon the expertise of professionals and facilitate the involvement of all the appropriate professionals in this work.

Multidisciplinary teams

Paediatric and adult oncology units pride themselves on their multidisciplinary team (MDT) approach to work. It has been recognized that an MDT has both the advantage of collaborative teamwork and the ability to take a comprehensive view of the patient. Such a team would have the availability of a range of skills, and provide mutual professional support. Burke and colleagues[6] describe an important number of areas of multidisciplinary teamwork – role definition, leadership, clinical responsibility, accountability, and understanding between the professions. These can be seen in many teams in the oncology setting. However, the paediatric and adult disciplines have very different ways of working.

In an adult oncology unit within a major cancer centre, the MDTs are shaped by the people required to treat the person with a specific type of malignancy. For example, a person with breast cancer would have her case reviewed and treatment planned by the Breast MDT. This team normally consists of a specialist surgeon, medical oncologist, clinical oncologist, radiologist, research nurse and pathologist, all with specific expertise in breast diseases. Other experts would be included in the MDT for supportive care of the patient, including a nurse specialist working alongside the ward and clinic nurses. The psychosocial needs of the patient would be assessed and the opinions of appropriate professionals obtained when required.

The paediatric model is somewhat different, having a philosophy of care that is family-centred rather than disease-centred, and is more holistic in its approach. Indeed, it is often seen as the gold standard of multidisciplinary working. However, it is clear that paediatric oncology units receive far fewer referrals per year compared with adult oncology services, thus possibly allowing more time and resources to be dedicated to the holistic approach.

For the child or young adult with cancer, coming through paediatric services, the team would include paediatric and nursing personnel, a surgeon, anaesthetist(s), a social worker, a dietician, a pharmacist, a physiotherapist, a psychologist, a psychiatrist, radiographers, radiologists, data managers and activity coordinators and teachers. These all generally meet weekly to discuss the care of the young patient and the family. Separate meetings may occur in which the psychosocial needs of the patient and his or her family are addressed, and for discussion of medical aspects. Within this model, many of these professionals would attend both meetings, providing the more holistic approach. Other professionals may also be involved and their opinions and input sought, from pain management or dental care teams, for example.

In order to successfully achieve such a development in the care of teenagers and young adults, many professionals from different disciplines will need to be able to work together, and in essence merge to form new MDTs. This may well give rise to controversies, not least of which will be the fact that professionals will need to cross the great paediatric–adult divide.

The scope of the problem is this: can effective team working be established by drawing together the two disciplines – adults and paediatrics – whilst maintaining close working relationships and causing minimal conflict? It is clear that these professionals have a lot to learn from each other and it is recognized that there are many advantages of collaborative teamwork. These include continuity of care, the ability to take a comprehensive view of the patient, the availability of a range of skills and mutual support and education.[6]

So, can such a team be developed which will manage to keep the patient and family needs in the centre of the model in order to create a seamless service?

How can we achieve this ideal model? It is important when developing new services that experiences are shared, and this includes the successes and failures. Only when we reflect and share can we truly learn. The following account is from a team who are well on the road to developing a comprehensive service, but have by no means reached the ultimate goal. There have been many positive experiences and some difficult issues, some of which will be described.

The aims

The initial aim was 'to develop services for teenagers and young adults with cancer in Yorkshire, UK'. The challenge was that this service needed to span the Paediatric Oncology Unit (POU) and the Adult Oncology Unit (AOU), which are geographically and structurally very different from each other.

The structure at the start consisted of two very separate physical areas of the hospital and models of working. The POU, with around 150 new referrals a year, functioned very well with one fully comprehensive MDT. The AOU, with around 700 new referrals a year, was made up of many disease-specific MDTs (Fig. 22.1).

Whilst developing such a new team, one is struck by the significance of overlapping circles, as taught to young children when they first start to learn mathematics (Fig. 22.2). In this example the differences and the similarities between a cat and a cougar are shown. The young pupil will be taught that the information in the overlapping section is the information relevant to both animals. A similar pattern of overlapping circles could be described for the teenager with cancer, and the overlapping needs of the MDT from both adult and paediatric medicine. This would create a far more complicated, yet intrinsically workable, pattern.

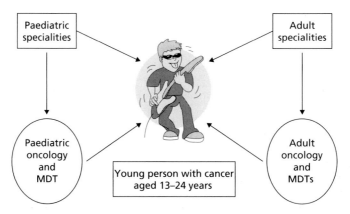

Fig. 22.1 Pathway of care for the teenager and young adult in many centres.

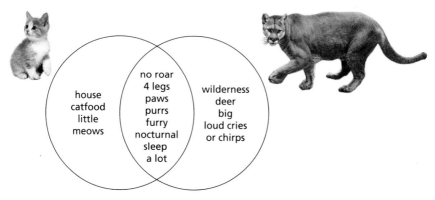

Fig. 22.2 Model of overlapping circles.

This is seen in the current model of cancer centres, where there are paediatric and adult cancer MDTs. Each of these teams has some expertise in the care of the young person and their family/carers, and every professional has something to offer to create such a team. So this became another aim for us – to develop a team with the expertise to work at the centre of the speciality of two oncology divisions. It was thought that this should be an all-encompassing MDT drawing in the expertise from all disciplines, yet with the professionals from those disciplines firmly maintaining their roots in both areas (Fig. 22.3).

A nest

The development gathered momentum in 1998 by the creation and subsequent opening of the Teenage Cancer Trust Unit (TCTU). This is a six-bedded unit geographically adjacent to the POU. A core team of nurses and a supportive team were established (Table 22.1) and the guidelines for the unit and the philosophy of care were developed. It was imperative that a safe place was created for these young people – somewhere that the patients were not afraid to leave, nor too frightened to return, safe in the knowledge that it would always be there for them. The team on the unit were not immediately experts in caring for teenagers and young adults with cancer, as all of them initially

Table 22.1 Identify the team

- Professionals who need to be wholly committed to the project
- Need to be a team who can work well together
- They need to have a mixture of skills . . . knowledge, compassion, enthusiasm, sense of humour, innovation and patience
- Must be a multiprofessional team
- Needs to adapt to change – with leaders who are adept at managing it

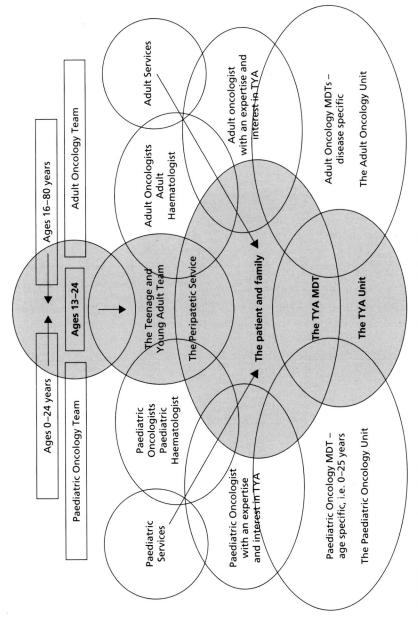

Fig. 22.3 Suggested model of teamwork for teenagers and young adults with cancer.

Paediatric Oncology Team

Adult Oncology Team

Ages 0–24 years

Ages 16–80 years

Ages 13–24

The Teenage and Young Adult Team

The Peripatetic Service

The patient and family

Adult Services

Adult Oncologists
Adult Haematologist

Adult oncologist with an expertise and interest in TYA

Adult Oncology MDTs – disease specific

The Adult Oncology Unit

The TYA MDT

The TYA Unit

Paediatric Services

Paediatric Oncologists
Paediatric Haematologist

Paediatric Oncologist with an expertise and interest in TYA

Paediatric Oncology MDT – age specific, i.e. 0–25 years

The Paediatric Oncology Unit

had been drawn from the POU. They undoubtedly learned on the job, and there was a huge learning curve for all involved.

A first major step in linking the two disciplines was the addition to the team of a medical specialist registrar (SpR) working on the TCTU as a part of training in medical oncology. The SpRs work on the unit for 1 year and those who have had the experience have all expressed it to be very worthwhile and positive. This has been ongoing since 1998, and has been perceived as highly beneficial to both areas in terms of learning from each other. It also ensures that future consultant medical oncologists return to their own areas with some insight into the care of this group of patients.

After 2 years the referrals to the unit had increased by 266%; it was found that the six beds were not enough, and at times 15 were needed. There was also the added pressure of other oncologists within our region wanting to refer patients to the unit. This was difficult to manage in terms of capacity but it was also difficult to establish good referral guidelines due to the different array of young people and diseases we were seeing.

Model of care

It was anticipated that a model of care would be developed and that this would make the running of the unit simpler! However, it was soon apparent that, if patients within the defined age group (13–24 years) were going to be admitted, then some would be seen with adult-type cancers, which might make such a development difficult. Whenever possible patients were given a choice as to where they would wish to be cared for, on the understanding that the constraints on bed space might limit this. Within the first 4 years many referrals were received, not all of them with a paediatric malignancy; therefore, not all of them had a paediatric oncologist or haematologist as their primary physician (Table 22.2). Some examples are given below.

- A 16-year-old male with an osteosarcoma
  Consultant: paediatric oncologist
  Place of care: the Teenage Cancer Trust Unit
- A 13-year-old male with colon cancer
  Consultant: paediatric oncologist with adult oncologist (gastrointestinal)
  Place of care: the Teenage Cancer Trust Unit

Table 22.2 Patients admitted to the TCTU, 2000–2003: aged 13–24 years

Sarcoma	51 patients
Hodgkin's disease	23 patients
Leukaemia	20 patients
Non-Hodgkin's lymphoma	14 patients
Germ cell tumours	13 patients
Carcinoma	13 patients
CNS tumours	11 patients
Malignant melanoma	2 patients

- A 20-year-old male with metastatic malignant melanoma
  Consultant: adult oncologist (melanoma)
  Place of care: the Teenage Cancer Trust Unit (patient choice)

The biggest challenge was coordinating the work of a vast array of professionals who brought with them the expertise with which to treat the range of diseases with which these patients present. Patients with a variety of adult-type cancers were admitted who required the disease expertise of an adult oncologist whilst being cared for in a teenage unit, sited within the POU! Because many new professionals were referring to the unit, the team on the TCTU were dealing on a daily basis with many disciplines, many teams, opinions/personalities, different practices and protocols, varied patterns of care and many egos! All of this needed tact and diplomacy, whilst always remembering to keep the patient at the centre of all developments.

The reality therefore became clear that there did not seem to be a single model of care. The referral pathways were all very different. Every team involved had very different ways of working and adjustments needed to be made to adapt to those. The unit had to ensure that they presented a united front to the patient and their family regardless of how difficult the team may have found the different situations. What developed was a single, equitable model of delivery of care, tailor-made for the young patient and their family/carers, keeping the patient central to all that we do. This model must allow them equal access to services and support regard-less of their disease referring physician or place of care. It should also provide them with access to the diagnostic and therapeutic expertise pertinent to them and the disease for which they are being treated.

The visiting teams were invited to become a part of the unit culture, invited to come to ward rounds and meetings when their patients would be discussed, invited to any social functions held on the ward by the patients, and were generally introduced to the concept of holistic care of each patient.

This was a difficult but very exciting time. The small innovative unit was becoming the focus for the development of teenage and young adult cancer services in Yorkshire, and a good reputation was developing. But, along with this came enormous pressure for the team to 'get it right'. They learned how to foster, nurture and respect professional relationships, understanding that if difficulties arose with the working relationship then the referrals might cease; this would be ultimately detrimental to the care of the young people and to the development of services.

A virtual unit

It soon became apparent that there were many young people who were diagnosed with cancer who could not be admitted to the unit due to the lack of beds and staff to care for them. There were no immediate plans, or space to create a larger physical unit. The referrals received were far greater than anticipated. It soon became clear that the supportive care offered to all young people within the region was not equitable. At this stage a solution was proposed: to set up a peripatetic service for all teenagers and young adults with cancer aged between 13 and 24 years from within our catchment area. The Teenage and Young Adult (TYA) Service was born!

The Teenage and Young Adult Service

The service now has six central members, a Macmillan Clinical Nurse Specialist, a Sargent Social Worker, an Oncology Nurse Specialist, a Candlelighters Trust Activity Co-ordinator, a learning mentor and a MacMillan Clinical Psychologist. These professionals have developed a service that reaches out to all young people with cancer and their families and offers psychosocial, practical educational and peer support to the patient no matter where they are treated. The team sees all of the young people who go through the TCTU, and will follow them from diagnosis onward. Importantly, the services were increased so that the isolated young person not physically cared for on the TCTU nevertheless had access to personal and family support. The team also give the patients unprecedented peer support which is so pivotal to their care, in the form of social support groups, conferences and outings.

This service works alongside, not instead of, the disease specialist teams, and the new team found that very soon new patterns of care began to emerge. They are now being invited to go to other departments within the region and attend oncology outpatient departments to offer the TYA Service to the young people attending them. At times the service has been a valuable resource to the referring teams and many young people have benefited from their input. Here are two examples:

- A 22-year-old male with a Ewing's sarcoma
  Consultant: adult oncologist and adult clinical oncologist
  Place of care: Adult Oncology Unit and TYA Service support
- A 19-year-old student from China with Hodgkin's disease
  Consultant: a clinical oncologist
  Place of care: Teenage Cancer Trust Unit (inpatient), Adult Lymphoma Clinic (outpatient) and TYA Service support

The reality of developing such a service is that it has taken around 5 years to start seeing results. The team is now receiving more referrals, and eventually other professionals stopped seeing the new team as a threat. Instead they could see the benefit of having additional resources to call upon when they were working with young people. The TYA Service staff now attend the weekly Germ Cell Tumour Clinic and have fully integrated into that team; attendance has also been requested at the Adult Haematology Unit and lymphoma clinics around the region.

It was always anticipated that referrals would be slow in coming, but the team were happy to gain momentum gradually, leading eventually to the principle that all young people would be referred to the TYA Service from throughout the cancer centre.

This is now a developing service. We are still seeing the tip of the iceberg – a minority of patients. But what can be seen is a very slowly evolving change in direction, and the concept of having specific services for this age group is a much more realistic one now.

Developing a teenage and young adult multidisciplinary team

Several attempts have been made at developing an MDT solely for teenagers and young adults, but this has been fraught with difficulties. At the moment the medical staff do not have sessions specifically for teenagers and young adults, as it is not yet seen as a specialty. We have adult oncologists and paediatric oncologists, but, as yet, no one specifically for adolescents. This means that an individual's time is limited and setting up yet another MDT is a very difficult task!

Identifying the patients who should be discussed is not the difficulty; the difficulty arises because the young patients will also have been discussed previously at the disease/paediatric oncology-specific teams. For example, a 19-year-old man with an oesophageal tumour will have been discussed at the gastrointestinal cancer MDT yet cared for on the TCTU. Many will not have the time and resources to discuss him at yet another TYA meeting.

As a team it was felt that it was a requirement to know where the patients are, without taking ownership of them. For statistical purposes, their diagnosis, age, referral pathway and place of care needed to be known as this would then inform forthcoming business cases which would underpin future developments. For the purpose of providing an equal service to all patients known to the team, contact needed to be made with them and the support of the TYA Service offered. Therefore, an embryonic MDT has been formed. This meets every 2 weeks and is attended by a core team, i.e. a paediatric oncologist and a medical oncologist, both of whom have an interest in teenagers and young adults with cancer and are leading the development of services in their area; the TYA Service team; nursing staff from the two units; and the MDT coordinator from the cancer centre. If a patient whose care is being led by another oncologist is to be discussed, the consultant involved would be invited to the meeting. If this was not possible a member of the TYA MDT would go to the disease-specific MDT for that patient, discuss the patient there, and then feed back into the TYA meeting. This has ensured cross-pollination of knowledge and working practices.

The formation of the TYA MDT is now at the centre of the development of the care of young people in the cancer centre. It is now a place for referrals, discussion and dissemination of knowledge and for identifying patterns of care. It is also a forum for discussing treatments and the controversies that surround those who care for patients with such complex problems, of which there are obviously many. It is hoped that it will continue to grow and develop.

More beds!

With the increase in referrals, the need for more beds became apparent. Hospitals throughout the country are in a state of financial flux and the reality is that there is very little in the way of money to aid new developments. However, a big breakthrough was the acceptance of a business case which outlined the need for finance to develop our services further. This enabled the team to create further beds, but also – and more importantly – it showed that the Trust was at last recognizing the need for additional services for these young people. As a result, three additional beds on the adult oncology ward have been developed, which run alongside the six beds on the TCTU.

The three extra beds on the AOU will be run with the TYA Service working in collaboration with the nursing and medical staff that runs the adult service on a day-to-day basis. Rotation of nursing and medical staff is planned between this new 'unit' and the six beds on the TCTU, and any developing issues will be addressed and resolved by the overall team. The total of nine beds gives greater flexibility of bed space and movement and it also allows the purchasers to be further reminded of the needs of young people with cancer.

The team has also worked very closely with national and local charities in order to develop the TYA Service and the unit. These collaborations have been central to all developments, and without them much of what has been done would not have been possible. Future plans now include the development of two ten-bedded units, which, due to geographical constraints within the hospital, have to be split between the adult oncology wing and the children's wing. The ideal would be to run it as one unit on two sites, with one management structure. The process has started in order for this to happen, but it still has a long way to go.

Lessons learned

The first thing to recognize is that change takes a very long time, especially when it involves the amalgamation of two disparate disciplines. Other professionals may regard this attempt at cross-pollination as a breakaway group, which may create negativity and evoke professional jealousies and insecurities. These issues are not easy to handle. However, from a reflective standpoint it is advisable to involve everyone in the original teams, continually tell them what is happening and the rationale for doing so, and encourage open, honest discussion.

Many will challenge the need for such services to be developed, especially as there is very little in the way of research to inform decision-making. It is advised that you take the doubters with you and involve them in making the decisions.

It is certain that in order to develop and/or improve services you need to have a champion for the cause. This person, or team of people, should be employed with the sole aim of developing services, and, importantly, should have the time, space and knowledge with which to do it. They could provide the initial bridge with which to start proceedings and initiate movement that brings people 'on board'.

There is no doubt that the voice of the patients and their families should be heard, and they are the best of advocates for special services. Throughout this whole experience it was ensured that the patients were given a voice and a choice in their care and their treatment. This has helped to inform and underpin everything that has been done. Most information about the need for specific services is purely anecdotal at the moment, but when you listen you will hear that many patients' journeys have been made easier by such developments. It would be very easy for the patient to be caught up between professionals and it is imperative that we, as professionals, prevent that happening and make it as easy as possible for the patient. There is no doubt that 'ownership' of patients can cloud professional judgement. Creating teams such as these will discourage professional ownership and help ensure that the patient is at the centre of his or her care.

Conclusion

Confusion may occur about whether it is best to treat the patient in a disease-specific unit, adult units, a paediatric unit or a teenage and young adult unit. Through trial and error we have found that it is possible to amalgamate all of the expertise and care for them under one umbrella. This has by no means been a trouble-free experience, but it has certainly provided the starting point from which to further develop services for this special group of patients.

Much more research is needed if we are to truly persuade the immovable doubters, and this must surely be the next step. Amalgamating experiences and proving the need for specialist services will take us all a step nearer to our goal.

References

1 Lewis IJ. Cancer in adolescence. In: Malpas JS, ed. *British Medical Bulletin: Cancer in Children.* London: Royal Society of Medicine Press, 1996: 887–897.
2 Hollis R, Morgan S. The adolescent with cancer – at the edge of no-man's land. *Lancet Oncol* 2001; **2**: 43–48.
3 Souhami R, Whelan J, McCarthy JF, Kilby A. Benefits and problems of an adolescent oncology unit. In: Selby P, Bailey C, eds. *Cancer and the Adolescent.* London: BMJ Publishing Group, 1996: 276–283.
4 Evans M. Interacting with teenagers with cancer. In: Selby P, Bailey C, eds. *Cancer and the Adolescent.* London: BMJ Publishing Group, 1996: 251–263.
5 Department of Health. *A policy framework for commissioning cancer services. A report by the Expert Advisory Group on Cancer to the Chief Medical Officers of England and Wales.* London: DoH, 1995.
6 Burke D, Herman H, Evans M *et al.* Educational aims and objectives for working in multidisciplinary teams. *Australas Psychiatry* 2000; **8**: 336.

CHAPTER 23

The next 10 years in biomedical science and care for teenagers and young adults with cancer

P. Selby, A. Shah, R. Yates and M. Leahy

Introduction

The last decade has seen significant progress in the development of care for teenagers and young adults (TYA) with cancer in the UK. The technical advances that have been made in the treatment of many of the uncommon cancers which are seen in this age group are beginning to be matched by service improvements. We must ensure that high-quality technical care is provided more uniformly and also that it is given in a supportive setting that allows young people to handle the difficulties that arise from the diagnosis of cancer and its treatment. The coming 10 years will see further technological advances. The applications of modern molecular biology to the diagnosis and prognosis of patients with cancer, and the rapid advances in sophisticated imaging, will improve the precision and effectiveness of diagnosis and treatment. New treatments are being developed now which are targeted more accurately against cancers and result in less, although still some, toxicity. Vaccine strategies and gene therapy remain credible research initiatives with considerable promise for patient benefits to come. These technological advances will be added to the existing treatments and allow us to be optimistic about improved outcomes for TYA with cancer.

In this chapter we will consider several aspects of future trends in cancer in TYA, in biomedical sciences, and in the care that will be important for TYA with cancer. Across this very broad topic we will concentrate on:
- trends in the incidence and mortality of cancer in TYA in Great Britain over the last 30 years as a means of predicting changes in the coming 30 years
- what needs to be done to ensure that we organize care for young people with cancer effectively

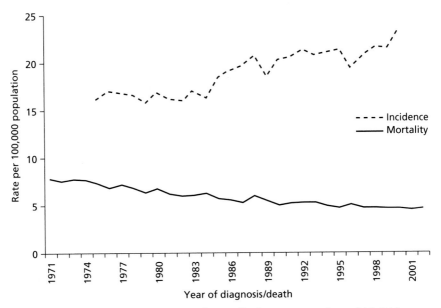

Fig. 23.1 Trends in cancer incidence and mortality in young people aged 15–24 in Great Britain between 1971 and 2002.

- the impact of modern biomedical science on these patients, particularly looking at (i) genomics and proteomics; (ii) drug development; and (iii) psychosocial sciences and the impact of new biomedical science upon them.

Trends

Figure 23.1 shows the trends in cancer incidence and mortality rates in young people aged 15–24 in Great Britain between 1971 and 2002.[1–7] It can be seen that the incidence rate has increased from approximately 16 per 100,000 per year to approximately 24 new cases per 100,000 per year between 1975 and 2000. This is an increase of 45% over the period. More encouragingly, there has been a steady fall in mortality, from 8 deaths per 100,000 population in 1971 to approximately 5 per 100,000 in 2002, a fall of 41% over the period. These data demonstrate clearly that outcomes for young people with cancer have improved as a result of more effective interventions of all kinds.

The impact of treatment is disease-specific and no global statements can be made. However, the overall improvement in mortality, when faced with a rising incidence, is a great compliment to the many professions and organizations that have been involved in providing for the diagnosis, treatment and support of young people with cancer in recent decades.

Figure 23.2 breaks these figures down, and the trend is seen to be occurring in both young men and young women. When data on individual cancers are examined, the increasing incidence is noticeable for testicular cancer

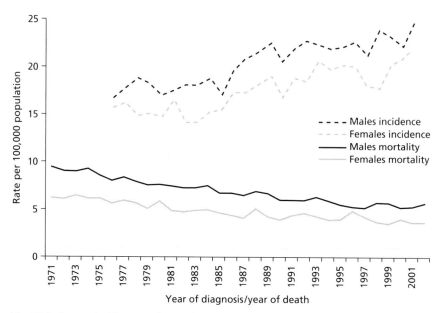

Fig. 23.2 Cancer incidence and mortality rates per 100 000 population in people aged 15–24 by sex, Great Britain, 1971–2001.

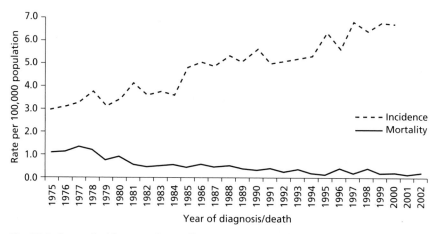

Fig. 23.3 Cancer incidence and mortality rates per 100,000 population for testicular cancer in people aged 15–24, Great Britain, 1975–2002.

(Fig. 23.3), ovarian cancer (Fig. 23.4), brain tumours, non-Hodgkin's lymphoma, melanoma (Fig. 23.5), thyroid cancer (Fig. 23.6) and invasive cancer of the cervix. There is no consistent increasing trend in colonic cancer, leukaemia or Hodgkin's disease (Fig. 23.7). Most of these trends are recognized across

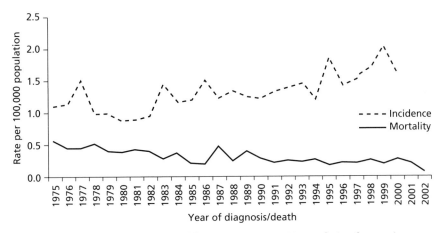

Fig. 23.4 Cancer incidence and mortality rates per 100,000 population for ovarian cancer in women aged 15–24, Great Britain, 1975–2002.

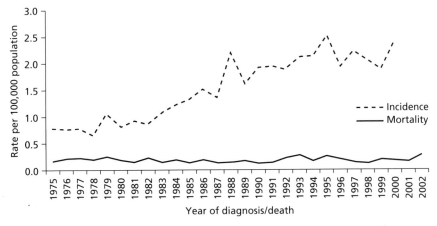

Fig. 23.5 Cancer incidence and mortality rates per 100,000 population for malignant melanoma in people aged 15–24, Great Britain, 1975–2002.

all age groups affected with those tumour types, but the frequency and consistency of the rising incidence in young people with cancer does require specific comment. These cancers, with the exception of cancer of the cervix and malignant melanoma, are not broadly associated with specific environmental factors. Concerns about exposure of young people to environmental risk factors exist, but specific aetiological environmental factors have not been identified.

Survival has improved in most cancers in this age group, not surprisingly considering the increasing incidence and decreasing mortality trends since 1971.

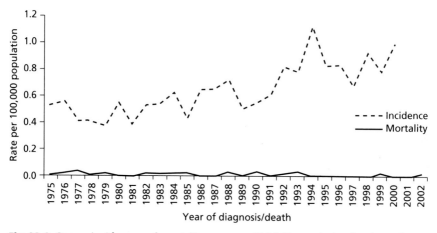

Fig. 23.6 Cancer incidence and mortality rates per 100,000 population for thyroid cancer in people aged 15–24, Great Britain, 1975–2002.

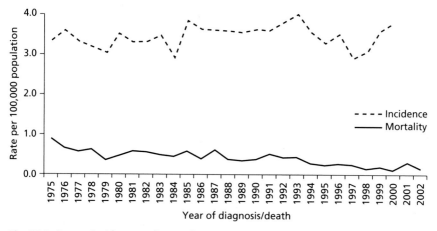

Fig. 23.7 Cancer incidence and mortality rates per 100 000 population for Hodgkin's disease in people aged 15–24 in Great Britain, 1975–2002.

This can be demonstrated directly by comparing relative 5-year survival for 15- to 24-year-olds in England and Wales in six successive calendar periods. The first five of these (1971–1975, 1976–1980, 1981–1985, 1986–1990, 1991–1995) have 5-year follow-up data (Table 23.1) but the final cohort (1996–1999) collects data for 4 years with 5-year follow-up to 2001. Over the 30 years covered by these data, survival has improved substantially for most cancers in this age group. Significant improvements in relative 5-year survival are demonstrated for young men and young women with Hodgkin's disease, non-Hodgkin's lymphoma, leukaemia, brain tumours, melanoma, breast cancer and ovarian and testicular cancers. Improvement in relative survival for carcinoma of the

Table 23.1 Relative survival to 5 years after diagnosis of 15- to 24-year-olds diagnosed between 1971 and 1999, England and Wales

Cancer	Sex	Period of diagnosis								
		1971–1975			1976–1980			1981–1985		
		n	Rate	95% CI	n	Rate	95% CI	n	Rate	95% CI
Hodgkin's	Male	664	73.2	69.6, 76.4	633	80.5	77.2, 83.4	660	82.6	79.5, 85.3
disease	Female	436	80.1	76.1, 83.6	508	84.2	80.7, 87.1	569	87.5	84.5, 90.0
Non-Hodgkin	Male	241	35.6	29.6, 41.6	233	45.5	39.0, 51.8	267	54.1	47.9, 60.0
lymphoma	Female	132	45.9	37.2, 54.1	112	46.8	37.2, 55.7	138	56.7	48.0, 64.5
Leukaemia	Male	345	12.2	9.0, 15.9	400	22.0	18.1, 26.1	402	31.0	26.5, 35.5
	Female	254	15.9	11.8, 20.6	252	23.7	18.7, 29.1	244	35.6	29.7, 41.6
Brain	Male	209	38.8	32.1, 45.3	228	44.3	37.7, 50.6	261	52.2	46.0, 58.1
	Female	183	36.0	29.1, 42.9	159	41.2	33.5, 48.7	204	56.5	49.4, 63.0
Colon	Male	41	47.5	31.6, 61.8	38	71.1	53.7, 82.9	48	51.9	36.9, 65.0
	Female	56	74.5	60.8, 84.1	59	79.2	66.2, 87.6	32	56.5	37.9, 71.5
Melanoma	Male	81	59.2	47.6, 69.1	85	62.1	50.8, 71.6	139	65.6	57.1, 72.9
	Female	161	77.1	69.7, 82.9	186	77.5	70.8, 82.9	252	82.2	76.9, 86.5
Thyroid	Male	21	89.8	64.5, 97.4				38	92.4	77.6, 97.5
	Female							150	98.1	93.9, 99.4
Breast	Female	95	45.7	35.4, 55.4	108	53.0	43.1, 61.8	93	52.6	42.0, 62.2
Cervix	Female	122	65.0	55.8, 72.7	190	79.0	72.5, 84.2	202	72.7	66.0, 78.3
Ovary	Female	183	57.0	49.5, 63.8	184	63.4	56.0, 70.0	196	77.2	70.7, 82.5
Testis	Male	418	54.5	49.5, 59.1	502	70.5	66.2, 74.3	722	85.0	82.1, 87.4
		1986–1990			1991–1995			1996–1999		
Hodgkin's	Male	692	84.3	81.3, 86.8	606	89.1	86.3, 91.4	405	93.3	89.3, 95.8
disease	Female	617	86.0	83.0, 88.5	568	91.3	88.7, 93.4	389	94.5	90.3, 96.8
Non-Hodgkin	Male	351	66.5	61.2, 71.2	329	66.2	60.7, 71.0	230	68.6	61.5, 74.7
lymphoma	Female	178	71.8	64.5, 77.8	176	70.9	63.5, 77.0	128	67.5	58.5, 74.9
Leukaemia	Male	410	41.3	36.5, 46.1	386	43.4	38.3, 48.3	277	50.5	43.8, 56.9
	Female	248	49.8	43.4, 55.9	285	47.5	41.6, 53.2	179	42.4	33.6, 51.0
Brain	Male	296	56.5	50.6, 61.9	322	59.3	53.7, 64.5	210	56.8	48.2, 64.4
	Female	250	61.4	55.0, 67.1	220	58.0	51.2, 64.3	170	58.9	50.2, 66.6
Colon	Male	35	44.7	27.8, 60.3	35	60.2	42.1, 74.2	36	60.2	42.1, 74.2
	Female	40	67.0	50.1, 79.3	40	64.8	47.9, 77.5	40	84.3	56.8, 95.0
Melanoma	Male	190	79.3	72.8, 84.5	210	80.3	74.2, 85.1	162	85.1	77.6, 90.2
	Female	386	88.7	85.1, 91.5	454	90.9	87.8, 93.2	294	95.4	91.6, 97.5
Thyroid	Male	54	92.7	81.3, 97.2	47	98.0	85.4, 99.7	52	98.1	86.1, 99.7
	Female	169	98.3	94.6, 99.5						
Breast	Female	132	65.0	56.1, 72.5	113	62.8	53.1, 71.0	157	77.3	65.1, 85.7
Cervix	Female	238	80.8	75.1, 85.3	203	83.3	77.4, 87.8	145	80.0	72.5, 85.7
Ovary	Female	217	80.2	74.2, 84.9	222	82.4	76.6, 86.8	205	87.3	81.3, 91.5
Testis	Male	922	88.5	86.2, 90.5	868	91.9	89.9, 93.6	777	95.2	93.1, 96.6

CI, confidence interval.

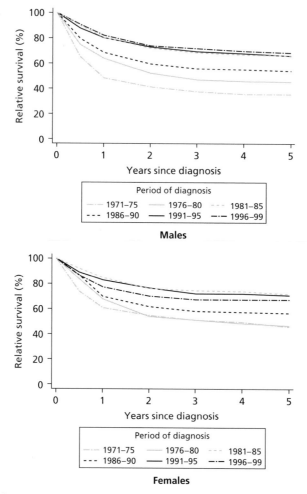

Fig. 23.8 Relative survival to 5 years after diagnosis from non-Hodgkin's lymphoma; aged 15–24 years.

cervix is substantial and just at the margins of significance, but for thyroid cancer and colon cancer the numbers are too small to draw conclusions. Relative survival to 5 years after diagnosis in the 1996–1999 period has decreased for young women with non-Hodgkin's lymphoma, leukaemia and cervical cancer and for both sexes with brain tumours compared with rates seen between 1986 and 1995. Examples of these data for non-Hodgkin's lymphoma and ovarian and testicular cancer are shown in Figs 23.8 and 23.9.

Falling mortality and improved survival result from different reasons in each cancer. In testicular cancer, Hodgkin's disease, non-Hodgkin's lymphoma and leukaemia, improvements in treatment, especially effective combination chemotherapy, play an important part in improved outcomes. For melanoma,

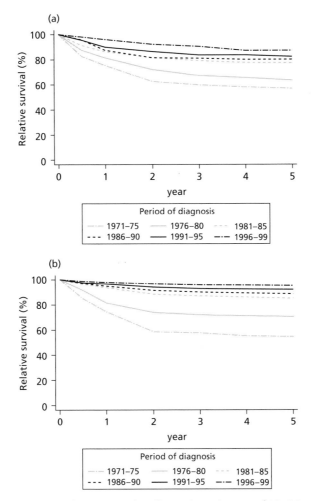

Fig. 23.9 Relative survival to 5 years after diagnosis: patients aged 15–24 years. (a) Ovarian cancer. (b) Testicular cancer.

the rising incidence without a rise in mortality is a reflection of changing stage distribution with an increasing proportion of new cases presenting with thin and therefore less dangerous tumours.

In breast cancer the data for incidence and mortality are shown in Fig. 23.10. There is a suggestion of a falling incidence and Table 23.1 shows improvement in survival. Explanations are complex, involving the efficacy of screening and the introduction of improved systemic therapies.

Thyroid cancer is an important cancer in this age group and is rising significantly in incidence, but treatment overall remains highly successful, with very low mortality despite the rising incidence (Fig. 23.6).

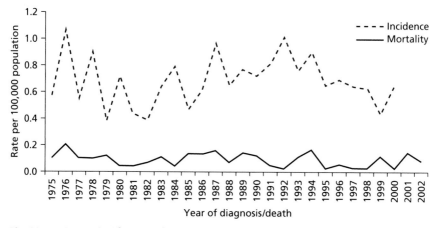

Fig. 23.10 Cancer incidence and mortality rates per 100 000 population for breast cancer in women aged 15–24, Great Britain, 1975–2002.

Table 23.2 Number of cases and 5-year survival in Europe

| | Crude | | | | Cancer type adjusted | |
| | Males | | Females | | Males | Females |
	No. of cases	5-year survival	No. of cases	5-year survival	5-year survival	5-year survival
Northern Europe	2013	78.7	1763	83.7	78.0	83.4
UK	3129	72.9	2725	77.6	73.9	78.5
Central Europe	747	75.6	580	80.5	73.3	81.7
Southern Europe	1181	71.5	925	77.9	74.3	77.8
Eastern Europe	946	61.9	710	70.8	63.6	70.6
European pool	8016	73.1	6703	78.8	74.0	79.5

Similar data that would compare trends across all of Western Europe are not available, but a comparison of current frequency and outcomes was given by the EUROCARE Group.[8] The number of cases and 5-year survival across Europe are given in Table 23.2. A wide range of outcomes is seen.

The UK's performance is compared with that of Northern Europe (Denmark, Finland, Iceland, Norway and Sweden), Eastern Europe (Czech Republic, Estonia, Poland, Slovakia, Slovenia), Central Europe (Austria, France, Germany, The Netherlands, Switzerland) and Southern Europe (Italy, Malta, Portugal and Spain) in Table 23.2. The UK figures are less good than those for Northern Europe but close to those for Central Europe and the whole European average. Studies by the EUROCARE Group overall have suggested that UK outcomes are less satisfactory because of differences in the organization of health-care services, and suggest that there may be distinct opportunities to improve outcomes in the coming decade.

Overall, the following conclusions seem to be reasonably well supported by the UK and EUROCARE data.

- Cancer incidence in the 15–24 age group has increased by almost 50% in three decades.
- It will continue to increase overall by over 10% in the next decade.
- Mortality is falling and survival rates are rising and will continue to do so in the next 10 years.
- There is a rising incidence of testicular, ovarian and brain tumours, non-Hodgkin's lymphoma, melanoma and thyroid and cervical cancers.
- The incidences of colon cancer, leukaemia and Hodgkin's disease are stable.

The organization of care

In much the same way that the special needs of teenagers with cancer are not met ideally by paediatric oncology services, the special needs of young adults with cancer are not well addressed by routine adult oncology practice. Both groups of patients report a feeling of isolation when treated within a service designed mainly for a different peer group, and report much greater satisfaction when their treatment can be delivered in the context of their own peer group. This has led to the development of units in the UK specializing in the TYA age group, with the benefits discussed throughout this conference.

In the UK, adult oncology services have reorganized to provide care in cancer site-specific multidisciplinary teams. This has improved the expertise being offered to patients. The challenge that faces the development of TYA services for patients presenting with tumours more usually seen in the older age group (particularly epithelial tumours) is to provide the benefits of peer-specific care without compromising the involvement of the highly expert site-specific team, and without fragmenting care by introducing ambiguity in the lines of responsibility. A model is being developed for young adults with cancer which can incorporate site-specific advice on management but deliver care within a peer group setting with an expanded team that includes social work, specialist nurses and activity coordinators who work solely with this age group. This model will be fully developed and evaluated. Figure 23.11 summarizes the issues that have to be considered in planning care for TYA with cancer.

The pattern of the illnesses that affect the TYA age group is an important factor in the consideration of service organization. In paediatric oncology great strides have been made in recent decades to develop care which is technically excellent, multiprofessional in its nature and centralized to an extent that ensures that children with cancer are cared for by teams with the necessary technical, psychosocial and clinical expertise, usually in cancer centres and almost always in the centres recognized by the United Kingdom Children's Cancer Study Group (UKCCSG). The diseases that make up the paediatric oncology practices are, substantially, characteristic of that age group. The common adult cancers of the lung, breast, colon, ovary, uterus, bladder, kidney and head and neck are found only rarely in childhood.

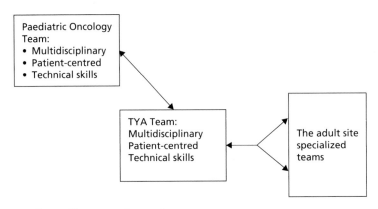

Fig. 23.11 How will we organize care?

In the TYA group between 15 and 24 years of age, the situation is more complex. Firstly, the diseases found in childhood occur usually less frequently in this age group. Secondly, some specific cancers occur with their highest incidence in this age group, notably osteosarcoma and Hodgkin's disease. Finally, particularly over the age of 20, the epithelial cancers which are characteristic of older people begin to occur infrequently but consistently. The practice of caring for TYA must take account of this complex case mix. Close working interfaces with paediatric oncology teams are clearly essential. Technical expertise in those cancers which make up the majority of cases in the TYA age group is also essential. Close working relationships with the specialist multiprofessional teams which care for the site-specific epithelial cancers of older people are also an absolute requirement.

These considerations suggest that the best care will be provided by a team working in a substantial centre which has an interface with paediatric oncology and an interface with a full range of expert multiprofessional teams caring for site-specific cancers in older age. Although patients need to be reviewed and their care influenced by this team, some of their care may be carried out on a shared basis with the cancer units surrounding these centres. The TYA team will deliver care for a substantial number of people and liaise with paediatric oncologists for another proportion of their population. They will also need carefully planned and close relationships with the multiprofessional site-specific adult teams to ensure that TYA patients can gain the benefits of the peer-based support available from the TYA team with its specialist knowledge of the issues surrounding the care of young people with cancer, as well as the technical and multiprofessional, commonly multimodality care which is the specialist and unique expertise of the site-specific adult multidisciplinary team.

Studies have shown an association between improved outcome for children and young people with cancer, not only in association with specialized models of care but also in association with an active programme of clinical trials which generate protocols for excellence in care as well as answering important scientific questions. It will be important to ensure that new service models for TYA with cancer incorporate an active commitment to clinical trials and clinical research. In the UK, a National Cancer Research Institute/National Cancer Research Network Clinical Studies Development Group is examining the best way to do so.

The impact of biomedical sciences on teenagers and young adults with cancer

A review of the future of biomedical sciences in the next 10 years is beyond the scope of this chapter. Advances in genomics and proteomics are rapidly being turned, as a result of technological developments which allow high throughput and highly parallel analysis of genomic and proteomic variables in tumours and patients, into a new kind of molecular pathology which will alter the diagnosis, prognostication and management of patients. The identification of novel targets for drug therapy is now moving forward equally quickly.

Genetic polymorphism in the patients and general population who are at risk of cancer is likely to prove an important factor both in the aetiology and the outcome of cancers, and our ability to do high-throughput genotyping will alter our approach to both diagnosis and treatment planning.

New biomedical sciences will not only influence the technological aspects of cancer care. Genetic polymorphism in neurotransmitter genes has been shown to be a powerful predictor of the emotional response of young people to adverse life events.[9] Although this needs confirmation and extension, it is likely that biomedical analysis using modern genotyping will allow us to identify young people who are at enhanced risk of serious emotional disorder during their diagnosis and treatment of cancer.

Improvements in diagnostic accuracy and classification are being made and will be essential for future analyses of trends.[10]

Conclusion

Trends show that cancer incidence in TYA is going to continue to increase and that there is therefore a pressing need to ensure that excellence in care is established and strengthened for all patients. However, trends also suggest that effective care is being provided and mortality is falling. Whilst this is a great compliment to those providing care for these patients, it does imply a pressing need to ensure that all patients have access to the best quality of care.

The next 10 years will see dramatic advances in biomedical sciences that will improve diagnosis and treatment in exciting new modes for young people with cancer. Whilst there is a great deal of work to be done, the trends for the next 10 years are such that we could see further substantial improvements in the care of TYA with cancer.

References

1 Office for National Statistics. *Cancer Statistics Registrations: Registrations of Cancer Diagnosed in 2000, England.* Series MB1, No.31. London: Office for National Statistics, 2003.

2 Office for National Statistics. *Mortality Statistics: Cause. England and Wales 2002.* London: TSO, 2003.

3 Welsh Cancer Intelligence and Surveillance Unit. *Cancer Incidence in Wales 1992–2001.* Cardiff: Welsh Cancer Intelligence and Surveillance Unit, 2002.

4 GRO for Scotland. *Annual Report of the Registrar General for Scotland 2002.* Registrar General for Scotland, 2003.

5 Information and Statistics Division, NHS Scotland. Scottish Health Statistics. http://www.show.scot.nhs.uk/isd/cancer/cancer.htm. ISD Online, 2003.

6 Northern Ireland Statistics and Research Agency. http:// www.nisra.gov.uk. NISRA, 2003.

7 Northern Ireland Cancer Registry. Cancer Incidence and Mortality. http://www.qub.ac.uk/nicr/commoncan.htm. Northern Ireland Cancer Registry, 2003.

8 Gatta C, Capocaccia R, De Angelis R, Stiller C, Coebergh JW and the EUROCARE Working Group. Cancer survival in European adolescents and young adults. *Eur J Cancer* 2003; **39**: 2600–2610.

9 Caspi A, Sugden K, Moffitt TE *et al.* Influence of life stress on depression: moderation by a polymorphism in the 5-HTT gene. *Science* 2003; **301**: 386–389.

10 Birch JM, Alston RD, Kelsey AM *et al.* Classification and incidence of cancers in adolescents and young adults in England 1979–1997. *Br J Cancer* 2002; **87**: 1267–1274.

Index